Principles of
Airway Management

Third Edition

Springer

New York
Berlin
Heidelberg
Hong Kong
London
Milan
Paris
Tokyo

Principles of Airway Management

Third Edition

Brendan T. Finucane, MBBCh, FRCPC
Professor and Program Director,
Department of Anesthesiology and Pain Medicine
University of Alberta
Edmonton, Alberta, Canada

and

Albert H. Santora, MD
Athens, Georgia, USA

With 283 Illustrations

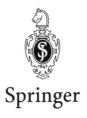

Springer

Brendan T. Finucane, MBBCh, FRCPC
Professor and Program Director
Department of Anesthesiology and Pain Medicine
University of Alberta
Edmonton, Alberta, Canada
btfinuc@shaw.ca

Albert H. Santora, MD
Athens, Georgia, USA

Library of Congress Cataloging-in-Publication Data
Finucane, Brendan T.
    Principles of airway management / Brendan T. Finucane, Albert H. Santora.—3rd ed.
    p. cm.
    Includes bibliographical references and index.
    ISBN 0-387-95530-5 (softcover : alk. paper)
    1. Airway (Medicine) 2. Trachea—Intubation. 3. Respiratory intensive care. 4.
    Anesthesiology. I. Santora, Albert H., 1952—II. Title.

RC732 .F56 2003
616.2—dc21   2002070729

ISBN 0-387-95530-5   Printed on acid-free paper.

Printed in the United States of America.

9 8 7 6 5 4 3 2 1   SPIN 10883418

www.springer-ny.com

Springer-Verlag New York Berlin Heidelberg
A member of BertelsmannSpringer Science+Business Media GmbH

To
Pat and Donna Finucane
and
Mary and Crissy Santora

Preface

Any man's death diminishes me, because I am involved in Mankind
—John Donne

In 1988 Belhouse and Dore[1] estimated that as many as 600 people died every year from complications of airway management in the developed world. The tragedy of this statistic was that most of these deaths were preventable. Information on airway-related topics has increased exponentially since we published the first edition of this book. In the past 10 years, almost 2000 English-language publications have been published on airway management, reflecting an increase in interest and change in this vitally important topic. We also have reason to believe that the number of deaths from airway mismanagement is declining at least in North America (ASA Closed Claims Study).[2]

When we first conceived this book, our intended audience was medical students. Then, we realized that other students and even seasoned practitioners of airway techniques might also benefit from it. In addition, trainees in anesthesiology, respiratory therapy, nurse anesthesia, as well as interns and residents involved in acute-care activity and emergency medicine technicians would also find much to learn. Thus, we published the second edition in 1996 with this expanded target audience in mind.

Why is a third edition needed? Because there is no other concise, comprehensive textbook available on airway management. Further, the growing number of publications on the subject indicates a growing interest in the field. Finally, it is difficult to remain current in this field because of the rapid rate of change in technology. It is difficult to imagine that the laryngoscope could be obsolete in perhaps twenty years time. The advent of the laryngeal mask has changed the practice of anesthesia, reduced the need for laryngoscopy and intubation, and may partly explain the declining death rate from airway problems all over the world.

This new edition has some important changes. We have expanded the discussion in most of the chapters. In addition, the chapters on airway management and CPR have been updated. The chapters on airway equipment, fiberoptic intubation, the "difficult airway," complications of airway management, and surgical approaches to airway management have been significantly changed. We have dedicated a new chapter to the laryngeal mask airway. The bibliography has been expanded to include the most up-to-date citations, with a special emphasis on the scientific aspects of airway management.

In the past two decades, the field of airway management has made great progress. We do not consider ourselves authorities on every aspect of the subject, but we have learned a great deal about this topic in our 60 years or so of combined experience. Anesthesiologists agree that there is no such thing as a "simple anesthetic." Similarly, there is no such thing as a "simple airway." We have all experienced the unheralded laryngeal spasm in the child emerging from anesthesia and are impressed by the rapidity of desaturation in those cases. Airway management is the backbone of our specialty, and we have a responsibility to disseminate the most up-to-date information to our colleagues on the front lines, not just in anesthesia, but in all disciplines that deal with the airway.

Brendan T. Finucane, MBBCh, FRCPC
Albert H. Santora, MD

References

1. Belhouse CP, Dore C. Criteria for estimating likelihood of difficult endotracheal intubation with the Macintosh laryngoscope. Anaes Intensive Care 1988;16:329-337.
2. ASA Closed Claims Project Lessons Learned. FW Cheney, MD; 1996 Annual Refresher Course Lectures; Oct 19-23, 1996.

Acknowledgments

We would like to acknowledge Pat Crossley for her tireless efforts to meet important deadlines, Steve Wreakes for his excellent photography, Gisele Goudreau and Marilyn Blake for their willingness to pose for photographs at short notice, and Marilyn Blake for her secretarial support.

Contents

1
Anatomy of the Airway

Knowledge of anatomy is essential to the study of airway management. First, anatomical considerations are helpful in diagnosing certain problems, such as the position of a foreign body in a patient with airway obstruction. Second, since some procedures involved in establishing and maintaining an airway are performed under emergency conditions, little if any time may be available for reviewing anatomy. Third, in many procedures involving the airway, such as intubation, anatomical structures are only partially visible. As a result, one must recognize not only the structures in view but also their spatial relationship to the surrounding structures. This chapter reviews basic airway anatomy, discusses some clinical correlates, and includes a comparison of the pediatric and adult airway.

The Nose

The nose is a pyramidal-shaped structure projecting from the midface made up of bone, cartilage, fibrofatty tissue, mucous membrane, and skin. It contains the peripheral organ of smell and is the proximal portion of the respiratory tract. The nose is divided into right and left nasal cavities by the nasal septum. The inferior portion of the nose contains two apertures called the anterior nares. Each naris is bounded laterally by an ala, or wing. The posterior portions of the nares open into the nasopharynx and are referred to as choanae. One or both of these apertures are absent in the congenital anomaly choanel atresia.[1] Infants are compulsive nose breathers at birth and therefore may suffocate if the condition is not corrected.

The nose has a number of important functions, including: respiration, olefaction, filtration, humidification, and is a reservoir for secretions from the paranasal sinuses and the nasolacrimal ducts.

Anatomically, each side of the nose consists of a floor, a roof, and medial and lateral walls. The septum forms the medial wall of each nostril and is made up of perpendicular plates of **ethmoid** and **vomer** bones and the **septal cartilage** (Fig 1.1). The bony plate forming the superior aspect of the septum is very thin and descends from the **cribriform plate** of the ethmoid bone. The cribriform plate may be fractured following trauma. Head injury victims should be questioned about nasal discharge, which may be cerebrospinal fluid (CSF). Nasal intubation and the passage of nasogastric tubes are relatively contraindicated in the presence of basal skull fractures.[2] The lateral walls have a bony framework attached to which are three bony projections referred to as conchae or turbinates (Fig. 1.2). The upper and middle conchae are derived from the medial aspect of the ethmoid; the inferior concha is a separate structure. There are a number of openings in the lateral nasal walls that communicate with the paranasal sinuses and the nasolacrimal duct.

A coronal section of the nose and mouth shows the location and relationships of the nasal structures more clearly (Fig. 1.3). Considerable damage can be inflicted on the lateral walls of the nose by forcing endotracheal tubes into the nasal cavity in the presence of an obstruction.

FIGURE 1.1. The nasal septum
(sagittal).

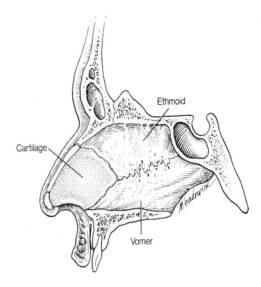

Nasal endotracheal tubes or airways should be well lubricated, and vasocon-
stricting solutions should be applied to the nasal mucosa before instrumentation.
When introducing a nasal endotracheal tube into the nostril, the bevel of the tube
should be parallel to the nasal septum (see Fig. 7.20, page 205) to avoid disruption of the conchae.

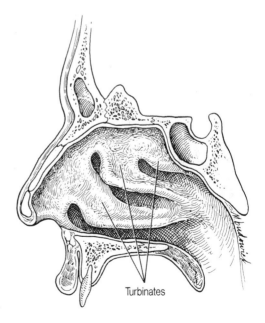

FIGURE 1.2. The lateral nasal wall.

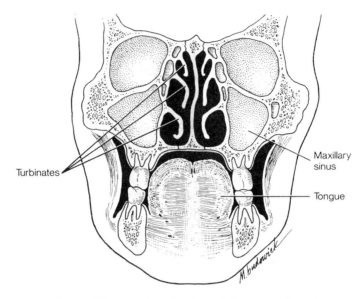

FIGURE 1.3. Coronal section through the nose and mouth.

Oral Cavity

The mouth, or oral cavity (Fig. 1.4), is divided into two parts: the vestibule and the oral cavity proper. The vestibule is the space between the lips and the cheeks externally and the gums and teeth internally. The oral cavity proper is bounded anterolaterally by the alveolar arch, teeth, and gums; superiorly by the hard and soft palates; and inferiorly by the tongue. Posteriorly, the oral cavity communicates with the palatal arches and pharynx.

Uvula

In the posterior aspect of the mouth, the soft palate is shaped like an *M,* with the uvula the centerpiece. This structure is a useful landmark for practitioners involved in airway management.

Tonsils

The tonsils are collections of lymphoid tissue engulfed by two soft tissue folds, **pillars of the fauces.** The anterior fold is called the palatoglossal arch, and the posterior fold the palatopharyngeal arch (see Fig. 1.4). The lingual tonsil is made up of lymphoid nodules found posterior to the sulcus terminalis and has a cobblestone appearance. Hypertrophy of the lingual tonsil can cause airway obstruction.[3]

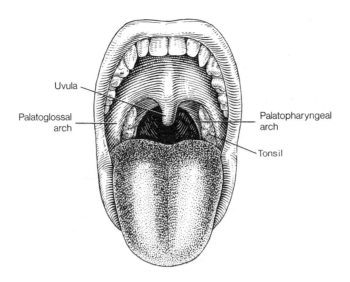

FIGURE 1.4. The oral cavity.

Tongue

The tongue is a muscular organ used for speech, taste, and deglutition. It is attached to the hyoid bone, mandible, styloid processes, soft palate, and walls of the pharynx. In an unconscious patient the oropharyngeal musculature tends to relax and the tongue is displaced posteriorly, occluding the airway. Since the tongue is the major cause of airway obstruction, it is an important anatomical consideration in airway management. Its size in relation to the oropharyngeal space is an important determinant of the ease or difficulty of tracheal intubation.

Nerve Supply to the Tongue

The sensory and motor innervation of the tongue is quite diverse and includes fibers from a number of different sources.

Sensory fibers for the anterior two thirds are provided by the lingual nerve. Taste fibers are furnished by the chorda tympani branch of the nervus intermedius (from the facial nerve [VII]). Sensory fibers for the posterior third come from the glossopharyngeal nerve (IX). In addition, some sensory innervation is provided by the superior laryngeal nerve (Fig. 1.5).

The Macintosh laryngoscope is inserted into the vallecula during laryngoscopy and theoretically, at least, is less likely to elicit a vagal response because the innervation of the vallecula is provided by the glossopharyngeal nerve. The Miller blade, on the other hand, is advanced toward the inferior surface of the epiglottis during laryngoscopy. The inferior surface of the epiglottis is innervated by the superior laryngeal nerve. Therefore, one is more likely to encounter vagal stimulation during laryngoscopy with a Miller blade.

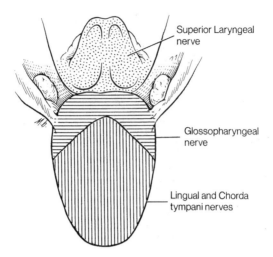

FIGURE 1.5. Sensory innervation of the tongue.

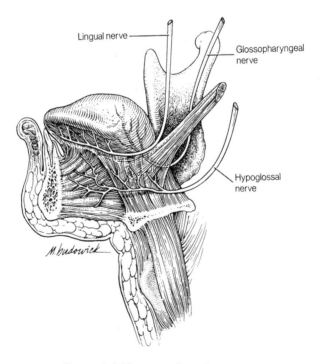

FIGURE 1.6. Nerve supply to the tongue.

The major motor supply is from the hypoglossal nerve (XII) (Fig. 1.6), which passes above the hyoid bone and is distributed to the lingual muscles. Since this nerve is very superficial at the angle of the mandible, it is prone to injury during vigorous manual manipulation of the airway.

Pharynx

The pharynx is a musculomembranous passage between the choanae and posterior oral cavity and the larynx and esophagus. It extends from the base of the skull to the inferior border of the cricoid cartilage anteriorly and the lower border of C6 posteriorly. It is approximately 15 cm long. Its widest point is at the level of the hyoid bone and the narrowest at the lower end where it joins the esophagus. Figures 1.7 and 1.8 should make it easier to visualize this structure. In a normal conscious patient the gag reflex may be elicited by stimulating the posterior pharyngeal wall. The afferent and efferent limbs of this reflex are mediated through the glossopharyngeal (IX) and vagus (X) nerves.

Prevertebral Fascia

The prevertebral fascia extends from the base of the skull down to the third thoracic vertebra, where it continues as the anterior longitudinal ligament. It also extends laterally as the axillary sheath (Fig. 1.9). Abscess formation, hemorrhage

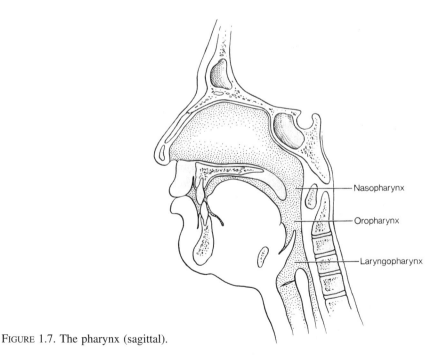

FIGURE 1.7. The pharynx (sagittal).

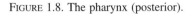

FIGURE 1.8. The pharynx (posterior).

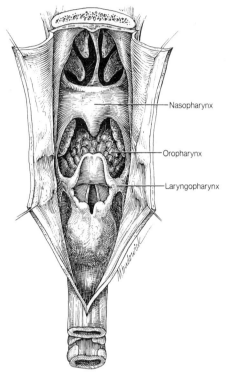

Nasopharynx

Oropharynx

Laryngopharynx

FIGURE 1.8. The pharynx (posterior).

following trauma, or tumor growth may cause swelling in this area and lead to symptoms of airway obstruction.

Retropharyngeal Space

The retropharyngeal space is a potential space lying between the prevertebral fascia and the buccopharyngeal fascia and allows some movement of the larynx,

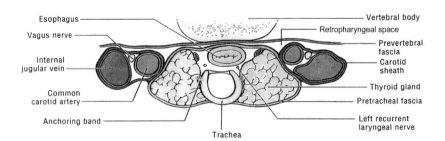

Esophagus

Vagus nerve

Internal jugular vein

Common carotid artery

Anchoring band

Trachea

Vertebral body

Retropharyngeal space

Prevertebral fascia

Carotid sheath

Thyroid gland

Pretracheal fascia

Left recurrent laryngeal nerve

FIGURE 1.9. Transverse section of the neck showing the prevertebral fascia and the retropharyngeal space.[4] (Altered with permission of the author.) (From Moore K. Clinically Oriented Anatomy, 3rd Edition. Baltimore: Lippincott Williams & Wilkins, 1992, with permission.)

pharynx, trachea, and esophagus during deglutition (Fig. 1.9). It is limited above by the base of the skull and inferiorly by the superior mediastinum. Pus posterior to the prevertebral fascia may penetrate the fascia, enter the retropharyngeal space, and cause airway obstruction.

Larynx

The larynx is the organ of phonation and is located in the anterior portion of the neck. It is a boxlike structure 4 to 5 cc in volume made up of cartilages, ligaments, muscles, and mucous membrane. In adults it is situated in the anterior portion of the neck at the level of C3 through C6. The larynx is shorter in women and children and is situated at a slightly higher level. The larynx is one of the most powerful sphincters in the body.

Laryngeal Cartilages

The larynx consists of three single cartilages: the epiglottis, the thyroid, and the cricoid; and three paired cartilages: the arytenoids, the corniculates, and the cuneiforms.

Single Cartilages

Epiglottis

The epiglottis, a well-known landmark to those performing intubation, is shaped like a leaf (Fig. 1.10). At its lower end it is attached to the thyroid cartilage by the thyroepiglottic ligament. Its upper, rounded, part is free and lies posterior to

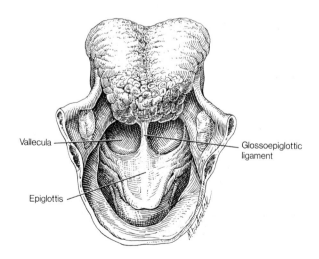

FIGURE 1.10. The epiglottis (posterior).

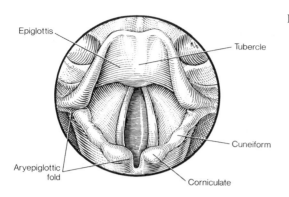

FIGURE 1.11. The glottis.

the tongue, to which it is attached by the median glossoepiglottic ligament. The epiglottis is attached to the hyoid bone anteriorly by the hyoepiglottic ligament. Small depressions on either side of this ligament are referred to as the valleculae. There is a recognizable bulge in the midportion of the posterior aspect of the epiglottis called the tubercle (Fig. 1.11). During swallowing, as the laryngeal muscles contract, the downward movement of the epiglottis and the closure and upward movement of the glottis prevent food from entering the larynx. When the epiglottis becomes acutely inflamed and swollen (in association with acute epiglottitis), life-threatening airway obstruction may occur.

Thyroid Cartilage

The thyroid cartilage (Fig. 1.12) is a shieldlike structure best visualized diagrammatically. Anteriorly the two plates come together to form a notch that is more prominent in men than in women. The reason for the prominence of Adam's apple in males is that the angle at which the thyroid laminae meet is much more acute and the anteroposterior diameter of the laminae is greater. These gender differences are usually evident by the age of 16. At the posterior aspect of each lamina there are horns on the superior and inferior aspects. The inferior horn has a circular facet that allows it to articulate with the cricoid cartilage.

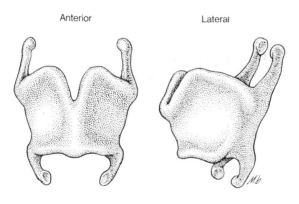

FIGURE 1.12. Thyroid cartilage.

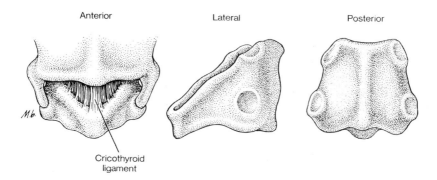

Anterior   Lateral   Posterior

Cricothyroid
ligament

FIGURE 1.13. The cricoid cartilage and cricothyroid ligament, or membrane.

Cricoid Cartilage

The cricoid cartilage is shaped like a signet ring, with the bulky portion placed posteriorly (Fig. 1.13). It has articular facets for its attachment with the thyroid cartilage and the arytenoids (Fig. 1.14). It is separated from the thyroid cartilage by the cricothyroid ligament, or membrane.

It is very important to be able to identify the cricoid cartilage because the cricothyroid ligament, or membrane, is contiguous with it inferiorly (Fig. 1.15). In acute airway obstruction, the cricothyroid membrane may be penetrated with a needle, knife, or tube and connected to an oxygen source. This procedure is called cricothyrotomy and is usually the first surgical procedure performed to relieve asphyxiation. Downward pressure on the cricoid cartilage is required to prevent passive regurgitation of gastric contents during induction of anesthesia in nonfasting patients and in emergency situations. This is also known as Sellick's maneuver.[5]

The hyoid bone, which is not part of the larynx proper, is attached to the thyroid cartilage by the thyrohyoid ligament (Fig. 1.15). The stylohyoid ligament, which is attached to the styloid process and the hyoid bone, frequently becomes

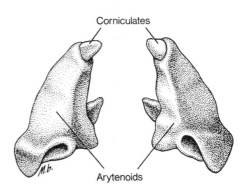

Corniculates

FIGURE 1.14. The arytenoids and corniculates.

Arytenoids

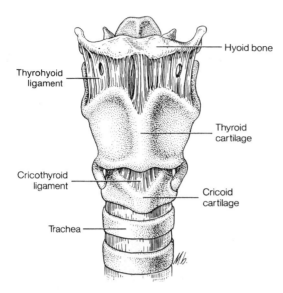

Thyrohyoid ligament

Cricothyroid ligament

Trachea

Hyoid bone

Thyroid cartilage

Cricoid cartilage

FIGURE 1.15. The larynx (anterior).

calcified in a significant number of individuals and may interfere with ability to see the larynx during intubation attempts. The inferior horn of the thyroid cartilage, joined by the cricothyroid ligaments, articulates with the cricoid cartilage bilaterally (Figs. 1.16 and 1.17). Cricothyrotomy is performed by penetrating this ligament.

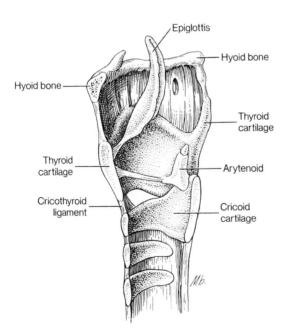

Epiglottis

Hyoid bone

Hyoid bone

Thyroid cartilage

Thyroid cartilage

Cricothyroid ligament

Arytenoid

Cricoid cartilage

FIGURE 1.16. The larynx (sagittal).

FIGURE 1.17. The larynx (posterior).

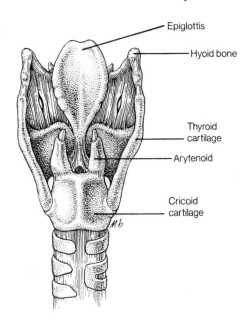

Epiglottis

Hyoid bone

Thyroid
cartilage

Arytenoid

Cricoid
cartilage

Paired Cartilages

The arytenoids are triangular structures located on the posterosuperior aspect of the cricoid cartilage. The corniculate cartilages are attached to the superior aspect of the arytenoids (see Figs. 1.16 and 1.17). The cuneiform cartilages are small and spheroidal, embedded within the aryepiglottic fold on each side (see Fig. 1.11).

Laryngeal Cavity

The space between the true vocal cords and the arytenoid cartilages is referred to as the rima glottidis. This landmark divides the larynx into two parts: the upper compartment extends from the laryngeal outlet to the vocal cords and contains the vestibular folds and the sinus of the larynx; the lower compartment extends from the vocal cords to the upper portion of the trachea (Fig. 1.18). The glottis refers to those structures at the level of the rima glottis. The term *glottis* is frequently misused to refer to the opening.

Fractures of the larynx occur from time to time following trauma. Boxers and hockey players are particularly vulnerable. Victims sometimes present with acute airway obstruction.

Piriform Sinus

There is a space between the epiglottis and the aryepiglottic folds medially, and the hyoid bone, thryohyoid ligament, and thyroid cartilage laterally, referred to

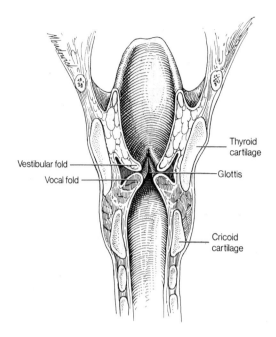

FIGURE 1.18. The larynx (coronal).

Vestibular fold

Vocal fold

Thyroid cartilage

Glottis

Cricoid cartilage

as the piriform sinus recess, or fossa (Fig. 1.19). Occasionally fish bones and other organic material may be entrapped in this recess, giving rise to symptoms of dysphagia.

Nerve Supply to the Larynx

The larynx is innervated by two branches of the vagus: the superior laryngeal and the recurrent laryngeal nerves.

Superior Laryngeal Nerve

The superior laryngeal nerve arises from the ganglion nodosum and descends inferiorly and medially to reach the internal side of the larynx. It communicates with the cervical sympathetics, passing between the greater horn of the hyoid bone and the superior horn of the thyroid cartilage, and divides into an external (motor) branch that descends to supply the cricothyroid muscle (Fig. 1.20) and an internal (sensory) branch that pierces the thyrohyoid membrane; it then divides into upper and lower branches that supply the mucous membrane of the base of the tongue, pharynx, epiglottis, and larynx.

Recurrent Laryngeal Nerve

The recurrent laryngeal nerve arises from the vagus nerve and loops around the subclavian artery on the right side and the aortic arch on the left side behind the ligamentum arteriosum. After ascending between the trachea and esophagus, it passes behind the thyroid gland and innervates all of the intrinsic muscles of the

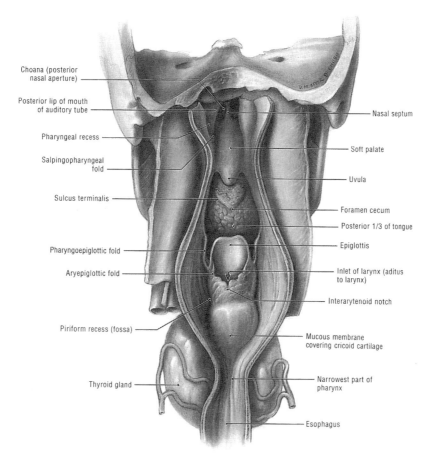

Choana (posterior nasal aperture)

Posterior lip of mouth of auditory tube

Pharyngeal recess

Salpingopharyngeal fold

Sulcus terminalis

Pharyngoepiglottic fold

Aryepiglottic fold

Piriform recess (fossa)

Thyroid gland

Nasal septum

Soft palate

Uvula

Foramen cecum

Posterior 1/3 of tongue

Epiglottis

Inlet of larynx (aditus to larynx)

Interarytenoid notch

Mucous membrane covering cricoid cartilage

Narrowest part of pharynx

Esophagus

FIGURE 1.19. The larynx (posterior) showing the piriform recess, or sinus. (From Moore K. Clinically Oriented Anatomy, 3rd Edition. Baltimore: Lippincott Williams & Wilkins, 1992, with permission.)

larynx except the cricothyroid. In addition, it supplies sensory branches to the mucous membrane of the larynx below the vocal cords.

In the event of bilateral recurrent laryngeal nerve damage (secondary to thyroidectomy, neoplasm, or trauma), the action of the superior laryngeal nerve is unopposed. Consequently, contraction of the cricothyroid muscle bilaterally results in adduction of the vocal cords and acute airway obstruction, necessitating tracheostomy. Complete paralysis of the recurrent laryngeal and superior laryngeal nerves simultaneously is characterized by a midway positioning of the vocal cords, often referred to as the cadaveric position, and frequently seen following the administration of neuromuscular drugs. A reflexive, forceful contraction of all the laryngeal muscles, as commonly occurs when a foreign body lodges in the larynx, is referred to as laryngospasm. Although laryngospasm normally serves a protective function, in such cases it may exacerbate an existing airway obstruction.

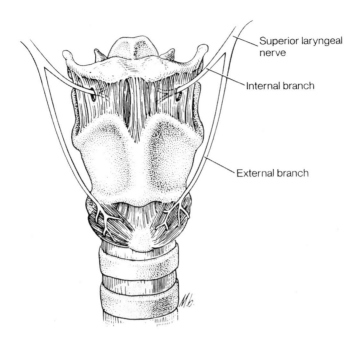

Superior laryngeal
nerve

Internal branch

External branch

FIGURE 1.20. Nerve supply to the larynx.

Trachea

The trachea is a tubular structure, about 15 cm long in adults, extending from the cricoid cartilage to the bronchial bifurcation. It has an outer diameter of 2.5 cm. On transverse section, it is shaped like the letter *D,* with the straight portion posterior. Structurally, it consists of 16 to 20 *C*-shaped cartilages joined by fibroelastic tissue and closed posteriorly by the trachealis muscle. At about the level of the fifth thoracic vertebra, the trachea bifurcates into right and left mainstem bronchi. The right mainstem bronchus appears (more than the left) to be a vertical continuation of the trachea; furthermore, the right upper lobe bronchus has its origin just about 2 cm from the carina, compared to the left, which arises about 5 cm from the carina. For these reasons, aspiration of food, liquids, or foreign bodies is far more likely to occur on the right side, and right mainstem intubations are far more common than left.

Comparative Anatomy of the Adult and Infant Airways

Before discussing how the anatomy of the airway varies with age, we should first define what we mean by "adult," "child," and "infant." An adult is an individual aged 16 or older, a child is between the ages of 1 and 8, and an infant is 1 year of age or less. At age 8 the larynx of the child closely resembles that of an adult except in size.

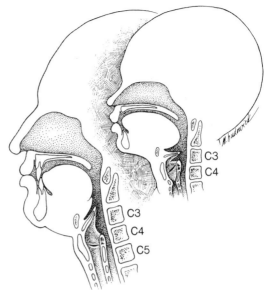

FIGURE 1.21. Comparison of
the adult and pediatric airways.

Any clinician involved in the management of airway problems should be cognizant of the infant airway. The differences between the adult and infant airway are not all explained by the age-associated changes in airway diameter (Fig. 1.21). There are differences in structure and function as well as size, involving the head, nose, tongue, epiglottis, larynx, cricoid, trachea, and mainstem bronchi.[5,6]

Head

In proportion to the rest of the body, the infant's head is much larger than the adult's. This is significant in that, in the absence of muscle tone, the weight of the infant's head forces the cervical spine to assume a more flexed position, which tends to induce airway obstruction.

Nose

The infant's nostrils are smaller in relation to the trachea than are the adult's. It is interesting to note that the infant is a compulsive nose breather during most of the first year of life. However, this is a functional difference rather than an anatomical one.

Tongue

The infant's tongue is proportionately larger than that of the adult's. Lack of muscle tone in the tongue and mandible allow the tongue to "fall back," obstructing the flow of air during inspiration and expiration. Posterior displacement of the tongue is the most common cause of airway obstruction in infants (as well as in adults). Respiratory efforts in the presence of diminished muscle tone tend to pull the tongue in a ball valve-like fashion over the airway, further contributing to obstruction.

Larynx

The larynx is situated at a higher level in relation to the cervical spine in infants (see Fig. 1.21). At birth, the rima glottidis lies at the level of the interspace between the third and fourth cervical vertebrae. Upon reaching adulthood, it lies one vertebra lower. The infant's vocal cords are concave and have an anteroinferior incline. In adults the vocal cords are less concave and lie more horizontally.

Cricoid Cartilage

The airway of the infant is narrowest at the level of the cricoid cartilage. In contrast, the adult airway is narrowest at the rima glottidis.

Epiglottis

The epiglottis in infants is remarkably different from that in adults. It is relatively longer, more omega shaped (Ω), and less flexible. In infants the hyoid bone is firmly attached to the thyroid cartilage and tends to push the base of the tongue and epiglottis toward the pharyngeal cavity; consequently, the epiglottis has a much more horizontal lie than in adults.

Trachea and Mainstem Bronchi

The major conducting airways are both narrower and shorter in infants, leaving less room for error in positioning endotracheal tubes. The trachea of a premature infant may be as short as 2.0 cm. In infants the bifurcation of the trachea (into right and left mainstem bronchi) projects at an angle of about 30° from the tracheal axis, whereas the left mainstem bronchus projects at an angle of about 47°.[8,9] In adults the angle between the right mainstem bronchus and tracheal axis is more acute[9] (Fig. 1.22). Therefore, endotracheal tubes inserted too far into the trachea are more likely to enter the right mainstem bronchus than the left in both adults and infants.

The salient anatomical differences between the infant and adult airways are summarized as follows: The infant's larynx is situated at a much higher level than the adult's. The infant's tongue is relatively larger, and the epiglottis is omega shaped, longer, and stiffer. The narrowest part of the infant's laryngeal airway is at the level of the cricoid cartilage, whereas that of the adult is at the rima glottidis. In infants the right mainstem bronchus is less vertical than in adults. The most significant difference between the adult larynx and the infant larynx is that the overall diameter of the adult's airway is 10 to 12 mm wider

FIGURE 1.22. Comparison of the adult and pediatric tracheae and bronchi.

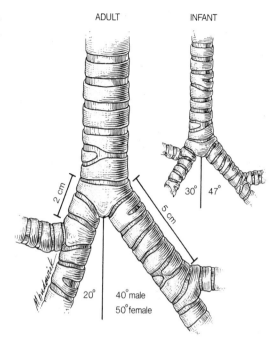

than that of a newborn. If the internal diameter of a neonate's larynx measures 4 mm at the level of the cricoid cartilage, a 1 mm circumferential reduction in this diameter (caused by either trauma or infection) will reduce the overall cross-sectional area of the airway by approximately 75%. A similar reduction in the diameter of the adult airway will reduce the cross-sectional area by about 44% (Fig. 1.23).[11]

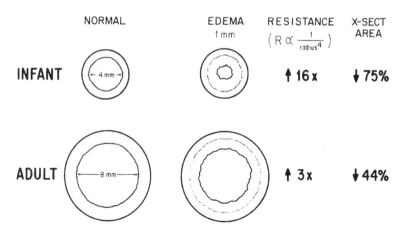

FIGURE 1.23. Comparative effects of airway edema in the infant and adult. (From Cote C, Todhes D. A Practice of Anesthesia for Infants & Children, 3rd Edition. New York: WB Saunders, 2001, with permission.)

Summary

Inspired air enters the body via the nasal and oronasal cavity and then passes into the pharynx. Subsequently, it flows beneath the inferior surface of the epiglottis and into the laryngeal inlet. Within the larynx, whose framework consists of the thyroid and cricoid cartilages, it traverses the space between the vocal cords and the rima glottidis. It then leaves the larynx and continues down the trachea, which bifurcates into the right and left mainstem bronchi, leading to the lungs.

The basics of anatomy presented in this chapter can serve as a foundation for learning how to manage airway problems. If nothing else, a knowledge of anatomy will help you to recognize what you are seeing when inserting a laryngoscope into a patient's mouth.

References

1. Ferguson CF. Pediatric Otolaryngology. In: Kendig EL, ed. *Disorders of the Respiratory Tract in Children.* 2nd ed. Philadelphia: WB Saunders; 1972.
2. Benummof JL, Sniderson LJ. *Anesthesia and Perioperative Complications.* 2nd ed. St. Louis: Mosby; 1999:5.
3. Jones DL, Cohle SD. Unanticipated difficult airway secondary to lingual tonsillar hyperplasia. *Anesth Analg.* 1993;77:1285.
4. Moore KL. *Clinically Oriented Anatomy.* 3rd ed. Baltimore: Williams & Wilkins; 1992.
5. Sellick BA. Cricoid pressure to control regurgitation of stomach contents during induction of anaesthesia. *Lancet.* 1961;2:404.
6. Eckenhoff JE. Some anatomic considerations for the larynx influencing endotracheal anesthesia. *Anesthesiology.* 1951;12:407.
7. Smith RM. *Anesthesiology for Infants and Children.* 4th ed. St. Louis: CV Mosby; 1980.
8. Kubota Y, et al. Tracheobronchial angles in infants and children. *Anesthesiology.* 1986;4:374, 376.
9. Brown TCK, Fisk GC. *Anesthesia for Children.* 1st ed. Oxford: Blackwell Scientific Publications; 1979:3.
10. Collins VJ. *Principles of Anesthesiology.* Philadelphia: Lea & Febiger; 1966:351.
11. Ryan JF, et al. *A Practice of Anesthesia for Infants and Children.* New York: Grune & Stratton Inc.; 1986:39.

Suggested Readings

Clemente CD. *Gray's Anatomy of the Human Body.* 30th ed. Philadelphia: Lea & Febiger; 1984.
Fellis H, McLarty M. *Anatomy for Anesthetists.* 2nd ed. Edinburgh: Blackwell Scientific Publications; 1969.
Lee JA. *A Synopsis of Anesthesia.* 7th ed. Baltimore: Williams & Wilkins; 1973.
Moore, Keith L. *Clinically Oriented Anatomy.* 3rd ed. Baltimore: Williams and Wilkins; 1992.

2
Basic Airway Management and Cardiopulmonary Resuscitation (CPR)

CPR AND PRECAUTIONS AGAINST THE
TRANSMISSION OF DISEASE
    Transmission of disease from CPR mannequins
SUMMARY

Almost 1 million deaths occur in North America each year as the result of cardiovascular disease (nearly 50% of deaths from all causes), including approximately 500,000 deaths due to coronary artery disease (CAD).[1] Sudden death related to CAD is the most prominent medical emergency in the United States today. Furthermore, a significant number of fatalities due to motor vehicle accidents and other traumatic events are precipitated by upper airway obstruction secondary to central nervous system (CNS) depression.[2] Many of these might be averted by appropriate and timely emergency intervention, including cardiopulmonary resuscitation (CPR). Since many preventable deaths occur outside the hospital, all health professionals should become competent in basic airway management and CPR.[3] (It has also been suggested[4] that operators of facilities where large crowds gather [e.g., factories, schools, office buildings, stadiums] should provide training for security and other personnel in the techniques of CPR and the use of an automated external defibrillator). Even in a hospital setting, the ancillary equipment and experienced personnel may not be available immediately in an emergency situation, and time should not be lost waiting for their arrival. Except in cases of hypothermia (in which the brain's decreased rate of oxygen consumption can prolong survival), patients will suffer irreversible hypoxic encephalopathy if CPR is delayed for more than 4 to 6 minutes after cardiopulmonary arrest. Therefore, timing is critical; the clinician must always be prepared to deliver basic life support.

In 1992, the American Heart Association (AHA)[5] presented an update of the training guidelines originally published in 1974, and reissued in 1980 and 1986, for cardiopulmonary resuscitation and emergency cardiac care. While emphasizing the need to identify risk factors and focus on primary prevention of cardiovascular disease in order to improve outcomes, the **chain of survival** concept was introduced. There are four links in this chain: (1) early access, (2) early CPR, (3) early defibrillation, and (4) early advanced cardiac life support (ACLS).

The most recent guidelines on emergency cardiac care (ECC) and CPR were published in *Circulation* in 2000.[6] These guidelines were internationally developed, science based, evidence based, and contain important new changes.

Etiology of Upper Airway Obstruction

When the patency of the airway is compromised, the amount of air entering or leaving the lungs is diminished. There are numerous causes of upper airway obstruction, but for the sake of clarity, they will be classified into two broad groups: CNS and peripheral.

CNS Causes

CNS depression from any cause leads to diminished tone in the mandibular muscles, resulting in airway obstruction by the tongue. Following are causes of CNS depression:

Decreased cardiac output (e.g., acute myocardial infarction, cardiac tamponade, congestive heart failure, ventricular tachycardia or fibrillation, hypovolemic shock, septic shock, massive pulmonary embolism)

Cerebral ischemia

Head trauma

Drug overdose (e.g., alcohol, barbiturates, opiates, cocaine, and combinations of these)

Hypoxemia/hypercarbia (e.g., chronic obstructive pulmonary disease, adult respiratory distress syndrome, pneumonia, pulmonary embolism)

Anesthesia

Metabolic derangements (e.g., hypoglycemia, hyperglycemia, hyponatremia, hypernatremia, hypokalemia, metabolic acidosis, uremia, hepatic encephalopathy)

Hypothermia

Hyperthermia

Peripheral Causes

Any disease or condition that allows encroachment on the upper airway is included in this category. Most causes fall under the following headings:

Congenital anomalies (e.g., Treacher Collins)

Infections (e.g., epiglottitis, croup, retropharyngeal abscess)

Tumors and mass lesions (benign, malignant) (e.g., thymoma; carcinoma of the oropharynx, larynx, and esophagus; aortic aneurysm)

Trauma

Drowning

Foreign body

Burns

Gas and smoke inhalation

Anaphylaxis (secondary to bee stings, pollen, food, drugs)

Laryngospasm

Bilateral vocal cord paralysis (secondary to trauma, thyroidectomy, or neoplasm)

The Tongue As a Cause of Airway Obstruction

The tongue is attached firmly to the mandible, hyoid bone, and epiglottis by a number of muscles and ligaments. In the normal conscious state, tone in these muscles prevents the tongue from encroaching upon the airway (Fig. 2.1). However, with altered consciousness the tone in these muscles decreases, allowing the tongue to gravitate toward the posterior pharyngeal wall and cause airway obstruction.

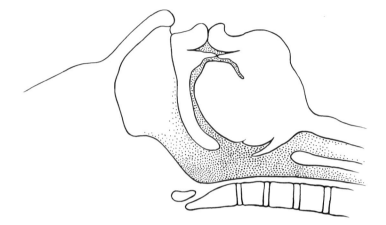

FIGURE 2.1. Tongue position in a conscious supine adult.

Three other factors contribute to airway obstruction by the tongue. First, in the comatose state the cervical spine adopts a semiflexed position, narrowing the distance from the tongue to the pharynx. Second, the epiglottis gravitates toward the glottis. Third, respiratory effort in the presence of airway obstruction pulls the tongue toward the airway (Fig. 2.2). Thus, the most common cause of upper airway obstruction is the tongue.

Basic Life Support

These guidelines apply to victims who are eight years or older. A different set of guidelines applies to those eight years old or younger.

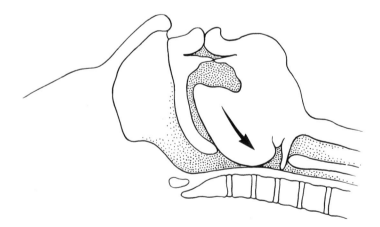

FIGURE 2.2. Tongue position in an unconscious supine adult.

Establishing Unresponsiveness and Calling for Help

Early Access

Upon encountering a collapsed victim, the rescuer must determine if the **environment is safe,** then quickly **assess** any injury and determine **unresponsiveness.**

If there is any evidence of trauma to the head or neck, suspect cervical spine injury and do not move the victim if at all possible, since there is the risk of exacerbating any spinal cord injury that may be present, which could lead to paraplegia or quadriplegia. If such a victim must be moved or rolled, try to control the head, neck, and torso as a unit. Furthermore, do not assume that all supine, motionless individuals are in need of CPR. Thus, you need to first **determine if the victim is unconscious** by gently tapping or shaking him and asking, "Are you all right?" Then, if he is responsive, **ask a few questions:**

1. Do you have neck pain?
2. Do you have numbness in your arms or legs?
3. Can you move your arms or legs?

If the victim is unresponsive, emergency medical services (EMS) should be activated in the United States (call 911). In other countries EMS is not activated unless there is evidence of apnea or absence of circulation and may be delayed until after initiation of rescue breathing. If there is more than one rescuer present, one rescuer remains with the patient while the other activates EMS. If a single rescuer is present and has determined that emergency care is needed, he should "phone first" in adult resuscitations (> eight years old).

Early CPR

It is then necessary to make sure the victim is properly positioned. For chest compressions to provide effective circulation, be sure that the victim is supine on a firm surface with the head below the level of the thorax. Then, kneeling beside the victim's shoulders, open the airway.

If cervical trauma is not suspected, place an unresponsive victim with spontaneous respirations in the **recovery position.** This involves rolling him or her onto one or other side to help protect the airway.

Airway

Determine if the victim is breathing. If the victim is facedown, he/she must be rolled as a unit into the supine position with arms by his/her side. The rescuer should position himself on one or other side and be prepared to start chest compressions and rescue breathing.

Maneuvers for Opening the Airway

Head Tilt/Chin Lift

The American Heart Association[5] has found that the head tilt/chin lift maneuver (Fig. 2.3) is the most effective technique for opening the airway of an unconscious victim as long as there is no evidence of head or neck trauma. (The head tilt/neck lift maneuver, although slightly easier to perform, is less effective and **not** recommended.) The head tilt/chin lift maneuver is achieved by placing one hand on the victim's forehead and tilting the head backward. The fingers of the other hand are placed firmly beneath the bony portion of the victim's chin, lifting it upward.

Vigorous pressure on the soft tissue structures beneath the chin can cause airway obstruction and should be avoided. The chin lift maneuver should be performed with the first two or three fingers and not the thumb (see Fig. 2.3). Dentures, if present, should not necessarily be removed, because they help maintain the normal contour of the mouth and facilitate rescue breathing.

Jaw Thrust

The jaw thrust maneuver is performed by gripping the angles of the mandible with both hands, one on each side, and pulling forward, while at the same time tilting the victim's head backward. When cervical spine injury is suspected, the modified jaw thrust maneuver, consisting of forward traction on the mandible without head tilt, is the method of choice for opening the airway, since it does not involve extension of the neck.

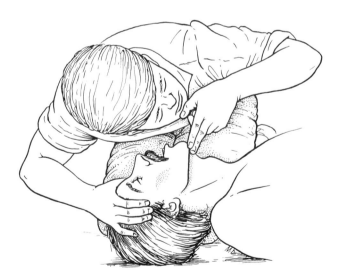

FIGURE 2.3. The head tilt/chin lift maneuver.

FIGURE 2.4. The triple airway maneuver.

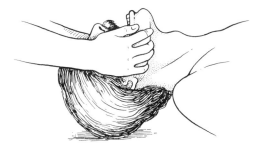

Triple Airway Maneuver (not included in recommendations)

This technique is a ramification or extension of the head tilt/jaw thrust maneuver. In addition to tilting the head backward and pulling the mandible forward, you retract the victim's lower lip with your thumb to open the mouth (Fig. 2.4). It is generally used by rescuers with advanced airway management skills.

Mandibular Displacement (not included in AHA recommendations)

The mandible can also be pulled forward by placing your thumb in the victim's mouth and your fingers beneath the chin and then lifting upward (Fig. 2.5). This maneuver is very effective in spontaneously breathing edentulous individuals, but it can be dangerous for the rescuer when the victim has teeth.

Determining Breathlessness (Look, Listen, and Feel)

After opening the airway, you must assess whether the victim is breathing spontaneously. This is done by placing your ear over the victim's mouth and (1) look-

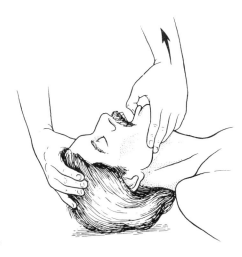

FIGURE 2.5. Mandibular displacement.

ing for the rise and fall of the chest, (2) listening for breath sounds, and (3) feeling for the exhaled air. If these signs are present, you should maintain a patent airway, and if there is no response, move the victim to the recovery position. However, if these signs are absent, the victim is not breathing adequately and you must begin resuscitation.

Rescue breathing will also be required if the victim is breathing inadequately. Gasping respirations (agonal) or respirations associated with retraction of the substernal region are signs of inadequate respiration and require augmented breathing.

Recovery Position

You may encounter a victim who is unresponsive yet breathing adequately. In that situation it is advisable to place the victim in the recovery position by turning them to one or other side.

Rescue Breathing (Single Rescuer)

Effective rescue breathing is best performed by occluding the nostrils with either your cheek or the same hand that you use to perform the head tilt maneuver (Fig. 2.6). The new AHA regulations recommend 2 to 5 initial breaths. The number of breaths varies across the world but is in the range of 2 to 5. Then you should attempt to give 10 to 12 breaths per minute and each breath should be given over a 2-second interval. The volume recommended is 10 ml/kg. You should take a deep breath before each rescue breath to maximize the amount of oxygen you deliver.

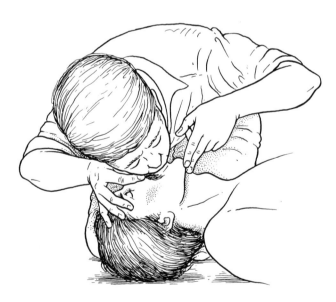

FIGURE 2.6. Rescue breathing.

FIGURE 2.7. Mouth-to-nose ventilation.

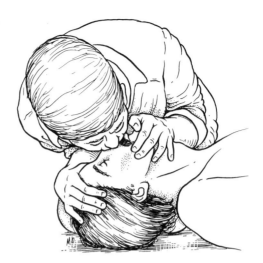

The technique of rescue breathing can be difficult to master and is best learned on a mannequin that shows the results on a printout. Effective rescue breathing requires correct head position, an airtight seal, and sufficient force to inflate the victim's lungs (i.e., cause a perceptible rise and fall of the chest). Adequate ventilation is not always possible, especially if a small rescuer is confronted with a large victim. Conversely, a large rescuer may use excessive ventilatory volumes in a child, causing barotrauma or gastric distention, leading to regurgitation and aspiration. If regurgitation does occur, turn the victim's head to one side, wipe out the mouth, and continue CPR.

When mouth-to-mouth ventilation is unsatisfactory for any reason, mouth-to-nose ventilation may be a viable alternative (Fig. 2.7). Mouth-to-mouth/nose ventilation may be necessary in children. Although the principles of basic airway management are similar in children, there are some differences, which will be discussed in the section on pediatric airway management. Finally, mouth-to-stoma ventilation may be required in patients with a tracheostomy (Fig. 2.8).

There are a number of other devices used for performing mouth-to-mouth breathing. These are:

Mouth to tracheostomy tube
Mouth to barrier device
Mouth to face shield
Mouth to mask
Bag-valve mask

These are listed for completeness.

Determining Pulselessness

Ventilation alone will not sustain an individual who has suffered a cardiac arrest. It is also essential to concurrently reestablish effective circulation for per-

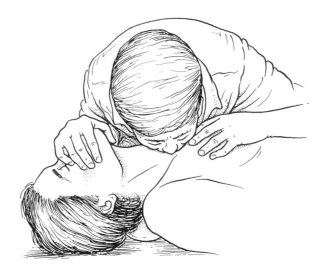

FIGURE 2.8. Mouth-to-stoma ventilation.

fusion of the vital organs. Focusing on one without the other is a futile exercise. Consequently, the next step in the resuscitation sequence is to assess whether the victim has effective circulation. This is best determined by palpating the carotid or femoral pulse. If a pulse is present but the patient is apneic, you should initiate ventilation at a rate of 12 per minute. However, if no pulse is detectable, cardiac arrest has occurred and the rescuer must begin external chest compressions.

If a layperson is a rescuer they are not expected to assess the circulation by performing the pulse check. This is a major change in the new guidelines. Studies have shown that laypeople wasted considerable time attempting to feel the pulse and that they failed to recognize the **absence** of a pulse in up to 10% of cases (false negative, or type II error). They also failed to diagnose the **presence** of a pulse in 40% of cases. These errors have serious consequences. In failing to recognize the absence of a pulse, victims were deprived of lifesaving measures (compressions and attachment of the automated external defibrillator [AED]). In failing to recognize the **presence** of a pulse (false positive, type I error) in up to 40% of cases the compressions are needlessly applied and the AED is attached. Therefore, instead of attempting to palpate the pulse a lay rescuer should look for other signs of circulation:

Look, listen, and feel for breathing or coughing
Look for signs of movement
If the above signs are absent, the rescuer should begin compressions

This assessment should take no longer than 10 seconds. If there is some doubt about your assessment of the circulation, begin chest compressions.

However, healthcare workers are expected to use the pulse check to determine the presence or absence of circulation.

External Chest Compressions

The mechanism whereby chest compression results in circulation of blood is somewhat controversial. There are two main theories. The **cardiac pump theory**[7] postulates that chest compression directly squeezes the heart between the sternum and the vertebral column. In contrast, the **thoracic pump theory**[8] maintains that chest compression increases the intrathoracic pressure, which is transmitted predominantly to the extrathoracic arteries, since they are much less collapsible than the extrathoracic veins. As a result, an arteriovenous pressure gradient is generated outside the thoracic cavity and blood flow occurs. These theories are not mutually exclusive, and it is likely that both may be operative.

To perform external chest compressions, place the heel of one hand over the victim's sternum, two finger-breadths above the xiphoid process, and the other hand on top of the first. Your arms must be straight, with the shoulders directly over the victim's sternum, so you are directing the vector of force vertically. To enhance the effectiveness of chest compressions, make each one a smooth motion, equal in duration to the relaxation phase. To minimize the risk of complications (listed below), maintain proper hand position at all times. For an adult, the depth of compression is 1.5 to 2 inches and the rate 80 to 100 per minute. In single-rescuer CPR, the compression:ventilation ratio is 15:2 (15 compressions and then 2 breaths). If CPR is generating some circulation, a second rescuer should be able to palpate a carotid pulse virtually synchronous with the chest compression.

Compression-Only CPR

Mouth-to-mouth breathing is unquestionably effective in CPR. However, some rescuers are reluctant to use it because of fear of contracting infectious diseases (hepatitis, acquired immunodeficiency syndrome [AIDS]). It is now accepted that CPR without mouth-to-mouth ventilation is better than no CPR at all.

Defibrillation

The majority of adults who present with sudden, witnessed, nontraumatic cardiac arrests are in ventricular fibrillation. The most important determinant of survival in this group is the time it takes to defibrillate the heart. With each minute lost the survival rate declines by 7% to 10%.

Limitations and Complications of CPR

Even when performed by experienced personnel, CPR is barely adequate to sustain life. First, exhaled air contains only 15% to 18% oxygen, which might be adequate were it not that the victim's arterial PO_2 is lowered substantially by the desaturation of mixed venous blood. Second, gastric distention is common and not only interferes with ventilation but also increases the risk of aspiration. Third, even with adequate chest compressions using standard CPR techniques, cardiac output is only 25% of normal. Luce and associates[8] have shown that in anesthetized dogs with electrically induced ventricular fibrillation who received conventional CPR, cerebral blood flow is only approximately 6% of normal and coronary blood flow 3% of normal.

In the past few years, many new techniques have been developed to improve circulation during CPR—including interposed abdominal compression, simultaneous ventilation and chest compressions, simultaneous ventilations and abdominal compressions, CPR with medical antishock trousers, and continuous abdominal binding.[5] Although these methods are still under investigation, some have resulted in marked improvement of cerebral blood flow, to 30% of normal, with only a slight increase in coronary blood flow.[9,10]

Furthermore, despite proper CPR technique, complications can occur—including rib and sternal fractures; costochondral separation; fat and bone marrow emboli; pneumothorax; hemothorax; gastric dilatation; aspiration; lung and myocardial contusions; pericardial tamponade; and lacerations of the gastroesophageal junction, aorta, spleen, and liver.[11]

Summary of Basic CPR

1. Establish unresponsiveness.
2. Determine that the environment is safe.
3. Do not leave the scene.
4. Call for help. Activate EMS (call 911).
5. Position the victim (preferably on a hard surface in the supine position). (In the event of head or neck trauma, do not move unless absolutely necessary. Control the head, neck, and torso as a unit.)
6. **Open airway** with head tilt/chin lift (except in suspected cervical spine injuries, when the modified jaw thrust maneuver is recommended).
7. **Determine breathlessness.** Look, listen, and feel for air exchange.
8. If spontaneous ventilation is occurring, turn victim to one side in the recovery position to minimize any risk of aspiration and then maintain patency of the airway.
9. If apneic, **deliver 2 slow breaths** (to 5 breaths).
10. If rescue breathing is unsatisfactory, reposition the head and attempt to ventilate again.
11. If rescue breathing is still unsatisfactory, suspect foreign body airway obstruction.
12. **Determine pulselessness.** Palpate the carotid or femoral artery (healthcare personnel only).
13. If a pulse is present, begin ventilations at a rate of 12 per minute. Each ventilation should be 1.5 to 2 seconds in duration.
14. If no pulse is present, begin **external chest compressions** at a rate of approximately 80 to 100 per minute. Perform cycles of 15 compressions and 2 ventilations, with each ventilation lasting 1.5 to 2 seconds.
15. After four cycles (1 minute), assess for return of pulse and spontaneous breathing. If absent, resume CPR. Thereafter, reassess the victim every few minutes. CPR should not be interrupted for more than 7 seconds.

16. In the pediatric population, **1 minute of CPR** is still recommended after initial assessment and before breaking to call EMS.

Foreign Body Airway Obstruction

Complete airway obstruction is a serious emergency that must be addressed as soon as possible. As already noted, the tongue is the most common cause of airway obstruction in unconscious patients. The epiglottis may contribute to obstruction caused by the tongue. Blood or solid food contents from the stomach may also obstruct the airway. It has been estimated that there are 1.2 deaths per 100,000 population from choking.[6]

In 1990, 2,000 people died from foreign body airway obstruction in the United States,[12] and 210 in Canada.[13] This condition has been labeled the "cafe coronary" because it occurs frequently in restaurants and the signs mimic those of an acute myocardial infarction. Typically, while eating, the individual suddenly stops breathing, becomes cyanotic, and loses consciousness. Factors that predispose to choking include ingestion of food while intoxicated or exercising, and, inadequate chewing of meat, especially in people wearing dentures. Most choking deaths occur in individuals who are aged 75 or older, or in children in the 1- to 4-year range. Meat, particularly steak and hot dogs, is the most common offending agent in adults, whereas children who often have more eclectic tastes, choke on a variety of organic and inorganic materials, ranging from peanuts to marbles to miniature toy trucks.

The diagnosis of foreign body airway obstruction should be considered in (1) any witnessed acute respiratory arrest and (2) any unwitnessed arrest wherein the rescuer cannot ventilate the victim despite repositioning the head.

The appropriateness of intervention in a conscious choking victim depends upon the adequacy of air exchange, which correlates with the degree of airway obstruction.

Partial Obstruction

In partial obstruction the narrowed portion of the airway still allows some air exchange to occur. Certain characteristic sounds may reveal the site of the obstruction. A crowing sound suggests obstruction at the vocal cords, a wheezing sound obstruction of the trachea or bronchi, and a gurgling sound regurgitation or aspiration. If there is adequate airflow, the victim can generate a powerful cough.

Since spontaneous coughing is more effective than any rescue maneuver in dislodging a foreign body, you should encourage rather than impede the victim's attempts to cough. In addition, you need to prevent the victim (who may be panic-stricken) from running out of sight (e.g., to the bathroom, where he might collapse and die unattended), and you should monitor him for signs of deteriorating respiratory status—a feeble cough, stridor, marked chest wall retractions, cyanosis, and ultimately loss of consciousness. The management of partial airway obstruction with poor airflow is the same as for complete airway obstruction.

Complete Obstruction

Complete airway obstruction is present when the victim cannot speak, cough, or breathe. Often the victim grips his throat—the universal distress signal for airway obstruction (Fig. 2.9). No signs of air exchange are detectable upon looking for chest movements, listening for breath sounds, and feeling for airflow. Efforts at inspiration are accompanied by marked chest wall retractions. In an apneic individual, complete obstruction is present when the lungs cannot be inflated by your ventilations.

Management of the Obstructed Airway— The Heimlich Maneuver

The Heimlich maneuver, alternatively described as subdiaphragmatic abdominal thrusts, is now considered the standard for relieving foreign-body upper airway obstruction in the adult.[13] Theoretically, it causes a sharp increase in intra-abdominal pressure, which in turn compresses the lungs. The resulting exhalation should be of sufficient force to expel an obstruction from the airway. The Heimlich maneuver may be performed on a conscious or an unconscious victim, who may stand, sit, or remain supine, and it may even be self-administered.

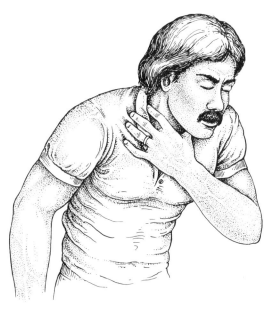

FIGURE 2.9. The universal sign of choking.

Conscious Victim

The conscious victim may be either standing or sitting when the Heimlich maneuver is carried out. (For the small rescuer the maneuver may be performed more easily with the conscious victim supine). Approaching from behind, encircle the victim's waist. Make a fist with one hand such that the thumb rests firmly on the abdominal wall in the midline slightly above the navel and well below the tip of the xiphoid process (Fig. 2.10A). Grip the fisted hand with your other hand (Fig. 2.10B) and rapidly apply an inward/upward thrust. Your hands must never rest on the xiphoid or lower ribs, lest internal organ damage may occur. Repeated thrusts should be delivered until the foreign body is expelled or the victim becomes unconscious.

The Heimlich maneuver may be self-administered by applying a fisted hand to the abdomen as just described and pressing it inward and upward. Alternatively, the victim may lean forcefully over the edge of a firm surface such as a railing or the back of a chair.

Unconscious Victim

The victim should be lying supine on a firm surface. Kneeling astride or beside him, place the heel of one hand in the midline between the xiphoid process and umbilicus (i.e., same hand position as above), the other hand on top of the first, and apply firm inward/upward pressure. Again, avoid contact with the xiphoid process and rib cage at all times.

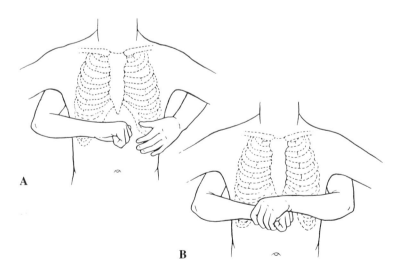

FIGURE 2.10. The Heimlich maneuver. **A.** Thumb facing inward in the midline between the navel and xiphoid process. **B.** Grip fisted hand and apply a firm inward/upward thrust.

Chest Thrusts

In markedly obese individuals, women in advanced pregnancy, and infants, the Heimlich maneuver is contraindicated and the **chest thrust** should be applied instead. (*Note:* In infants, a combination of chest thrusts and back blows is recommended [see Figs. 11.11 and 11.12].) In adults the hand position for the chest thrust is identical to that for chest compression during CPR (Fig. 2.11).

Finger Sweep

The finger sweep should be used only in an unconscious choking victim. Open the mouth by using the tongue/jaw lift (i.e., gripping the tongue and mandible between the thumb and fingers and lifting upward) and insert the index finger of your other hand alongside the cheek toward the larynx. Using a hooking motion, try to dislodge the foreign body into the mouth (Fig. 2.12). In performing this maneuver, remember that there is a risk of further impacting the object and exacerbating the airway obstruction.

Recommendations for the Conscious Choking Victim Who Becomes Unconscious (AHA Sequence)

1. Recognize the signs of choking.
   a. Universal distress
   b. Inability to speak

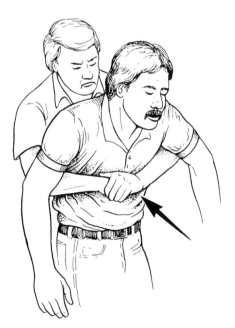

FIGURE 2.11. The chest thrust.

FIGURE 2.12. The finger sweep.

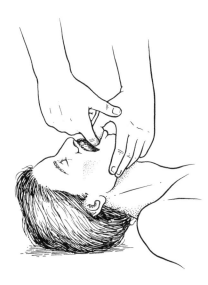

    c. Cyanosis
    d. Correct scenario
2. Call for help. Activate EMS (call 911).
3. If victim is conscious and able to speak, cough, and breathe, do not interfere with attempts to cough. Otherwise, use the Heimlich maneuver until successful or until the victim loses consciousness.
4. Place the victim in a supine position.
5. Open the mouth (tongue/jaw lift) and perform a "finger sweep."
6. Open the airway (head tilt/chin lift) and attempt to ventilate.
7. If unsuccessful, perform up to five Heimlich maneuvers.
8. Finger sweep.
9. Open the airway and attempt to ventilate.
10. Repeat steps 7 through 9 until successful, or until expert help arrives.

If the proper equipment is available, a qualified person should attempt to visualize the area with a laryngoscope and attempt to remove the foreign body with either a Magill forceps or a Kelly clamp. Failing this, a cricothyrotomy should be performed. (See Chapter 12.)

CPR and Precautions Against the Transmission of Disease

CPR is predominantly performed by healthcare workers and public safety personnel. The lay public is far less likely to perform CPR than healthcare workers. However, laypeople are more likely to perform CPR in the home.

The risk of disease transmission during mouth-to-mouth ventilation is minuscule. There are 15 reports of CPR-related infections reported in the literature between 1960 and 1998[5]. Organisms identified in these cases of CPR-related transmission include *Helicobacter pylori, Mycobacterium tuberculosis,* meningococcus, herpes simplex, shigella, streptococcus, salmonella, and *Neisseria gonorrhea*. There are no reports of human immunodeficiency virus (HIV), hepatitis B virus (HBV), hepatitis C, or cytomegalovirus infections. Despite these data, both lay personnel and healthcare workers are reluctant to perform CPR, and the reason for this reluctance is fear of contracting AIDS. In one survey, 5% of 975 questioned reported a willingness to perform mouth-to-mouth ventilation on a stranger. On the other hand, 68% were willing to perform chest compression alone if it was offered as an alternative.

Direct mouth-to-mouth ventilation will likely result in exchange of saliva between victim and rescuer. Saliva contaminated with HBV is not infectious to oral mucous membranes, such as through sharing musical instruments, even among HBV carriers. The risk of infection is far greater with airborne diseases such as tuberculosis. When a healthcare worker or layperson is exposed to tuberculosis following mouth-to-mouth respiration, the caregiver should have a skin test and should be tested again 12 weeks later.

During the past 10 to 15 years there has been a significant increase in the incidence of tuberculosis in North America.[14] Patients with AIDS are susceptible to opportunistic infections, which probably accounts for the unexpected increase in the number of patients with tuberculosis. In the United States between 1981 and 1988, there were 14,000 new cases.[15] The risk of developing tuberculosis from respiratory droplets is clearly far greater than the risk of developing AIDS.

Whenever possible, disposable airway equipment should be used, and gloves should be worn when available.[16] Furthermore, known carriers of hepatitis or persons who are HIV positive or have other infections should not teach CPR. In addition, prehospital emergency health care providers—including paramedics, emergency medical technicians (EMTs), police, and firefighters—should become skilled in the technique of bag-valve-mask ventilation.

Healthcare workers who have a duty to perform CPR on a regular basis should follow guidelines recommended by the Centers for Disease Control and Prevention (CDC) and the Occupational Safety and Health Administration (OSHA) and take precautions to protect themselves (i.e., use latex gloves and bag mask equipment with one-way valves).

Transmission of Disease from CPR Mannequins

The risk of disease transmission is extremely low during CPR training and there are no cases of CPR related infections in the literature up to the year 2000.[6] We still should make every effort to avoid the risk of infection by using cleansing agents and disinfectants after each use. Both external and internal parts of mannequins must be thoroughly cleaned after each use. There is no evidence that HIV can be transmitted by casual personal contact. The HIV virus is very delicate and is inactivated in less than 10 minutes at room temperature by a number of disinfectants. If current AHA and mannequin manufacturer recommendations are followed, the risk of HIV, HBV, bacterial, and fungal infection is extremely low.

Summary

Since time is of the essence in the prevention of cerebral hypoxia, the rescuer must always be prepared to perform CPR or relieve airway obstruction at a moment's notice, without using a bag/valve device (Ambu Bag), laryngoscope, or other sophisticated equipment. Cardiopulmonary resuscitation is best thought of as a series of alternating diagnostic and therapeutic steps. The first step (establishing unresponsiveness) is followed by maneuvers to open the airway (head tilt/chin lift, jaw thrust, triple airway maneuver, mandibular displacement). Subsequently, you need to assess whether the victim is breathing and, if necessary, initiate ventilations. Finally, if no pulse is palpable, external chest compressions must begin.

In managing a choking victim, you must assess whether the obstruction is partial or complete by evaluating the adequacy of airflow and the victim's ability to speak, cough, and breathe. The Heimlich maneuver (which may have to be repeated several times) proves effective in most cases of foreign-body airway obstruction. Be aware, however, that many of the maneuvers described in this chapter are controversial, especially those dealing with foreign-body airway obstruction, and the recommendations may change in the near future.

Now that basic resuscitation has been reviewed, the ensuing chapters will deal with evaluation of the airway and advanced techniques of airway management. **Remember:** In adults, call first; in children, call fast.

References

1. American Heart Association. *Heart and Stroke Facts.* 1991. Dallas: AHA 1992.
2. National Safety Council. *Accident Facts.* Chicago: NSC 1991.
3. American Heart Association. Standards and guidelines for cardiopulmonary resuscitation (CPR) and emergency cardiac care (ECC). *JAMA.* 1986;255:2905.
4. Lund I, Skulberg A. Cardiopulmonary resuscitation by lay people. *Lancet.* 1976;2:702.
5. Part I: Introduction to the international guidelines 2000 for CPR and ECG. *Circulation.* 2000;102 (suppl 1, pts 1-10):1-3421.
6. Babbs CF. New versus old theories of blood flow during CPR. *Crit Care Med.* 1980;8:191.
7. Rudikoff MT, et al. Mechanism of blood flow during cardiopulmonary resuscitation. *Circulation.* 1980;61:345.
8. Luce JM, et al. Regional blood flow during cardiopulmonary resuscitation in dogs using simultaneous and nonsimultaneous compression and ventilation. *Circulation.* 1983;67:258.
9. Schwartz GR. Cardiopulmonary cerebral resuscitation: basic and advanced life support. In: *Principles and Practice of Emergency Medicine*. 2nd ed. Philadelphia: WB Saunders; 1986:247.

10. Atcheson SC, Fred HL. Complications of cardiac resuscitation. *Am Heart J.* 1975;89: 263.
11. National Safety Council. *Accident Facts.* Chicago: 1987.
12. Canadian Government Printing Bureau. *Statistics Canada.* Ottawa: 1990.
13. Heimlich HJ. A life-saving maneuver to prevent food choking. *JAMA.* 1975;234:398.
14. Update: Tuberculosis Elimination—United States, *MMWR.* 1990;39:153.
15. Montanex J, et al. The spectrum of pulmonary disease in patients with HIV infection. *Can J Infec Dis.* 1994;5 (suppl E).
16. Centers for Disease Control and Prevention. Recommendations for preventing transmission of infection with human T-lymphotrophic virus type III/lymphadenopathy-associated virus in the workplace. *MMWR.* 1985;34:681.

3
Basic Airway Management Equipment

The purpose of this chapter is to describe basic oxygen-delivery systems and the equipment for intubation and ventilation. Subsequent chapters will discuss the use of this equipment as well as the use of more sophisticated equipment and techniques.

Oxygen Sources

The primary goal of airway management is to oxygenate the patient. If oxygenation is inadequate, all other supportive care will fail. An understanding of the equipment and networks used for oxygen storage and delivery will help one to avoid making fundamental mistakes that could interfere with oxygenation.

Wall Oxygen

Commercially available oxygen is obtained from the fractional distillation of air and is at least 99% pure. It is stored either in liquid form or as a gas in large cylin-

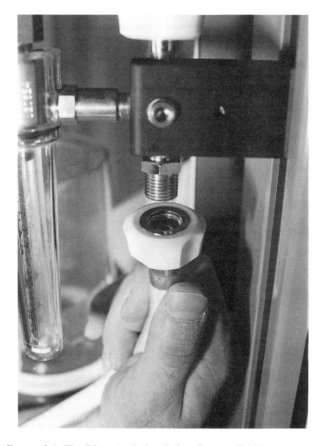

FIGURE 3.1. The Diameter Index Safety System (DISS) connector.

der reservoirs. Oxygen is piped throughout most hospitals to wall outlets. At an outlet, oxygen passes through a reducing valve at a pressure of 50 psi, which is maintained at all flow rates to every outlet. In addition, piping systems are arranged in defined zones throughout the hospital to allow the termination of oxygen delivery to a specific area while providing normal flow to other areas. This allows manual shutoff of a specified zone of outlets (e.g., in the case of fire in an isolated area). In the event of a central system failure, low-pressure alarms are activated throughout the hospital, alerting responsible individuals to take appropriate action. The standards for oxygen reservoir and piping systems are set forth by the National Fire Protection Association and the Compressed Gas Association.[1]

Each wall station is capped by an outlet, usually the Diameter Index Safety System (DISS) or quick-connect system (Figs. 3.1 and 3.2). To obtain oxygen at a reduced pressure and manageable flow rate, a flowmeter is connected to the outlet (Fig. 3.3). Flowmeters are either back-pressure compensated or non-back-pressure compensated, depending on the location of the needle valve that regu-

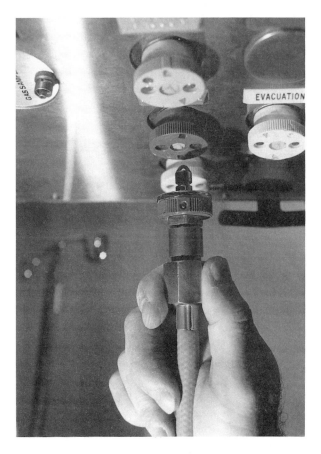

FIGURE 3.2. A modern oxygen quick-connect outlet.

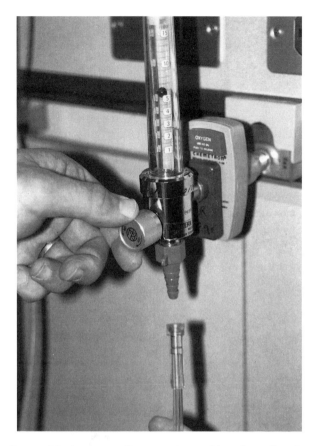

FIGURE 3.3. An oxygen flowmeter inserted into the wall outlet.

lates the flow. In a non-back-pressure compensated system the actual flow may be different from the indicated flow, owing to back pressure within the device. If in doubt as to which type of flowmeter is in use, consult the respiratory therapy department for details concerning the model used in a particular hospital.

From the flowmeter, oxygen tubing may be connected directly to the oxygen-delivery equipment, whether it is a self-inflating bag, a face mask, or nasal prongs. To ensure oxygen delivery from a wall outlet, follow these guidelines:

1. Be sure that the flowmeter is properly fitted in the wall outlet.
2. Check that the ball within the flowmeter is freely floating, then set the flow in liters per minute.
3. Inspect the oxygen tubing from the flowmeter, making sure that all connections are tight and the tube is not kinked or obstructed.
4. Listen for or feel oxygen flow at the mask or self-inflating resuscitation bag.
5. If there is any doubt about the nature or content of the gas coming from the wall outlet, use an O_2 analyzer for verification.

Tank Oxygen

Another type of oxygen storage system commonly used is the portable oxygen cylinder with an affixed regulator and flowmeter (Figs. 3.4 and 3.5). The regulator reduces the pressure within the system to 50 psi for delivery through the flowmeter. Unfortunately, there is not an international color code for oxygen cylinders. This is potentially dangerous when physicians move from one country to another. In the United States, oxygen cylinders are **green** and carry various markings that document the manufacturer and inspection dates. The common E cylinder is pressurized to between 1800 and 2400 psi at 70°F and 14.7 psi absolute (atmospheric pressure) and contains 659 liters of oxygen; therefore, the cylinder will last approximately 1 hour at a flow rate of 10 liters per minute.

To ensure oxygen flow from a portable tank, follow these guidelines:

1. Check that the seal is in place between the cylinder valve and regulator yoke.
2. Make sure that all connections are tight between the cylinder valve and regulator yoke.
3. Open the cylinder valve with a key or wrench (Fig. 3.6).
4. Read the pressure on the regulator pressure gauge.
5. Open the flowmeter and check for flow in liters per minute.

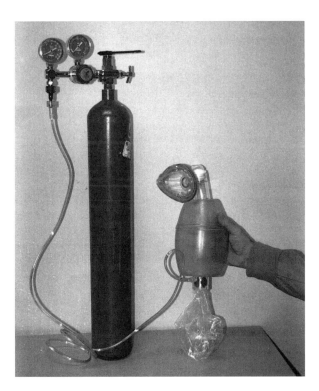

FIGURE 3.4. An oxygen E cylinder, showing the regulator and flowmeter.

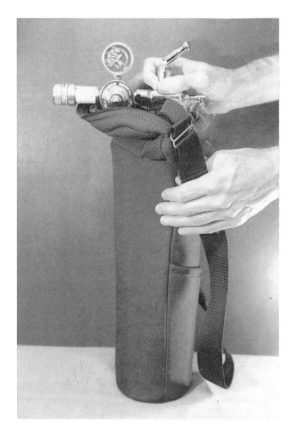

FIGURE 3.5. A portable oxygen tank for transportation.

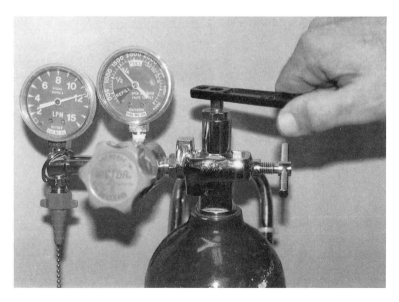

FIGURE 3.6. The tank wrench used to open an E cylinder.

6. Inspect the oxygen tubing from the flowmeter and make sure that it is connected to the mask or self-inflating resuscitation bag and is unobstructed.

As simple as these suggestions seem, in an emergency it is easy to overlook fundamental details that could interfere with oxygen flow.

Vacuum Suction Apparatus

Occasionally secretions, vomitus, and blood may interfere with gas exchange. For these reasons a suction apparatus is necessary for airway management. Suction may be obtained from a wall or portable vacuum source (Fig. 3.7).

Suction tubing may be attached either to a flexible catheter (Fig. 3.8A) or a rigid tonsillar tip (Fig. 3.9A). Both types should be immediately available to the person managing the airway. The flexible catheter is useful for decompressing the stomach and suctioning the esophagus, pharynx, and endotracheal tube (Fig. 3.8B). The tonsillar tip is useful for rapid suctioning of large volumes of fluid from the oropharynx (Fig. 3.9B). Both types, however, can induce laryngospasm, mucosal damage, or bradycardia, so care must be exercised whenever they are being used. In addition, rigid tonsillar suction tips can damage the teeth, and overzealous suctioning can dislodge an endotracheal tube. Finally, prolonged suctioning can lead to deoxygenation. Thus, suctioning should be limited to less than 10 seconds per application and 100% oxygen should be delivered in the intervals between applications.

Recent publications warn that traditional suction equipment, even the Yankauer tip suction, is not big enough to clear common particulate material in vomitus.[2] Therefore, larger-diameter suction tubing and tips should be available to the

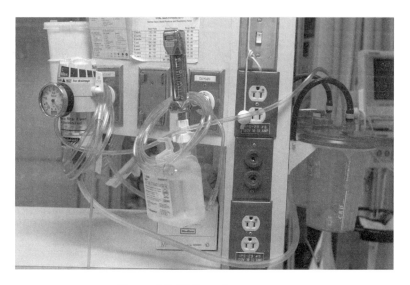

FIGURE 3.7. Wall suction apparatus.

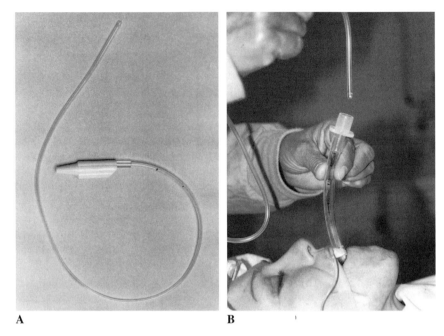

A   B

FIGURE 3.8. **A.** A flexible suction catheter. **B.** The catheter can be used to clear secretions from an endotracheal tube or the patient's upper airway.

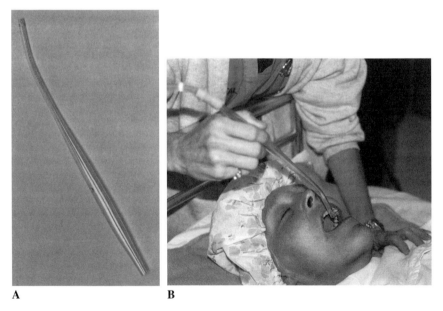

A   B

FIGURE 3.9. **A.** A rigid tonsillar suction tip. **B.** The tip can be used to remove large volumes of fluid from a patient's upper airway.

airway manager. Contact the sales representatives of airway equipment manufacturers to review the latest suction system modifications and design improvements.

Oxygen-Delivery Systems for Spontaneously Breathing Patients (Nasal Cannulae/Oxygen Masks)

Many patients who do not require ventilatory support need supplemental oxygen, particularly those with pneumonia, postoperative atelectasis, or cardiac disease. In patients with normal hemoglobin concentration and cardiac output, the goal of oxygenation should be to achieve an oxyhemoglobin saturation of at least 90%.

In the spontaneously breathing patient, the simplest method to supplement oxygen is with nasal cannulae (prongs) (Fig. 3.10) or a nasopharyngeal catheter.

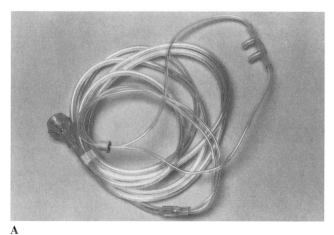

A

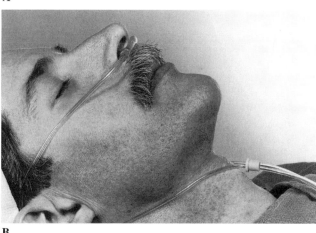

B

FIGURE 3.10. **A.** Nasal prongs. **B.** In use.

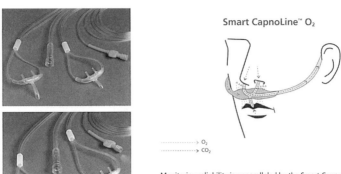

Smart CapnoLine™ O₂

····· → O₂
····· → CO₂

Monitoring reliability is unparalleled by the Smart CapnoLine™
ability to collect EtCO₂ samples from either the nose or the mouth.
The waveform display is uninterrupted by a change in patient's
breathing patterns.

FIGURE 3.11. Smart Capnoline™ (Oridion Capnography, Inc., Boston, MA, with permission.)

These are lightweight and usually well tolerated, and they do not allow rebreathing of expired air. The actual FiO_2 delivered is variable and depends upon the flow rate and the fraction of inspired oxygen.[3] The monitoring of $PETCO_2$ with nasal oxygenating systems is becoming more common, especially if the patients are receiving "conscious sedation." Many nasal oxygenation–CO_2 sampling systems are available. Be aware that different systems are tolerated differently by patients and that CO_2 sampling is affected by oxygen flow rates. Woda et al.[4] reported that the Hospitak (HOS) nasal cannula (Lindenhurst, NY) is well tolerated and that CO_2 sampling is not affected by respiratory rate and the oxygen flow rates tested (2-6 L/min). Another nasal cannula–CO_2 sampling system is the Smart CapnoLine™ O₂ (Oridion Capnography Inc., Boston, MA). Carbon dioxide monitoring can be performed by operating room analyzers or the portable Microcap™ (Oridion) monitor (Figs. 3.11 and 3.12). Future studies will care-

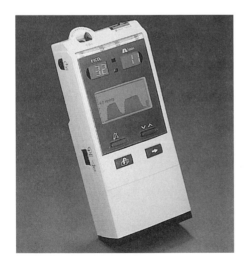

FIGURE 3.12. Microcap™ (Oridion Capnography Inc., Boston, MA, with permission.)

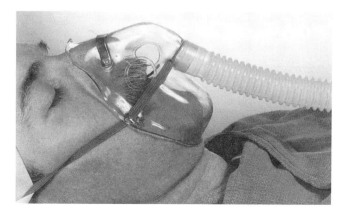

FIGURE 3.13. A simple oxygen mask in use.

fully document how accurately various nasal sampling systems reflect true $PETCO_2$ and how well nasal PCO_2 correlates with $PaCO_2$.

Nasal cannulae and modified oxygen masks (with the top cut off just above the insufflation holes and other "custom" designs) are sometimes used to supply oxygen to patients whose lower face (including the nose) is covered by surgical drapes, such as for eye surgery. There is debate in the literature as to the best oxygen delivery system. Adding a system to suction CO_2 from under the drapes, to decrease $FiCO_2$ and increase patient comfort, should be considered along with oxygenation systems.[5–10]

A plastic mask may also be used. Commonly used masks are called simple, Venturi (air entrainment), partial rebreathing, and nonrebreathing (Figs. 3.13 to 3.15). The Venturi is designed to deliver specified percentages of oxygen (Table 3.1), depending upon the size of the entrainment ports and/or the jet of oxygen. All of these masks can be used on spontaneously breathing patients who are alert

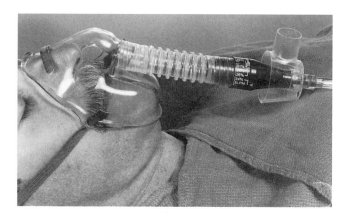

FIGURE 3.14. A Venturi oxygen mask in use.

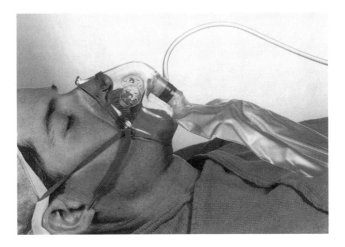

FIGURE 3.15. A partial rebreathing oxygen mask in use.

TABLE 3.1. Oxygen therapy

Delivery device	Flow rate (liters/min)	Percent O$_2$*
Nasal catheter	1 to 8	30 to 50
Nasal cannula	1 to 8	22 to 50
Simple mask	6 to12	35 to 60
Partial rebreathing	6 to 12	60 to 90
Non-rebreathing	6 to 8	Up to 100
Venturi	(See instructions for partial mask)	24, 28, 35, 40
Oxygen reservoir mask	10 to 16	90

*Approximate ranges for adults
Source: Compiled from Hunsinger DL, et al., 1980,[11] and from McPherson SP, 1981[12] and Waldau, et al.[13]

enough to protect their airway from the aspiration of secretions or vomitus. If a patient cannot protect his airway (e.g., because he is obtunded or does not manifest a gag, cough, or swallow reflex), an endotracheal tube must be inserted. All the masks illustrated are made of plastic and equipped with a head strap for support. The type of mask used depends on the desired FiO$_2$.

Oxygenation and Ventilation Systems (For Patients Requiring Ventilatory Assistance)

The remainder of this chapter describes different types of equipment used to support the patient who has lost control of his airway. Patients in this category may be obtunded, perhaps from drugs, hypoxia, or anesthesia, or are, for some reason, unable to maintain adequate gas exchange and oxygenation. This section reviews the use of airways, masks, resuscitation bags, and intubation equipment.

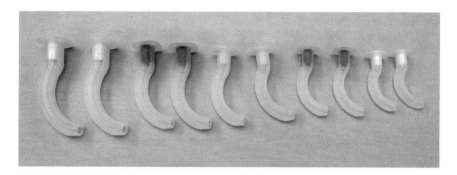

FIGURE 3.16. Oral airways (commonly made of plastic).

Airways

A patient's oropharynx can become occluded when the tongue falls posteriorly. This obstruction is often relieved by repositioning the head or anteriorly displacing the mandible. If these maneuvers are unsuccessful, an artificial airway may be inserted either orally or nasally and will usually provide a route through and around which ventilation can be maintained. However, the jaw lift maneuver is usually required even with a nasal or oral airway in place.

Oral Airway

The first oral airway was described by Hewitt in 1908.[14] Oral airways come in different lengths and designs (Fig. 3.16). They may be inserted easily behind the tongue that has been anteriorly displaced by a wooden tongue blade or a finger (Fig. 3.17). Alternatively, they may be inserted into the mouth by pointing them

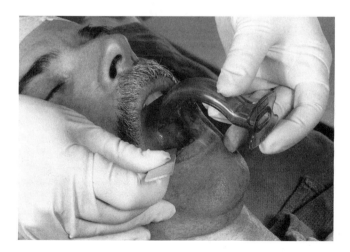

FIGURE 3.17. An oral airway can be inserted over the tongue that has been displaced by a wooden tongue blade.

initially toward the hard palate (Fig. 3.18A), and then advancing the airway and simultaneously rotating it 180° so that the tip slides behind the tongue into the hypopharynx (Fig. 3.18B). This maneuver can cause trauma to the lips, teeth, or oralpharyngeal mucosal surfaces.

Oral airways can stimulate the gag and vomit reflexes and should therefore be used only in patients whose protective reflexes have been obtunded, or who have been anesthetized. Also, it must be stressed that the insertion of an oral airway may not relieve soft tissue obstruction. Often, atlantooccipital joint dorsiflexion is necessary, even after the airway is in place.[15]

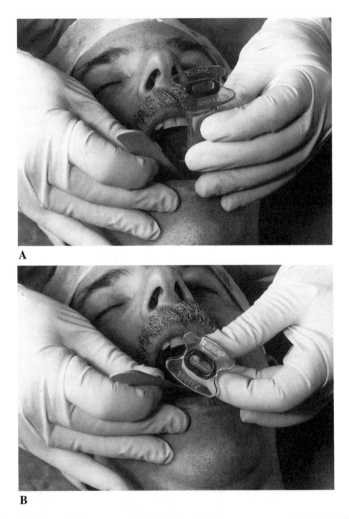

A

B

FIGURE 3.18. The oral airway can also be inserted using a two-step method. **A.** Step one: The tongue is depressed and the airway tip angled toward the roof of the mouth. **B.** Step two: The airway is rotated 180° so its tip slides into the hypopharynx.

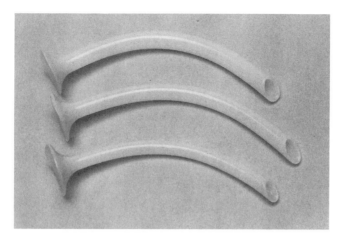

FIGURE 3.19. Nasal airways (trumpets). The most commonly used are made of soft plastic or rubber.

Nasal Airway

Nasal airways are manufactured in various diameters and lengths (Fig. 3.19). Care must be taken to ensure that airway has a ring, cone, or pin through its proximal end so that it does not slip into the esophagus or trachea. (Fig. 3.20). It should be inserted gently, through a passage that has been lubricated with viscous lidocaine or K-Y Jelly and should be advanced perpendicularly (not

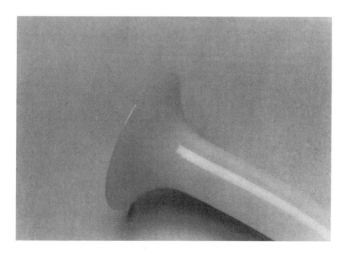

FIGURE 3.20. The distal end of the nasal airway should have a cone or ring on it so that it does not slip into the pharynx, esophagus, or trachea.

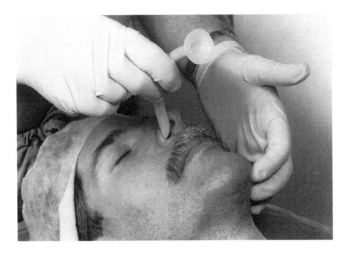

FIGURE 3.21. The nasal airway, well lubricated, is inserted parallel to the turbinates.

superiorly) against the turbinates (Fig. 3.21). If resistance to insertion is encountered, the other nostril or a smaller-sized airway should be tried. Remember that nasal airways can induce laryngospasm, epistaxis, or vomiting, and if left in place for a prolonged period, they can cause tissue necrosis. One should seriously consider using another type of airway if the patient has a basilar skull fracture.[16] If the airway is too long its tip can enter the esophagus or trachea.

Stoneham[17] commented that "the ideal position for the distal tip of the nasopharyngeal airway is within 1 cm. of the epiglottis tip" and that a 150-mm airway is appropriate for most male patients, while a 130-mm airway is suitable for most female patients. Stoneham also studied the position of the nasopharyngeal airway tip fiberoptically and noted that the tip's position did not change very much with flexion or extension of the head. Beattie[18] described the "modified nasal trumpet" maneuver. He prepared an airway by inserting a 15-mm adapter from a 7.5 or 8.0 endotracheal tube into the proximal end of a nasal airway that had been modified by cutting a "Murphy eye" into its distal end (Fig. 3.22). He then inserted the modified nasal airway and attached the distal end to an anesthesia machine circuit and attempted to ventilate the patient. If ventilation was unsuccessful, he pulled the nasal airway back 1 to 2 cm and attempted to ventilate again. He was able to provide ventilation easily to most patients. He described performing fiberoptically guided nasotracheal intubation through the other nostril with the modified airway in place used to ventilate and oxygenate the patient during the intubation. Those interested in the history of the oral and nasal airway should read the scholarly article by John McIntyre[19] that succinctly reviews the subject. He writes, "Currently for supraglottic airway management during general anaesthesia, four types of airway should be available: a Guedel (oral) airway, a nasopharyngeal airway, a

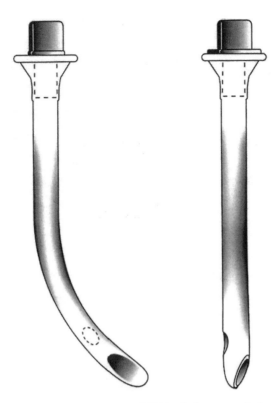

FIGURE 3.22. The modified nasal trumpet (MNT). Ordinary nasal airway with an endo-tracheal tube (ETT) connector wedged into the flared end. Also shown is an optional "Murphy eye," a fenestration cut (with scissors) into the distal end opposite and slightly proximal to the bevel. (Beattie, 2002,[18] with permission.)

laryngeal mask airway [LMA], and an airway specifically designed to facili-tate blind tracheal intubation." (See Chapter 13.)

Anesthesia Masks and Resuscitation Bags

Adequate ventilation and oxygenation can be maintained with a bag and mask system that is connected to an oxygen source (Fig. 3.23). The bag/valve/mask is the primary system utilized by clinicians involved in airway management. Ven-tilation and oxygenation can be maintained for long periods while other sup-portive therapy is initiated. Do not abandon the mask for intubation unless the added protection of a cuffed endotracheal tube is indicated. All too often, bag/mask ventilation is neglected or underutilized and intubation becomes the main priority of the individual managing the airway, occasionally to the detri-

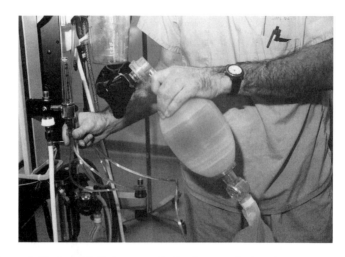

FIGURE 3.23. A self-inflating resuscitation bag attached to the oxygen source.

ment of the patient. Mask ventilation should be maintained until all intubation equipment is on hand and checked out.

Masks

There are many shapes and sizes of anesthesia/resuscitation masks (Fig. 3.24). A mask should fit over the bridge of the nose, cheeks, and chin to produce an airtight seal. If a seal is difficult to establish, reshaping the mask's malleable perimeter or selecting a different-sized mask may be helpful. The mask should be pressed against the nasal bridge with the thumb while the index finger exerts downward pressure on the base of the mask over the chin. The little finger should engage the angle of the mandible. With the hand thus positioned, one can lift the

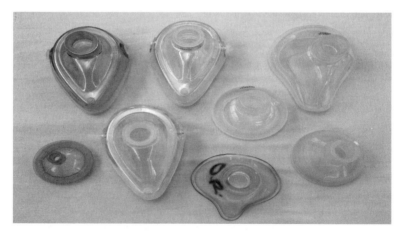

FIGURE 3.24. Anesthesia resuscitation masks. These come in a variety of sizes, shapes, and materials.

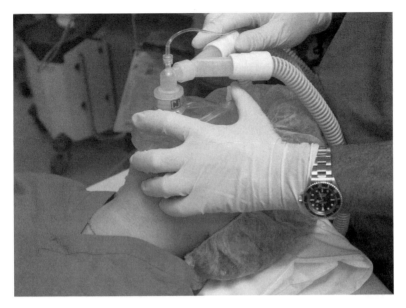

FIGURE 3.25. Proper mask fit. Note the position of the hand, with two fingers holding the mask, and three lifting the mandible.

mandible upward to open the airway (Fig. 3.25). Although the grip must be tight, intermittent relaxation of one or two fingers at a time will prevent the hand and arm from tiring. Anesthetists often maintain mask airways for 1 to 2 hours after they have mastered the technique. All masks increase dead space, so larger tidal volumes are required. Note also that opaque masks may conceal vomit or secretions within the mouth; thus, clear masks are preferable. Perhaps the masks of the future will be designed with more attention to anatomical considerations.

A variety of devices have been used to assist with mask fit and the maintenance of a patent airway. Most have been used in the operating room by anesthesiologists. Some are of simple design, such as the head strap, others more complex (Fig. 3.26). Be aware that the use of a mask with or without supporting devices can cause nerve or eye injury.

Many authors describe **two-person** or **two- or three-handed**[20–22] mask ventilation when one operator has trouble maintaining a mask fit with one hand and providing positive pressure ventilation with the other. These maneuvers are performed with one person applying the mask with two hands and providing jaw lift while the other ventilates the patient. The person ventilating the patient can also help to position the mask on the patient's face with a free hand. Two-person mask ventilation is often effective when one-person ventilation is not.

Manual Resuscitation Bags

It is preferable to use a self-inflating manual resuscitation bag/valve/mask device so that in the event of oxygen system failure, at least room air can be delivered.

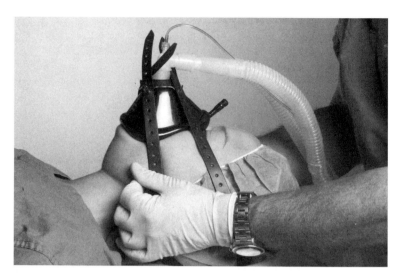

FIGURE 3.26. To improve the fit, a mask may be supported by a head strap.

The bag/valve device should have standard fittings for connection to an endotracheal tube or face mask (15 mm inside, 22 mm outside, diameter delivery port) (Fig. 3.27). A self-inflating system can deliver enriched oxygen mixtures when connected to an oxygen storage tank or wall outlet. The valves of the system should be designed to function during either spontaneous or controlled positive-pressure ventilation. To avoid the development of high airway pressures, pediatric bag/valve devices should be fitted with a 25 to 30 cm H_2O release valve. All systems should

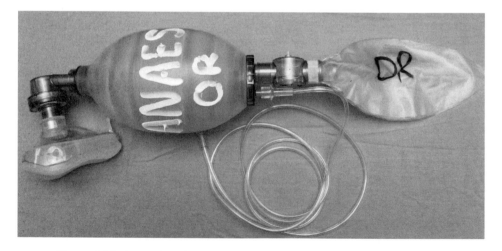

FIGURE 3.27. A complete mask/resuscitation bag/oxygen reservoir/tubing system.

also be able to accept a positive end-expiratory pressure (PEEP) valve and should be designed so that either a tube-type reservoir or a reservoir bag can be fitted to deliver high FiO_2. Before use, check the valves for proper operation and gas flow and make sure that the plastic connections are properly secured.

Summary

The basic equipment required to oxygenate and ventilate a patient includes an oxygen source, an oral or nasal airway, a face mask, a resuscitation bag, and a reliable suction apparatus. One must master the technique of manual airway support using these relatively simple and inexpensive pieces of equipment before advancing to more sophisticated airway management techniques.

Equipment for Endotracheal Intubation

This section describes the laryngoscope and various types of laryngoscope blades, endotracheal light sources, the endotracheal tube, and stylets used for intubation.

Laryngoscope

Although intubation can be accomplished without a laryngoscope ("blind" intubation), one of the best ways to ensure proper tube placement is to see the tube pass between the vocal cords.

The laryngoscope consists of a handle and a blade (Fig. 3.28). The handle houses the batteries that power the light. Conventional laryngoscope blades are fitted with a small light that screws into an outlet on the blade. Newer blades are fitted with a fiberoptic light-delivery channel, the light source may be housed in the handle of the laryngoscope. The surface of the handle is usually machined to afford a rough surface for improved grip. The top of the handle has a fitting into

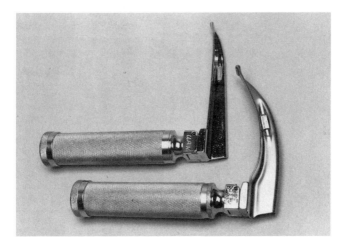

FIGURE 3.28. Laryngoscopes.

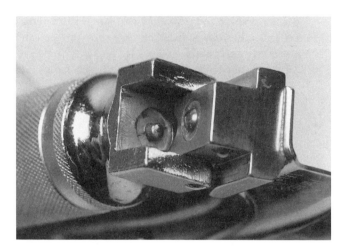

FIGURE 3.29. To ensure good contact and bright illumination, the electrical connections of the laryngoscope handle and blade must be clean.

which the blade is secured and through which electricity is supplied to the bulb. The electrical contacts should be clean and the batteries fresh (Fig. 3.29).

Laryngoscope blades are designed to enter the mouth, displace the soft tissues, elevate the epiglottis (either directly [straight blade] or indirectly [curved blade with the tip in the vallecula]), and expose the vocal cords. There are many types of blades (Fig. 3.30). Some are of ingenious design to facilitate difficult intubation, such as the Siker mirror blade, the Huffman prism, and the Bellhouse blade. Many of these specialty blades are described in Chapter 8. In an article addressing laryngoscope blade design and function, John McIntyre[23] evaluates many types

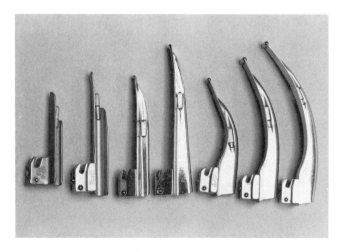

FIGURE 3.30. Laryngoscope blades.

of laryngoscope blades and suggests anatomic findings that should trigger the intubationist to consider a particular blade design. Dr. McIntyre writes, "Selection of the laryngoscope for the task must be based on problems identified at clinical examination, the patient's history, and an intuitive matching of a laryngoscope that appears to have characteristics that will offset these factors. . . . Thus, an axiom for anaesthesiologists is: 'Examine your patient, understand laryngoscopes, learn how to use them.' " This is sound advice reflecting years of study and experience. One needs to become familiar with only two basic designs—the straight blade (Miller) and the curved blade (MacIntosh). In a recent analysis of laryngoscope blade shape and design, the authors state[24]: "Since the advent of tracheal intubation in anesthesia, at least 50 descriptions of laryngoscope blade designs have been published, and many more designs exist unpublished."

The "ultimate" blade has not been designed, but more study of the shape, size, and classification of laryngoscope blades is under way, and in the future, selection of the best blade for intubation in the widest variety of clinical scenarios should be more predictable, based upon scientific data rather than traditional clinical bias and anecdote.[24–28]

One should become familiar with one or two simple designs of blades before graduating to the more sophisticated varieties. The laryngoscope blade has four main features: a light source (or fiberoptic channel), a spatula for compression or manipulation of soft tissue, a flange to help guide the tube, and a tip to contact and support the epiglottis or vallecula for exposure of the vocal cords. To ensure good electrical or fiberoptic contact, the end of the blade that mates with the handle should be clean. The light source should be tightly secured so that the bulb produces constant illumination and is not dislodged in the oropharynx. All resuscitation trays should contain at least two laryngoscope handles with a variety of straight and curved blades.

One needs to keep in mind the observations of Bucx et al.[29], Tousignant and Tessler,[30] and Fletcher[31] when using fiberoptic laryngoscopes. These scopes are designed with the light source in the handle of the scope. The light is transmitted toward the tip of the blade with a fiberoptic channel. Fiberoptic laryngoscopes are made by many manufacturers such as Heine (Herrsching, Germany), Medicon (Tuttlingen, Germany), Penlon (Abingdon, UK), Riester (Jungingen, Germany), and Upsher (Foster City, CA).[29] When new and functioning optimally, the light intensity directed toward the airway is bright and focused. However, these authors report that sterilization and handling of the blades can compromise the quality and intensity of the light directed into the airway. The quality of the light produced with traditional scopes can also be altered with cleaning and handling, and the bulbs and batteries need to be checked on a regular basis.

Laryngoscopes with a "levering" tip have been introduced into practice. These scopes employ a Macintosh blade with a hinged tip that can be "levered" upward, causing the tip to exert more force to the vallecula, a maneuver that purportedly will more efficiently elevate the epiglottis. It is postulated that less lifting need be applied to the scope and that neck movement can be minimized. Avoiding neck movement might make laryngoscopy safer for patients with cervical spine pathol-

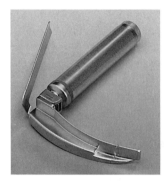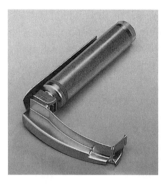

FIGURE 3.31. The Heine CL flexible tip laryngoscope blade. (Heine USA Limited, Dover, NH, with permission.)

ogy. Two such scopes are the McCoy Levering Laryngoscope (Penlon Ltd., Abingdon, UK)[32] and the Heine CL (Corazzelli-London) Flexible Tip Laryngoscope Blade (Heine USA Ltd., Dover, NH) (Fig. 3.31). The utility of this design of laryngoscope blade is still under investigation. Some authors report that it is useful when neck extension is limited or undesirable.[32,33] Others report that the McCoy blade can be used to facilitate fiberoptic intubation even if the laryngoscopic view is not significantly improved.[34,35] The reports of Randell et al.[36] and Ochroch and Levitan[37] suggest that laryngoscopic visualization is more improved by external tracheal manipulations ("B.U.R.P." maneuver) than by utilization of the McCoy scope for patients placed in the "sniff" position for elective intubation. McCoy et al.[38] reported that the force applied to the pharyngeal tissues was less with his blade than that applied with a traditional Mac 3 laryngoscope. One case report by Usui et al.[39] documents arytenoid dislocation in a patient intubated with a McCoy scope. (This injury is reported with standard blade designs also.) Future study will more clearly define the role of this laryngoscope blade design.

Another new instrument is called the Flexiblade™ laryngoscope (Arco Medic Ltd., Israel) (Fig. 3.32). The Flexiblade™ is composed of three basic parts, described by Yardeni et al.[40] to be "1. A flexible steel blade with a pushing rod rigidly attached to the front. 2. A base for the blade that includes a trigger, whereby a force is applied directly to the rear of the pushing rod, and transmitted to the tip of the blade causing its 'bending' in its middle part. 3. A standard handle." Yardeni et al.[41] write, "The device is designed to facilitate orotracheal intubation with the patient's head in the neutral position." These same authors declare that the blade is easy and safe to use and that it "seems that it has a special place in difficult intubation."[40] Future study will define the blade's utility and efficacy. Care should be taken to reassemble the blade properly after cleaning.[42]

In concluding this section on laryngoscopes and blade design, one is encouraged to become familiar with the use of standard Macintosh and Miller blades before experimenting with blades of more sophisticated design.

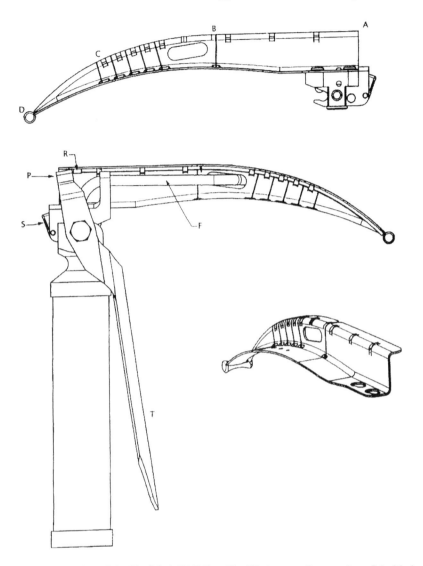

FIGURE 3.32. Design of the Flexiblade™. BC = Flexible intermediate portion of the blade, R = rod, F = fiberoptic, P = pusher, and T = trigger (Arco Medic Ltd., Israel,[41] with permission.)

Alternative Light Source

The more sophisticated airway tray might contain an alternative light source—a headlight,[43] pen light,[44] a pocket flashlight,[45] or a high-intensity external fiberoptic light source.[46] These devices have been used to illuminate the airway when the primary light source (on the laryngoscope blade) has failed because of loose connections, weak batteries, blood covering the bulb, or poor illumination.

Endotracheal Tube

The endotracheal tube is one of the most essential tools for airway management. Despite the fact that tracheal intubation is often lifesaving, both the technique and tubes themselves can be hazardous to the patient. An understanding of tube design and function is essential for safe application.

Compared to the normal airway, an endotracheal tube increases the resistance to gas flow. In certain cases it may also increase dead space. Tubes are calibrated in external and internal diameters (mm), and in length (cm). To prevent excessive airway resistance, a tube should not become kinked or sharply bent. Also, whenever possible, straight or large-bore connectors should be used in the circuit from the tube to the resuscitation bag. Modern tracheal tubes are usually made of polyvinyl chloride, or medical-grade silicone rubber. Since many chemicals are involved in the manufacture of plastic tubes, tissue toxicity from the tubes themselves has long been a concern. Most manufacturers now tissue-test their tubes and document the lack of tissue toxicity by printing "IT" (implant tested) or Z-79 (Z-79 Committee of the American National Standards Institute) on the tubes. Only tubes with these safety designations should be used. Endotracheal tubes should not be reused.

This section will describe some of the common types of tracheal tubes available as well as a few that are designed for special applications. Most tubes incorporate a high-volume, low-pressure cuff (Fig. 3.33). Cuff pressure should not exceed 25 torr (capillary pressure) lest mucosal ischemia or tracheal necrosis occur. Standard endotracheal tubes may be used for nasal and oral intubation. The tip of the tube is bevelled and should include a side port or Murphy eye (Fig. 3.34). The side port may allow ventilation even if the main port becomes occluded by the tracheal wall, blood clot, or secretions. The other end of the tube is fitted with a standard 15-mm adapter for connection to a resuscitation bag or

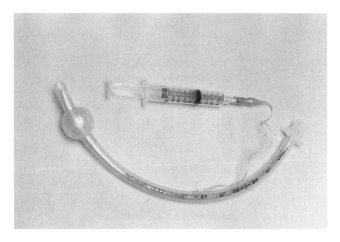

FIGURE 3.33. Standard endotracheal tube with inflated cuff. (Nellcor Puritan Bennett Inc., Pleasanton, CA, with permission.)

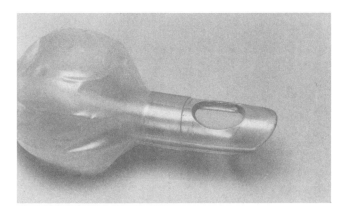

FIGURE 3.34. Tip of a standard endotracheal tube, demonstrating the Murphy eye or side port.

ventilator. The cuff of the tube may be inflated by injecting air into the valve, which is attached to a side port.

There are many special types of endotracheal tubes—Endotrol; armored, or wire-reinforced Anode; double-lumen endobronchial, special tip designed, and uncuffed. The **Endotrol** tube is designed with a built-in stylet (Fig. 3.35). When its "trigger," or ring, is pulled, a thread running through a channel in the tube wall applies traction to the tip of the tube, causing the tube curvature to increase. Endotrol tubes are useful for "blind" nasal or difficult oral intubations. The **wire-reinforced Anode** tube is manufactured with a metal wire or nylon filament embedded into its wall (Fig. 3.36). This design has the advantage of resisting col-

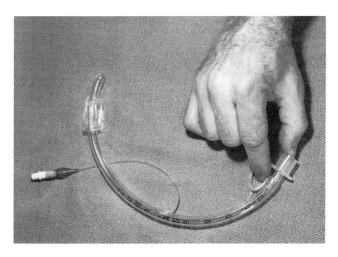

FIGURE 3.35. The Endotrol tube (Mallinckrodt), showing the ring, or "trigger", near its distal end. When the trigger is pulled, the curvature of the tube increases, thus lifting the tip of the tube. (Nellcor Puritan Bennett Inc., Pleasanton, CA, with permission.)

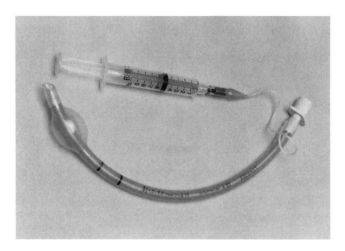

FIGURE 3.36. The Anode, wire-reinforced or armored, endotracheal tube (Mallinckrodt). (Nellcor Puritan Bennett Inc., Pleasanton, CA, with permission.)

lapse or kinking. Since the tube is very flexible in its longitudinal axis, a stylet is needed for intubation. The tube can be used orally, nasally, or through a tracheostomy stoma. Certain manufacturers do not incorporate a bevel or Murphy eye in its tube design. A **double-lumen endobronchial tube** is used when one-lung anesthesia or isolation of the lungs is desired, (Fig 3.37). Its indications are discussed in Chapter 6. Older designs of this tube include the Gordon-Green, Carlens, White, Bryce-Smith, and Robert-Shaw.[47] Newer, disposable, clear plastic designs are now available. Since these are often difficult to insert, however, and can easily occlude the right or left bronchus, an anesthesiologist should always be consulted

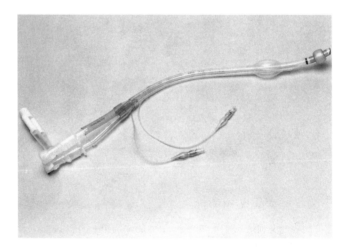

FIGURE 3.37. The double-lumen endobronchial tube (Mallinckrodt). (Nellcor Puritan Bennett Inc., Pleasanton, CA, with permission.)

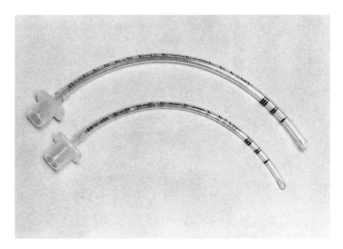

FIGURE 3.38. Uncuffed pediatric endotracheal tubes. (Nellcor Puritan Bennett Inc., Pleasanton, CA, with permission.)

before they are used. **Uncuffed tubes** are generally inserted in pediatric patients (Fig. 3.38). Cuffs are not necessary in most children under 8 years of age because the narrowest portion of a small child's airway is at the cricoid cartilage and an uncuffed tube of appropriate size should afford a reasonable seal at this level.

Recent articles document that cuffed endotracheal tubes are safe to use in pediatric patients. The old dogma of using only uncuffed tubes in children is no longer accepted by many practitioners.[48–50]

An article by St. John,[51] which reviews recent advances in artificial airway management, describes some interesting new equipment. The Hi-Lo Evac Endotracheal Tube (Mallinckrodt Inc., St. Louis, MO) incorporates a dedicated suction lumen and channel that can be used to clear secretions below the cords and above the balloon. These secretions may increase the risk of pulmonary infection in long-term intubated patients. St. John also presents a section on endotracheal cuff design and describes an ultrathin-walled tube that has a "no pressure" intraglottic cuff of unique "gill" design. This tube is described by its developers in various articles.[52,53] Newly designed tubes and cuffs have been introduced that will hopefully make ventilation easier (less airway resistance) and decrease the likelihood of pressure-related trauma and injury to the mouth, larynx, or trachea.

One should consider the **orientation and shape of the tip** of the endotracheal tube, especially if one has difficulty passing a standard tube through the vocal cords over a fiberoptic scope or a gum bougie. West et al.[54] described an experimental tube that had the bevel reversed and found that it was very easy to pass over a bougie under "simulated" difficult airway conditions. A tube manufactured by Parker Medical (Englewood, CO) is called the Parker Flex-Tip™ (Fig. 3.39). This tube has its bevel pointing toward the back of the tube. It also has a smooth, "hooded" tip that could facilitate passage of the tube through the glottic opening.

Much is written concerning the pressures exerted against the mucosal surfaces by the tube and its cuff. An article by Brimacombe et al.[55] warns that indirect meth-

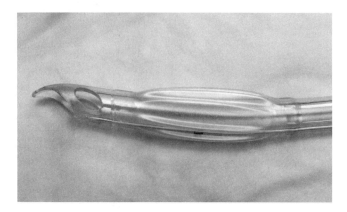

FIGURE 3.39. The Parker Flex-Tip™ endotracheal tube. Note the bevel pointing to the back of the tube and the "hooded" tip of the tube's distal end (Parker Medical, Englewood, CO, with permission.)

ods to measure mucosal pressure, such as cuff pressure, are of "moderate predictive value" and may not accurately reflect true mucosal pressure. These investigators also remind us that mucosal pressures vary at different anatomic levels and with different head movements. When evaluating manufacturer's claims with respect to the mucosal pressure exerted by various designs of airway equipment, verify that the methods used to measure mucosal pressure are accurate and precise.

In the future, manufacturers of endotracheal tubes will incorporate new materials and design features into their products to make them more useful and safer. An example of one such feature is a cuff impervious to nitrous oxide that could limit pressure buildup in the cuff during an operation. Articles by Fujiwara et al.[56] and Karasawa et al.[57] describe the Trachelon™, a gas barrier–type endotracheal tube (Terumo Co., Ltd., Tokyo), with such a cuff design. The authors of the second article suggest that cuff compliance, rather than N_2O impermeability, may be responsible for lower cuff pressures developed when N_2O is used.

Equipment for Selective Lung Ventilation

New equipment has been developed that is used to provide selective lung ventilation and/or isolation. It is beyond the scope of this book to describe this advanced equipment. Mention should be made of the **Arndt Endobronchial Blocker** (Cook Critical Care, Bloomington, IN) and the **Univent Tube** (Vitaid Ltd., Lewistown, NY). Both of these devices have been studied and described extensively in recent literature dealing with advanced airway management techniques.

Stylet

A stylet is a malleable metal or plastic stent over which an endotracheal tube is passed (Fig. 3.40). It allows the curvature of the tube to be altered to facilitate a difficult intubation (Fig. 3.41).

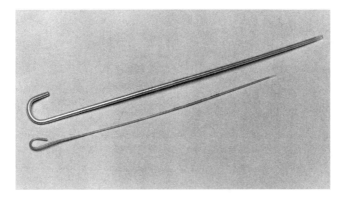

FIGURE 3.40. Stylets.

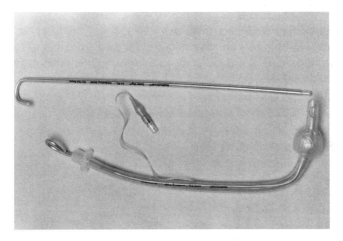

FIGURE 3.41. When used in an endotracheal tube, the stylet will hold its hockey-stick configuration to assist in directing the tube toward the airway when the larynx is not readily visible.

Withdrawal of the stylet may cause the tip of the endotracheal tube to move anteriorily, a maneuver documented by Stix and Mancini.[58] This anterior movement could help direct the tube through an anteriorly positioned glottis.

Other Useful Airway Tools

One's arsenal of basic airway equipment should include a gum elastic bougie, various intubating catheters such as the Aintree catheter,[59] Magill forceps,[60] and possibly mouth gags or other mouth-opening devices used by ear, nose, and throat (ENT) surgeons.[61] Consult an experienced instructor when learning to use this equipment.

Pulse Oximetry and Capnography

The pulse oximeter is used to document the level of oxyhemoglobin saturation in capillary tissue and the capnograph is used to measure end-tidal CO_2 as expired from the lungs. These monitors are used routinely in the operating room, recovery room, emergency room, and the intensive care unit. Practitioners of airway management must learn to apply the monitors correctly and to interpret the data properly. These monitors can be used to help diagnose various anatomic abnormalities as well as mechanical problems with oxygenation/ventilation equipment. One may learn about these monitors (and their limitations and problems) in formal anesthesiology and intensive-care medicine textbooks.

Equipment Problems

Rule No. 1: Any piece of equipment can break or fail
Rule No. 2: Have backup equipment immediately available

The literature is replete with articles and letters describing examples of equipment failure. It is important to check equipment before use and to have backup equipment immediately available if an instrument fails or breaks. Any piece of equipment can fail. The following list summarizes problems the airway manager may encounter.

Oxygen Source

Failure of the central oxygen piping system
Plumbing and piping errors that allow gasses other than oxygen to be delivered
    from the oxygen outlet
A broken flowmeter[62]
A contaminated oxygen tank[63]
Occluded or obstructed oxygen tubing
Scavenging system failures[64,65]

Endotracheal Tube

Obstruction by a wall defect, membranes, or other manufacturing flaw[66–69]
Leaks[70–72]
Cuff herniation or rupture[73]
Cracks, leaks, or obstruction of the cuff-inflation valve[74]
A malfunction that makes it difficult to deflate the cuff[75,76]
Kinking or dislodgment by another device (e.g., a suction catheter)[77]
Fire (with laser surgery)
A broken or slipped 15-mm adapter[78,79]

Laryngoscope

A broken handle or blade[80–85]
Short-circuiting that leads to excessive heating of the handle[86,87]

Dead batteries
A dead or loose lightbulb[88]

Stylet

Direct tissue damage
Fracture if the plastic coating with pieces is left in the airway[89]
Broken in the airway[90]
Bent so as to obstruct the cuff side-port

Anode or Wire-Reinforced Tube

Deformation/obstruction (e.g., a patient bites and bends the wires in its wall)[91]
Bubbles forming in the wall and causing obstruction[92]
A faulty cuff[93]

Oral Airways

Irritation of salivary duct, causing transient sialadenopathy[94]
Manufacturing defects[95]

Nasal Airways

Cannula displaced submucosally[96]

"The Dedicated Airway" and the "Ideal Airway Device"

Charters and O'Sullivan[97] define the "dedicated airway" to be "an upper airway device dedicated to the maintenance of airway patency while other major airway interventions are anticipated or in progress." Charters[98] lists the features one may expect from the "ideal airway device." These authors remind us that the development of equipment traditionally used in airway management has evolved empirically. The designs are not necessarily based on observations derived from anatomic or physiologic scientific study. They recommend that future design considerations should reflect new knowledge obtained from controlled research designed to define upper airway anatomy and physiologic function.

Summary

A visit to the anesthesiology or respiratory therapy department in **advance** of an emergency will allow you to become familiar with all the equipment available. In an emergency such avist can save time, minimize anxiety, and ultimately benefit patients. Important rules to follow are:

1. Learn to examine the airway quickly.
2. Know the various equipment options available for airway support and instrumentation.

3. Choose the correct piece of equipment for the job. Consider backup equipment and techniques.
4. Oxygen and suction should always be available.
5. Never leave the patient with an airway problem unattended.
6. If you encounter equipment failure, do not forget the basics. Utilize the bag/valve/mask.
7. If you are in doubt or if unanticipated difficulty is encountered with a patient's airway, get help immediately! No time can be wasted trying to prevent the irreversible sequelae of hypoxia!

References

1. Dorsch JA, Dorsch SE. *Understanding Anesthesia Equipment.* 2nd ed. Baltimore: Williams and Wilkins; 1984:16–17.
2. Vandenberg JT, Vinson DR. The inadequacies of contemporary oropharyngeal suction. *Am J Emerg Med.* 1999;17(6):611.
3. Ooi R, et al. An evaluation of oxygen delivery using nasal prongs. *Anaesthesia.* 1992;47:591.
4. Woda RP, et al. Cost-benefit analysis of nasal cannulae in non-tracheally intubated subjects. *Anesth Analg.* 1996;82(3):506.
5. Williams AR, Tomlin K. The modified bitegard: a method for administering supplemental oxygen and measuring carbon dioxide. *Anesthesiology.* 1999;90(1):338.
6. Livingston M. Questions use of nasal cannula for oxygen supplementatin during cataract surgery. *Anesthesiology.* 1999;91(4):1176.
7. Kurt I, et al. A simple and inexpensive nasal cannula to prevent rebreathing for spontaneously breathing patients under surgical drapes. *Anesth Analg.* 2001;93:667.
8. Schlager A, et al. Nasal application of oxygen does not prevent carbon dioxide rebreathing in spontaneously breathing patients undergoing eye surgery. *Br J Anaesth.* 1999;82(1):30.
9. Langer RA. Simple modification of a medium concentration (Hudson type) oxygen mask improves patient comfort and respiratory monitoring with capnography. *Anesth Analg.* 1996;83:193.
10. Guzeldemir ME. A mask for operations on and above the eye. *Can J Anaesth.* 1998;45(7):709.
11. Hunsinger DL, et al. *Respiratory Technology Procedure and Equipment Manual.* Reston, VA: Reston Publishing; 1980:chap 3.
12. McPherson SP. *Respiratory Therapy Equipment.* 2nd ed. St. Louis: Mosby; 1981:91.
13. Waldau T, et al. Evaluation of five oxygen delivery devices in spontaneously breathing subjects by oxygraphy. *Anaesthesia.* 1998;53:256.
14. Ball C, Westhorpe R. Clearing the airway—the development of the pharyngeal airway. *Anaesth Intensive Care.* 1997;25(5):451.
15. Marsh AM, et al. Airway obstruction associated with the use of the guedel airway. *Br J Anaesth.* 1991;67:517.
16. Muzzi DA, et al. Complication from a nasopharyngeal airway in a patient with a basilar skull fracture. *Anesthesiology.* 1991;74:366.
17. Stoneman MD. The nasopharyngeal airway. *Anaesthesia.* 1993;48:575.
18. Beattie C. The modified nasal trumpet maneuver. *Anesth Analg.* 2002;94:467–469
19. McIntyre JWR. Oropharyngeal and nasopharyngeal airways: (1880–1995). *Can J Anaesth.* 1996;43(6):629.

20. Wheeler M. The difficult pediatric airway. In: Hagberg CA, *Handbook of Difficult Airway Management*. Philadelphia: Churchill Livingstone; 2000:268.

21. Ward ME. A new look at the breath of life [editorial]. *Br J Anaesth.* 1992;69:339.

22. Benumof JL, ed. *Airway Management and Principles and Practice.* St. Louis: Mosby; 1996.

23. McIntyre JWR. Airway equipment. *Anesthesiology Clinics of North America.* 1995; 13(2):309.

24. Marks RRD, et al. An analysis of laryngoscope blade shape and design: new criteria for laryngoscope evaluation. *Can J Anaesth.* 1993;40:262.

25. Relle A. Laryngoscope design. *Can J Anaesth.* 1994;41:162.

26. Norton ML. Laryngoscope blade shape. *Can J Anaesth.* 1994;41:263.

27. McIntyre JWR. Tracheal intubation and laryngoscope design [editorial]. *Can J Anaesth.* 1993;40:193.

28. McIntyre JWR. Laryngoscope design and the difficult adult tracheal intubation. *Can J Anaesth.* 1989;36:94.

29. Bucx MJL, et al. The effect of steam sterilisation at 134-deg. C. on light intensity provided by fibrelight macintosh laryngoscopes. *Anaesthesia.* 1999;54:875.

30. Tousignant G, Tessler MJ. Light intensity and area of illumination provided by various laryngoscope blades. *Can J Anaesth.* 1994;41(9):865.

31. Fletcher J. Laryngoscope light intensity. *Can J Anaesth.* 1995;42(3):259.

32. Uchida T, et al. The McCoy levering laryngscope in patients with limited neck extension. *Can J Anaesth.* 1997;44(6):674.

33. Sugiyama K, Yoloyama K. Head extension angle required for direct laryngoscopy with the McCoy laryngoscope blade. *Anesthesiology.* 2001;94:939.

34. Asai T, et al. Use of the McCoy laryngoscope of fingers to facilitate fibrescope-aided tracheal intubation. *Anaesthesia.* 1998;53:903.

35. Aoyama K, et al. The McCoy laryngoscope expands the laryngeal aperture in patients with difficult intubation. *Anesthesiology.* 2000;92:1855.

36. Randell T, et al. The best view at laryngoscopy using the McCoy laryngoscope with and without cricoid pressure. *Anaesthesia.* 1998;53:536.

37. Ochroch EA, Levitan RM. A videographic analysis of laryngeal exposure comparing the articulating laryngoscope and external laryngeal manipulation. *Anesth Analg.* 2001;92:267.

38. McCoy EP, et al. Comparison of the Forces Exerted at Laryngoscopy; The Macintosh vs the McCoy blade. *Br J Anaesth.* 1995;75(2):241.

39. Usui T, et al. Arytenoid dislocation while using a McCoy laryngoscope. *Anesth Analg.* 2001;92:1347.

40. Yardeni I, et al. A clinical trial of a new laryngoscope with flexible blade: a comparison with Macintosh. *Br J Anaesth.* 1999;82(suppl 1):32.

41. Yardeni I, et al. A new laryngoscope with flexible adjustable rigid blade [letter]. *Br J Anaesth.* 1999;83(3):537.

42. Law BCW. Incorrect assembly of the flexiblade fibreoptic bundle. *Anaesthesia.* 2001;56:906.

43. Stowell DE. An alternative light source for laryngoscopy. *Anesthesiology.* 1994; 80:487.

44. Kubota Y, et al. Endotracheal intubation assisted with a pencil torch. *Anesthesiology.* 1988;68:167.

45. Przemeck M, et al. Mini flashlight as a spare light source for a failing fiberoptic laryngoscope. *Anesthesiology.* 1997;86(5):1217.

46. Arthurs GJ. Fibre-optically lit laryngoscope. *Anaesthesia.* 1999;54:873.

47. Miller RD, ed. *Anesthesia.* New York: Churchill Livingstone; 1981:940.
48. Khine HH, et al. Comparisons of cuffed and uncuffed endotracheal tubes in young children during general anesthesia. *Anesthesiology.* 1997;86:627.
49. Deakers TW, et al. Cuffed endotracheal tubes in pediatric intensive care. *J Pediatr.* 1994;125(1):57.
50. Fisher DM. Comparison of cuffed and uncuffed endotracheal tubes in young children during general anesthesia [editorial]. *Anesthesiology.* 1997;86(3):27A.
51. St John, RE. Advances in artificial airway management. *Crit Care Nurs Clin North Am.* 1999;11(1):7.
52. Kolobow T, et al. Design and development of ultrathin-walled nonkinking endotracheal tubes of a new "no pressure" laryngeal seal design. *Anesthesiology.* 1994;81: 1061.
53. Reali-Forster C, et al. New ultrathin-walled endotracheal tube with a novel laryngeal seal design: long-term evaluation in sheep. *Anesthesiology.* 1996;84(1):162.
54. West MRJ, et al. A new tracheal tube for difficult intubation. *Br J Anaesth.* 1996;76(5):673.
55. Brimacombe J, et al. Direct measurement of mucosal pressures exerted by cuff and non-cuff portions of tracheal tubes with different cuff volumes and head and neck positions. *Br J Anaesth.* 1999;82(5):708.
56. Fujiwara M, et al. A new endotracheal tube with a cuff impervious to nitrous oxide: constancy of cuff pressure and volume. *Anesth Analg.* 1995;81:1084.
57. Karasawa F, et al. Profile soft-seal cuff, a new endotracheal tube, effectively inhibits an increase in the cuff pressure through high complinace rather than low diffusion of nitrous oxide. *Anesth Analg.* 2001;92:140.
58. Stix MS, Mancini E: How a rigid stylet can make an endotracheal tube move. *Anesth Analg.* 2000;90:1000.
59. Maxwell LG, et al. The tongue depresser, COPA, and Aintree catheter: valuable tools in a complicated airway. *Am J Anesthesiol.* 2001;28:355.
60. Quinones FR, et al. Magill forceps: a vital forceps. *Ped Emerg Care.* 1995;11(5):302.
61. Ball C, Westhorpe R. Clearing the airway—mouth gags, wedges and openers. *Anaesth Intensive Care.* 1997;25(4):335.
62. Szocik JF. Preoperative Hypoxemia. *Anesth Analg.* 1992;76:681.
63. Coveler LA, Lester RC. Contaminated oxygen cylinder. *Anesth Analg.* 1989;69:674.
64. Hwang NC, Carvalho B. Hidden hazards of scavenging. *Br J Anaesthes.* 2000;84(6): 827.
65. Khorasani A, et al. Inadvertent misconnection of the scavenger hose: a cause for increased pressure in the breathing circuit. *Anesthesiology.* 92(5):1501, 2000.
66. Campbell C, et al. Manufacturing defect in a double-lumen tube. *Anesth Analg.* 1991;73:825.
67. Barst S, et al. An unusual cause of airway obstruction. *Anesth Analg.* 1994;78:195.
68. McLean RF, et al. Another cause of tracheal tube failure [letter]. *Can J Anaesth.* 1989;36:733.
69. McCoy E, Barnes S. A defect in a tracheal tube. *Anaesthesia.* 1989;44:525.
70. Gettelman, TA, Morris GN. Endotracheal tube failure: undetected by routine testing. *Anesth Analg.* 1995;81:1311.
71. Lewer BMF, et al. Large air leak from an endotracheal tube due to a manufacturing defect. *Anesth Analg.* 1997;85:944.
72. Saini S, Chhabra B. A tracheal tube defect. *Anesth Analg.* 1996;83:1129.
73. Patterson KW, Keane P. Missed diagnosis of cuff herniation in a modern nasal endotracheal tube. *Anesth Analg.* 1990;71:563.

74. Basagoitia JN, LaMastro M. Another complication of tracheal intubation. *Anesth Analg.* 1990;70:460.

75. Bourne TM, Tate K. Failed cuff deflation. *Anaesthesia.* 1990;45:76.

76. Heusner JE, Viscomi CM. Endotracheal tube cuff failure due to valve damage. *Anesth Analg.* 1991;72:270.

77. Saade E. Unusual cause of endotracheal tube obstruction. *Anesth Analg.* 1991;72:841.

78. Oystan J, Holtby H. Fracture of a RAE endotracheal tube connector [letter]. *Can J Anaesth.* 1988;35:438.

79. McCaskill KR. Polamedco endotracheal tubes. *Can J Anaesth.* 1993;40:577.

80. Desmeules H, Tremblay PR. Laryngoscope blade breakage during intubation. *Can J Anaesth.* 1988;35:202.

81. Smith MB, Camp P. Broken laryngoscope. *Anaesthesia.* 1989;44:179.

82. Vernon JM. A broken laryngoscope. *Anaesthesia.* 1990;45:697.

83. Jolly DT, et al. Fibreoptic laryngoscope blade [letter]. *Can J Anaesth.* 1998;45(4):382.

84. Paterson JG. Laryngoscope breakage. *Can J Anaesth.* 2000;47(9):927.

85. Norman PH, et al. Failure of a laryngoscope blade [letter]. *Anesth Analg.* 1998;86:448.

86. Siegel LC, Garman JK. Too hot to handle: a laryngoscope malfunction. *Anesthesiology.* 1990;72:1088.

87. Alexander PD, Meurer-Laban M. Rechargeable optima laryngoscopes. *Br J Anaesth.* 1995;74(6):724.

88. Hall DB. Takes a lickin' and keeps on tickin'. *Anesth Analg.* 1999;88:1421.

89. Larson CE. A problem with metal endotracheal tubes and plastic-coated stylets. *Anesthesiology.* 1989;70:883.

90. Fishman RL. Reuse of a disposable stylet with life-threatening complications. *Anesth Analg.* 1991;72:266.

91. Hoffman CO, Swanson GA. Oral reinforced endotracheal tube crushed and perforated from biting. *Anesth Analg.* 1989;69:552.

92. Populaire C, et al. An armoured endotracheal tube obstruction in a child. *Can J Anaesth.* 1989;36:331.

93. Wright PH, et al. Obstruction of armoured tracheal tubes: case report and discussion. *Can J Anaesth.* 1988;35:195.

94. Gupta R. Unilateral transient sialadenopathy: another complication of oropharyngeal airway. *Anesthesiology.* 1998;88(2):551.

95. Michelsen LG, Valdes-Murua H. An intubating airway with teeth. *Anesthesiology.* 2001;94:938.

96. Ickx BE, Lamesch F. Life-threatening upper airway obstruction caused by oxygen administration with a nasal catheter. *Anesthesiology.* 2000;92(1):266.

97. Charters P, O'Sullivan E. The "dedicated airway": a review of the concept and an update of current practice. *Anaesthesia.* 1999;54:778.

98. Charters P. Airway devices: where now and where to? *Br J Anaesth.* 2000;85(4):504.

4
Fiberoptic Airway Management Techniques

After more than two decades of clinical application, research, teaching, and equipment development, the utility of the flexible fiberoptic endoscope in airway management has been established. **Proficiency** with fiberoptic techniques, rather than **familiarity,** is now the standard of care, at least for advanced airway management practitioners. Proficiency does not imply guaranteed success in all circumstances. Rather, skillful utilization of fiberoptic techniques offers the practitioner an additional option when managing the airway.

Proficient use of fiberoptic airway management techniques requires training, extensive practice, and a thorough understanding of the equipment. Many publications deal with fiberoptic airway techniques, instrument design, and function. Recent textbooks on airway management include a section on fiberoptic techniques. Most notable among recent texts is Andranik Ovassapian's *Fiberoptic Endoscopy and the Difficult Airway,* 2nd ed.[1] Less detailed reviews are published by many authors. These are, nonetheless, comprehensive and practical. Excellent review articles include those by Fulling and Roberts[2] and Dierdorf.[3,4]

The development of manual skills should begin with two steps. First, attend a workshop that features extensive hands-on practice with mannequins and models. Contact the Society for Airway Management,[5] the American Society of Anesthesiologists,[6] or an academic anesthesiology department to ask for information concerning fiberoptic workshops. Secondly, refine manual skills by using the fiberoptic endoscope on human subjects. Seek a colleague who is a competent practitioner of fiberoptic techniques and work with him when first dealing with patients. The more you practice on patients with normal airways, the better prepared you will be to manage a patient with a difficult airway.

The primary purpose of this chapter is to describe **basic** fiberoptic airway management techniques. More sophisticated techniques will be discussed later in the chapter.

Applications

The flexible fiberoptic endoscope has many applications with respect to airway management (Table 4.1).

One of the major advantages of the fiberoptic endoscope is that it allows a thorough evaluation of abnormal or traumatized anatomy while the patient is awake, breathing spontaneously, and protecting his own airway. Both the proximal and distal airway can be evaluated. It is prudent to evaluate the airway while the patient is awake. While the patient breathes spontaneously, the practitioner can define airway options, gather special equipment, and summons assistants before administering anesthetics or muscle relaxants or proceeding with an awake fiberoptic intubation.

Implementation: Learning the Technique

Twenty-two years ago, Ovassapian and associates developed a training program based on a series of graduated written learning objectives to teach nasotracheal fiberoptic intubation.[1(p265)] Current teaching protocols and formal workshops utilize the graduated approach developed by these pioneers. Models and mannequins are used extensively to teach manual skills that are essential to efficient fiberoptic intubation.[1(chap15),2,10–12]

In the clinical setting, in addition to working with a competent colleague, a **"fiberoptic cart"** that contains all of the equipment necessary to perform fiberoptic intubation must be readily accessible.[13] (The contents of the cart will be described in detail later in the chapter.) Having the equipment immediately available saves time and encourages one to use the fiberoptic scope in the routine of daily practice.

You should be assured that fiberoptic intubation performed under the supervision of a competent teacher is safe, comfortable for the patient, and expedi-

TABLE 4.1. Applications of the fiberoptic endoscope in airway management

1. Diagnostic
     a. Evaluation of airway anatomy
     b. Evaluation of equipment placement (endotracheal, endobronchial, nasogastric tubes, LMA)
2. Therapeutic
     a. Tracheobronchial lavage[9]
     b. Removal of foreign bodies
     c. Oxygenation
3. Practical
     a. Endotracheal intubation
     b. Endobronchial intubation
     c. Endotracheal tube change[9(p166–175)]
     d. Special applications (retrograde wire placement, use with new airways, surgical airway management, critical care setting)

Sources: From Lefebvre and Stock, 1988,[7] Dellinger and Bandi, 1992,[8] and Clark et al., 1989,[9] Ovassapian.[1]

tious.[1(chap15),14–16] With this knowledge, you should plan to use the fiberoptic endoscope to perform "routine" intubations instead of using a laryngoscope. The more intubations you perform on patients with normal airways, the quicker proficiency will be attained. To maintain proficiency, the fiberoptic endoscope should be used on a routine basis. Both oral intubations, as well as nasal intubations when appropriate, should be practiced. Adult and pediatric patients should be included in the training schedule. Once you establish an organized and expeditious approach to learning the technique, your colleagues, other operating room personnel, and patients will accept your efforts to master this **essential technique.** The effort will prove beneficial when it is used to manage more difficult airways with which practitioners will certainly be confronted.

Many studies have been undertaken to define how many fiberoptic intubations must be performed before one develops reasonable competence. Fulling et al.[2] reported that residents required a median of **10** fiberoptic intubation attempts to reach a success rate of 90% on the first try. Many variables, though, exist in clinical practice, such as the patient's age, weight, airway anatomy, physical status, his mental state (awake, sedated, anesthetized, patient's level of cooperation), as well as the degree of emergency with respect to airway control, all of which need to be studied in order to establish the number of intubations that defines **proficiency.** Furthermore, standard goals need to be established. At the present time, the number of attempts it takes to gain **proficiency** has not been established.

Indications

Table 4.2 lists the indications for use of the flexible fiberoptic endoscope as an airway management tool.

One of the most important indications is the necessity to perform an awake intubation in a patient whose airway must be secured without the use of muscle relaxants, deep sedation, or general anesthesia. (See section on Awake Fiberoptic Intubation page 93).

Equipment

In addition to basic airway management equipment, the special equipment needed to perform fiberoptic intubation includes the following items:

1. Intubating airways
2. Masks/adapters
3. Endotracheal tubes
4. Light source
5. Fiberoptic endoscope
6. **"Fiberoptic cart,"** on which all equipment is stored.

TABLE 4.2. Indications for use of the fiberoptic endoscope in airway management

1. Routine intubations
2. Evaluation of the airway
   a. Existing pathology
   b. Trauma
   c. Abnormal anatomy
3. Therapeutic
   a. Bronchopulmonary lavage
   b. Removal of foreign bodies
   c. Oxygenation
   d. Confirmation of endobronchial, endotracheal, or nasogastric tube placement
4. Difficult intubation
   a. Anticipated
      i. History of difficult intubation
      ii. Abnormal anatomy
   b. Unanticipated
      i. Missed evidence of difficult intubation
      ii. Other causes
      iii. ASA Difficult Airway Algorithm (Adjunctive Airway Tool)[17]
   c. Compromised airway
      i. Pathology
      ii. Trauma
   d. Neck movement not desirable
      i. Unstable cervical spine
      ii. Vertebrobasilar artery insufficiency
   e. High risk of dental damage
5. Awake intubation with topical anesthesia with/without sedation

Source: Modified from Ovassapian, 1996.[1(p72)]

Intubating Airways

Special airways have been designed to facilitate fiberoptic intubation. These airways are used to displace the tongue anteriorly, to help guide the tip of the scope toward the glottis, and to protect the scope from the patient's biting, which could cause expensive damage to the instrument. Figures 4.1 to 4.3 illustrate three types of intubating airways.

The Ovassapian airway is designed with slitted tube guides that allow the endotracheal tube to be slipped off of the airway after intubation without removal of the 15-mm adapter (Fig. 4.4).

Chung[18] reported modification of the Williams airway by cutting a 7-mm slot in its anterior wall that would allow the airway to be slipped off the endotracheal tube after successful intubation.

One potentially helpful modification to the Ovassapian airway was reported by Aoyama et al.[19] They suggested that placing a black line along the midline of the pharyngeal surface of the airway will help orient the scope's placement during intubation (Figs. 4.5 to 4.6).

Ravindran[20] suggested that the black line could also help indicate whether the endoscope has been inserted properly along the airway's pharyngeal surface or improperly through a hole in the airway.

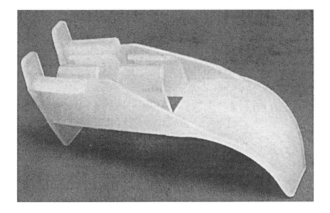

FIGURE 4.1. The Ovassapian fiberoptic intubating airway. (From Ovassapian, 1996,[1] with permission.)

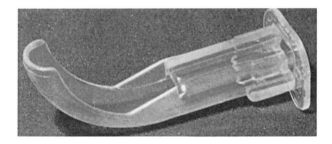

FIGURE 4.2. The Williams intubating airway. (From Ovassapian, 1996,[1] with permission.)

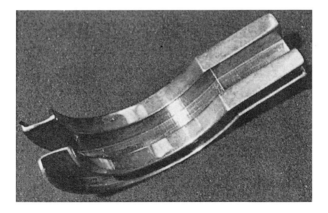

FIGURE 4.3. The Patil-Syracuse airway. (From Ovassapian, 1996,[1] with permission.)

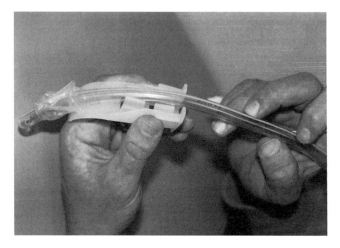

FIGURE 4.4. Slitted guides in the Ovassapian airway allow it to be removed easily after the endotracheal tube is in the trachea.

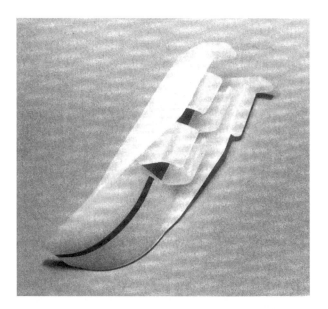

FIGURE 4.5. An Ovassapian airway with a black line placed on the midline of the pharyngeal surface. (From Aoyama, 1999,[19] with permission.)

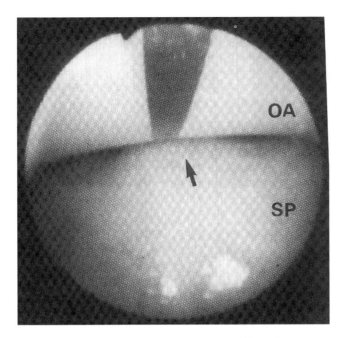

FIGURE 4.6. With the Ovassapian airway placed in the middle of the tongue, the view through the scope shows the line in the midline of the airway. In this picture the Ovassapian airway is identified (OA) and the soft palate with an (SP). The arrow points to the base of the uvula. (From Aoyama, 1999,[19] with permission.)

Goskowicz et al.[21] described the use of a modified baby bottle nipple as an airway to facilitate intubation in a 7-month-old infant. The nipple had an 8-mm hole cut into its lateral side at its distal end. A mark was placed on the hub of the nipple in line with the distal hole to assure inferior orientation of the hole (Fig. 4.7).

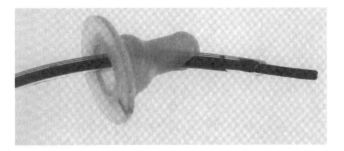

FIGURE 4.7. A 3.4-mm fiberoptic bronchoscope jacketed with a 4.0-mm internal diameter endotracheal tube placed through a modified standard nipple used as an intubating airway. (From Goskowicz, 1996,[21] with permission.)

Finally, Krensavage[22] suggested that one could consider using an oral obturator (mouth gag) to open the airway and displace the tongue during fiberoptic intubation.

Masks/Adapters

Specially designed masks and adapters are available that allow mask control of the airway while fiberoptic intubation or airway examination is being performed. A Portex adapter can be fitted onto the mask, or a hole may be drilled through a standard plastic mask, both of which allow passage of the fiberoptic scope. An airtight diaphragm can be formed over the hole with plastic dressing material through which a small hole is punctured to allow scope passage. Many authors have published descriptions of creative adaptations and modifications of equipment to augment use during fiberoptic intubation.[23–26] Beware that a number of problems have been reported involving fragmentation and separation of mask material and fittings that have endangered patients (Figs. 4.8 to 4.10).[27–29]

Endotracheal Tubes

Historically, most fiberoptically assisted endotracheal intubations have been performed utilizing standard-tipped endotracheal tubes. These tubes are beveled at the tip, though not tapered. Many recent papers report that different endotracheal tube tip designs may facilitate passage of the tube through the glottic opening as it is slipped over the endoscope. Three recent papers[30–32] report that the silicone-tipped, beveled tube that is supplied with the **Intubating Laryngeal Mask Airway** (Laryngeal Mask Company, UK) is easier to pass into the trachea than are standard, nonbeveled endotracheal tubes. In Europe, this tube is referred to as an

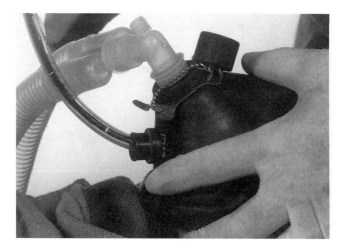

FIGURE 4.8. The Patil-Syracuse endoscopy mask.

FIGURE 4.9. Mask ventilation is maintained while passing the doscope through the diaphragm of a Portex adapter. The small aperature of the adapter allows the scope to pass easily for airway examination. An endotracheal tube up to 6.0 mm ID (cuffed) can be passed over the scope if the diaphragm has been removed.

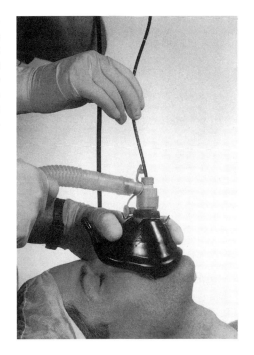

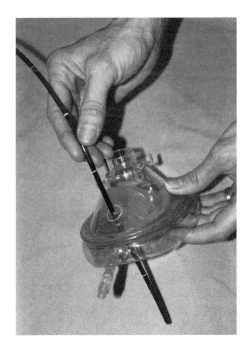

FIGURE 4.10. An endoscopy mask can be made by drilling a hole through a standard anesthesia mask and creating a diaphragm with a plastic film dressing.

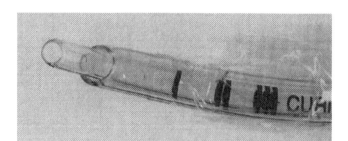

FIGURE 4.11. The double setup endotracheal tube configuration forms a "taper" by passing a 5.0-mm endotracheal tube through the tip of a 7.5-mm endotracheal tube. (From Rosenblatt, 1996,[34] with permission.)

Intavent Tube. In the United States, the intubating LMA system is called the **Fastrach** (LMA, North America) and the tube is called the **Fastrach Endotracheal Tube.** Finally, Jones, Pearce, and Moore[33] described the Moore tapered-tip endotracheal tube that was demonstrated to facilitate fiberoptic intubation because of its tip design.

Rosenblatt[34] tested the efficacy of the "double setup endotracheal tube," described by Marsh[35] to facilitate fiberoptic intubation (Fig. 4.11). His conclusion was that the tapered configuration to the intubating system, created by passing the tip of a 5.0-mm endotracheal tube through a 7.5-mm endotracheal tube, facilitated fiberoptic intubation. Note that a rather small diameter endoscope must be used with this technique, (3.5-mm outside diameter (OD) or smaller).

Brull[36] conducted a study comparing the flexometallic (anode) tube with a standard endotracheal tube and found that the flexible tube was easier to pass over a bronchoscope.

In contrast, Hakala et al[37] found an arode tube harder to pass. Suffice it to say, you should not force a tube into the trachea. If you are encountering difficulty passing the tube into the trachea, in spite of facilitating maneuvers, **consider selecting a tube with a different tip configuration.**

Light Source

Fiberoptic light sources are available from many manufacturers. Whichever is chosen, it should be fitted with an adapter specifically designed to accept the light cable from the scope in use (Fig. 4.12). Battery powered light sources are another option.

Fiberoptic Endoscope

Many fiberoptic endoscopes are available for use in airway management. When choosing an instrument, consider the following:

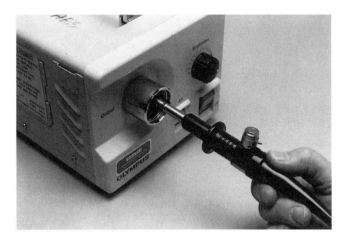

FIGURE 4.12. The light cable from the fiberoptic scope is plugged into the light source. (Olympus America, 2001,[38] with permission.)

1. Cost (up to $17,000, approximately)
2. Size
    a. Diameter
    b. Length
3. Angle of tip deflection
4. Field of view
5. Working ports (suction, instrumentation, oxygenation, drug injection)
6. Handle controls
7. Availability of adjunctive equipment
    a. Teaching attachments
    b. Video-photographic capability
    c. Light sources ($5,000, approximate cost)
8. Portability (battery source built into the scope)
9. Cleaning protocol
10. Customer service, repair service, and scope loan during the repair period; technical support, educational support by the manufacturer

The basic features of the fiberoptic endoscope are illustrated in Figure 4.13.

Tables 4.3 and 4.4 summarize design details of various scopes that are commercially available. Bronchoscopes, laryngoscopes, rhinoscopes, intubating laryngoscopes, and **"mobile"** or **portable** scopes, which have a battery, are included in the tables. (In general, the depth of field for the scopes listed is 35 to 50 mm and the light guide cable from the light source is 5 to 7 ft.)

The portable scopes are extremely utilitarian. They can be used independently in the intensive care unit (ICU), emergency room, or the operating room. They are lightweight and have excellent optics.

Finally, there are literature reports of scopes that are custom-made or modified that have been used to perform fiberoptic intubations.[40,41]

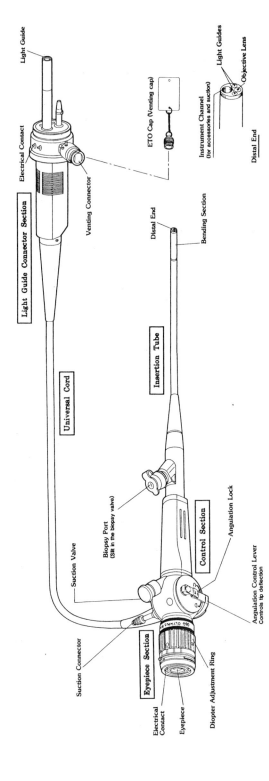

FIGURE 4.13. Components of a bronchofiberscope. Olympus BF-20 D series. The BF-30 series fiberscopes are similar in design to BF-20 series. Changes include improved optics and introduction of disposable suction valve and connector system. (Ovassapian, A., 1996,[1] with permission.)

TABLE 4.3. Olympus endoscopes

Model	Insertion tip diameter (mm)	Insertion cord length (mm)	Working port diameter (mm)	Tip deflection (degrees up/down)	Angle of view (degrees)
BF-P40	5.0	550	2.2	180/130	120
BF-3C40	3.6	550	1.2	180/130	120
BF-N20	2.2	550	N/A	160/90	75
LF-P	2.2	600	N/A	120/120	75
LF-T	5.2	600	2.6	180/130	120
ENF-P4	3.6	300	N/A	130/130	85
ENF-XP	2.2	300	N/A	130/130	75
ENF-L3	4.3	365	N/A	130/130	85
ENF-TD	5.0	365	2.2	130/130	85
ENF-L2	4.2	265	N/A	120/120	85
Portable scopes					
LF-DP	3.1	600	1.2	120/120	90
LF-TP	5.2	600	2.6	180/130	90
LF-GP	4.1	600	1.5	120/120	90
ENF-GP	3.6	300	N/A	130/130	85

Note: Olympus offers a rechargeable battery for its portable scopes.
Source: From Olympus America, 2001,[38] with permission.

TABLE 4.4. Pentax endoscopes

Model	Distal tip diameter (mm)	Working cord length (mm)	Working channel diameter (mm)	Tip deflection (degrees up/down)	Angle of view (degrees)
FI-7P	2.4	600	N/A	130/130	95
FI-10P2	3.4	600	1.4	130/130	90
FI-13-P	4.2	600	1.8	160/130	95
FB-8V	2.7	600	1.2	180/130	100
FB-10V	3.4	600	1.2	180/130	95
FB-15V	4.9	600	2.2	180/130	120
FB-18V	5.9	600	2.8	180/130	120
FB-19TV	6.2	600	3.2	180/130	120
FB-18Rx	5.9	600	2.2	180/130	120
FNL-7RP3	2.4	300	N/A	130/130	75
FNL-10RP3	3.4	300	N/A	130/130	75
FNL-15RP3	4.8	300	2.2	130/130	75
FNL-10RAP	3.4	350	1.2	130/130	95
FNL-13RAP	4.1	350	1.2	130/130	100
Portable scopes					
FB-15BS	4.8	600	2.0	180/130	100
FB-18BS	5.9	600	2.6	180/90	100
FNL-10RBS	3.4	300	N/A	130/130	75
FI-7BS	2.4	600	N/A	130/130	95
FI-9BS	3.0	600	1.2	130/130	90
FI-10BS	3.4	600	1.4	130/130	90
FI-13BS	4.1	600	1.8	160/130	95
FI-16BS	5.1	600	2.6	160/130	95

Source: From Pentax, 2001, with permission.[39]

You should contact a sales representative and arrange to have a demonstration of the various scopes that are under consideration for purchase. Most departments in which fiberoptic intubation is practiced have two scopes, one for adults and one for pediatric use. Serious consideration should be given to the purchase of a portable scope as well.

Fiberoptic Cart

A portable cart should be supplied with all of the equipment needed to perform fiberoptic intubation (Fig. 4.14). This cart should include trays or cabinets that protect the scopes from damage while in storage. **Contaminated equipment must be isolated from clean equipment.** The fiberoptic cart should contain items from Table 4.5.

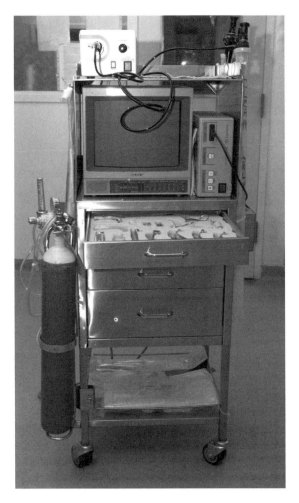

FIGURE 4.14. The "fiberoptic cart."

TABLE 4.5. Contents of the fiberoptic cart

1. Basic airway management equipment
2. Various sizes of syringes and needles including Loer Lok tipped syringes
3. Various sizes of intravenous needles/cannulae
4. Long cotton swabs, pledgets, forceps, long Q-tips
5. Gauze
6. Topical anesthetics
   a. Lidocaine 4%
   b. Lidocaine 1%
   c. Lidocaine 10%
   d. Benzocaine 20%
   e. Viscous lidocaine jelly or ointment 2% to 2.5%
7. Local anesthetics for nerve blocks and/or injection through the scope
   a. Lidocaine 1%
8. Nebulizer for topical application of local anesthetic to the airway
9. Vasoconstrictor agents
   a. Phenylephrine (Dristan 0.5%)
   b. Oxymetazoline (Afrin 0.05%)
10. Suctioning equipment
11. Oxygenation equipment
    a. Tubing
    b. Oxygen source
    c. Masks
    d. Nasal prongs
12. Fiberoptic intubating airways
13. Intubating masks/adapters
14. Fiberoptic light source
15. Fiberoptic endoscopes (protective trays or tubes for safe storage)
16. Photographic/video and teaching adapters if desired
17. **"Difficult airway equipment"** if so desired, including surgical and percutaneous cricothyroid-otomy equipment

Techniques of Fiberoptic Intubation

Fiberoptic intubation routed orally or nasally can be performed in the following settings:

1. Awake patient
2. Anesthetized patient (breathing spontaneously)
3. Anesthetized patient (apneic)

This applies to pediatric as well as adult patients. With the availability of small scopes, very small infants can be intubated with the techniques described in this section. More sophisticated techniques for the intubation of infants are described in detail by Ovassapian.[1(chap7)]

Awake Fiberoptic Intubation

One of the most important applications of fiberoptic intubation is the performance of an awake intubation in a patient whose airway should be secured

without the use of general anesthetics, heavy sedation, or muscle relaxants. Awake intubations are performed with the patient breathing spontaneously while he protects his airway, both with respect to muscular support of his neck as well as handling secretions and other fluids.

In the middle of the last decade, writers debated whether it was more appropriate to perform fiberoptic intubation with the patient "awake"[42] or "anesthetized".[43] Now, it has become apparent that the **proficient** practitioner of fiberoptic airway management needs to have mastered **both techniques.** The choice of one technique over the other should be based on the clinical setting, not the limited training or experience of the practitioner.

Table 4.6 lists some of the indications to perform **awake** fiberoptic intubation.

Fiberoptic intubation of an awake patient may be easier than intubating an anesthetized patient for the following reasons.[1(p75)]

1. The awake patient can swallow secretions and help clear the airway.
2. The tongue does not tend to fall back against the pharyngeal wall and obstruct the view of the endoscopist.
3. The awake patient can breathe deeply and phonate, maneuvers that help the endoscopist to visualize the glottis when the anatomy is compromised.
4. Spontaneous ventilation and adequate oxygenation gives the endoscopist more time to secure the airway.

Awake fiberoptically assisted intubation can be accomplished quickly and comfortably for the patient. The steps to be taken are listed in Table 4.7.

When choosing the route of intubation (nasal or oral), you must consider pathologic and anatomic distortions of the airway as well as the level of cooperation

TABLE 4.6. Indications for awake fiberoptic intubation

1. When it would be **safer** to establish a secure airway with the patient breathing spontaneously
   a. Difficult or impossible mask ventilation predicted
   b. Difficult or impossible intubation predicted
      i. History of difficult intubation
      ii. Congenital or acquired craniofacial abnormalities
      iii. Airway tumors/masses/infections
      iv. Cervical spine disease, trauma, instability, inflexibility
      v. Airway trauma
      vi. Morbid obesity
   c. High risk for aspiration of gastric contents
2. When a neurological examination is needed after intubation
   a. Unstable cervical spine
   b. Vertebrobasilar arterial insufficiency
3. When it is advantageous for the patient to position himself in the operating room after intubation
4. Outside of the operating room if the patient is very unstable physically
   a. Ventilatory failure
   b. Severely ill patient

Source: From Ovassapian, 1996,[1] with permission.

TABLE 4.7. Steps to perform awake fiberoptic intubation

1. Assess the airway
2. Decide to perform an awake fiberoptic intubation
3. Select the route
   a. Oral
   b. Nasal
4. Prepare for contingency interventions
5. Obtain the equipment: **Fiberoptic cart**
6. Educate the patient
7. Educate assistants
8. Apply appropriate monitors
9. Administer supplemental oxygen
10. Administer antisialagogues to decrease airway secretions
11. Administer vasoconstrictors if nasal route selected
12. Administer sedation if appropriate
13. Anesthetize the airway
    a. Topical anesthetics
    b. Nerve blocks
    c. Transtracheal injection
    d. Through the endoscope
14. Perform the intubation
15. Verify correct tube position in the trachea
16. Further sedation/anesthesia/ventilation

of the patient. Any contraindications to nasotracheal intubation would be applicable to these considerations.

Educate the Patient

A cooperative patient can be intubated much easier than one who is restless or fighting. When faced with the prospect of being intubated awake, most patients are extremely apprehensive. Most, though, cooperate when they understand the reasons behind the decision to intubate awake. One needs to explain the reasons and the plan, assure the patient that his airway will be anesthetized, and remind the patient that his cooperation will facilitate the process. When appropriate, administer sedatives, analgesics, and amnestic medications.

Educate the Assistants

The person performing the fiberoptic intubation is the airway manager. He must be sure that his assistants know which monitors to watch, how to provide oxygen and suctioning, how to manipulate the patient's neck and mandible, how to assess the patient's level of consciousness, and how to administer medications. In some cases, a surgeon should be standing by, with all appropriate equipment and assistance, in case an emergency cricothyroidotomy is needed. The airway manager is responsible for maintaining a quiet, organized, communicative, and attentive team of assistants.

Monitoring the Patient

The following should be monitored before sedatives are administered and/or the intubation process begins:

1. Oxygenation
    a. Administer oxygen by face mask or nasal prongs
    b. Oxyhemoglobin saturation monitor applied to the patient
2. Blood pressure
3. Electrocardiogram (ECG)
4. Ventilation
    a. Precordial stethoscope
    b. Observe chest movements
5. Intravenous access
6. Level of consciousness: observation and talking to the patient. Sedation may cause hypoventilation, hypoxemia, or loss of the airway.

Oxygen Insufflation Through the Fiberoptic Endoscope

Hershey and Hannenberg[44] reported a case in which a patient who had undergone a fiberoptic intubation suffered a gastric rupture. They hypothesized that the rupture was due to oxygen injected through the endoscope into the esophagus. Ovassapian[45] stated that he did not recommend insufflation of oxygen through a scope to assist fiberoptic intubation. If you choose to insufflate oxygen during the intubation process, whether through the scope or with an independent catheter or airway, you should be aware that the oxygen flow might cause gastric distention, predisposing to injury or regurgitation.

Administer Antisialagogues

An antisialagogue drug should be administered before undertaking a fiberoptic intubation to help minimize airway secretions, thereby improving visualization.[46]

1. Atropine: 0.006 mg/kg IV or IM, or 0.012 mg/kg PO
2. Glycopyrollate: 0.003 mg/kg IV or IM, or 0.006 mg/kg PO
3. Scopolamine: Same as glycopyrollate

If scopolamine is administered as an antisialagogue, remember that it may cause significant CNS side effects, especially in older patients.[47] These side effects, including "motor incoordination, nausea and vomiting, hallucinations, shivering, fever, as well as dry mouth and skin," can be reversed with physostigmine.

Administer Vasoconstrictors

If a nasotracheal intubation is planned, consider administering a topical vasoconstrictor before beginning the intubation. If cocaine is used to provide topical anesthesia, no additional vasoconstrictor is necessary. The vasoconstrictor will

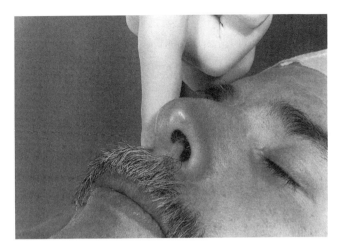

FIGURE 4.15. To assess patency of the nasal passage, compress the contralateral side and observe air movement. Test both sides and choose the more patent side through which to perform a nasal fiberoptic intubation.

serve to open the airway and decrease bleeding, which can obscure visualization. It has been customary to choose the nasal passage that is more patent through which to perform the intubation. To assess patency, ask the patient to breathe through each nostril while obstructing the other and note air movement (Fig. 4.15). More recently, Smith and Reid[48] suggested that a more appropriate way to choose the nostril for intubation would be to examine each nasal passage fiberoptically to define preexisting nasal pathology, such as septal deviation, and to select the more patent passage after visual examination.

After choosing the nasal passage, spray a topical vasoconstrictor into the nose.

1. Phenylephrine (Dristan 0.5%): 2 to 4 sprays
2. Oxymetazoline (Afrin 0.05%): 2 to 4 sprays

Administer Sedatives and Hypnotics

If appropriate, a patient should be sedated before an awake intubation is performed. Be extremely careful, though, when sedating a patient with a difficult or tenuous airway. If he stops breathing spontaneously, the situation may become critical if mask ventilation proves difficult or impossible. Furthermore, fiberoptic intubation may be more difficult if the patient is not breathing spontaneously.

Sedate the patient **incrementally and slowly.** Set a firm sedation endpoint, such as the following:

Attempt to establish a level of sedation at which the patient appears comfortable and relaxed while still cooperative, responsive to verbal commands, and breathing spontaneously.

The following **IV drugs** may be used to "sedate" the patient:

1. Midazolam (Versed): 0.01 to 0.03 mg/kg
2. Diazepam (Valium): 0.01 to 0.04 mg/kg
3. Fentanyl: 0.4 to 2.0 μg/kg
4. Morphine: 0.01 to 0.15 mg/kg

The benzodiazepines are also excellent amnestics. After their use, patients often do not remember the intubation process.

Administer Topical Anesthetics (Upper Airway Anesthesia)

For nasal intubations, the nasal passage, nasopharynx, oropharynx, and suproglottic structures must be anesthetized. For oral intubations, the tongue, oropharynx, and supraglottic structures must be anesthetized.

Nebulized (Aerosolized) Lidocaine

Various techniques have been described to apply aerosolized lidocaine to the airway.[49,50] Given time, the entire airway can be anesthetized with this method. One technique (Fig. 4.16) is illustrated using a simple nebulizer containing 4 to 6 ml of lidocaine 4%.

Topical Anesthetic Sprays and Ointments

The upper airway can be anesthetized with various combinations of local anesthetic sprays and ointments. Topical anesthetics are more effective when applied to a dry mucosal surface. (See Administer Antisialogogues, page 96)

Commonly used local anesthetics include the following:

1. Viscous lidocaine jelly or ointment: 2 to 2.5%
2. Lidocaine 2%
3. Lidocaine 4%
4. Lidocaine 10%
5. Cocaine 4%
6. Benzocaine 20%
7. Dyclonine 1%

To avoid systemic effects of these local anesthetics, do not exceed the recommended safe doses:

1. Lidocaine: 4 to 7 mg/kg
2. Cocaine: 1.5 to 3 mg/kg
3. Benzocaine: 10 mg/kg

You should consider that cocaine blood levels, after topical or intratracheal[51] administration, may remain elevated for a prolonged period of time.

With respect to benzocaine, Khorasani et al[52] documented that the dose of drug administered is dependent on the orientation and residual volume in the dis-

FIGURE 4.16. A nebulizer/mask system can be used to administer lidocaine to the entire airway to provide topical anesthesia.

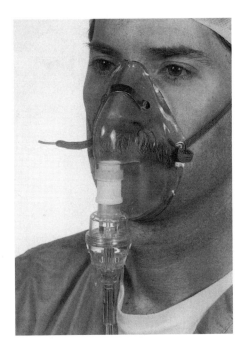

pensing canister. Ellis et al.[53] reported a case of **methemoglobinemia** after an unknown amount of benzocaine was used to anesthetize the airway in a 76-year-old woman who underwent fiberoptic intubation. In this case, the pulse oximeter reading dropped to 83% saturation and "cyanosis" was observed. A blood gas analyzed at that time revealed a PaO_2 of 502 mm Hg and a methemoglobin level of 24% (normal: 0.4% to 1.5%).

You should always monitor the patient for signs of local anesthetic toxicity!

Applying Topical Anesthetics

Many practical and effective methods have been described to apply topical anesthetics to the airway. A few are listed below:

1. Lidocaine gargle[54]: Two aliquats of 5 ml lidocaine 2% (gargle) and 20 ml of lidocaine 1.5% slowly instilled to the posterior tongue.
2. Lidocaine "toothpaste method"[55]: A "line" of lidocaine 5% ointment is placed down the middle of the patient's tongue while he is supine. He is instructed to oppose the tongue to the roof of his mouth, allowing the lidocaine to melt over the mucosal surfaces. A second "line" may be applied.
3. The lidocaine can be injected through the fiberoptic scope[56,57] directly onto the vocal cords and down the trachea.
4. Dyclonine gargle[58]: Two aliquats of dyclonine 1%, each 12.5 ml, for gargle. (Consider using dyclonine if the patient is "allergic" to common local anesthetics.)

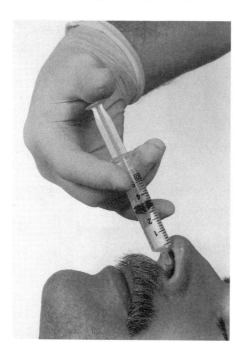

FIGURE 4.17. Initially, lidocaine 2% can be used to begin topical anesthetization of the nasal and nasopharyngeal mucosa.

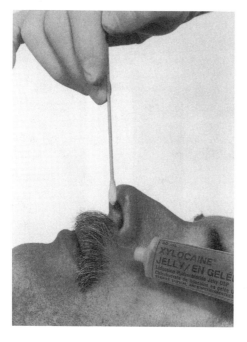

FIGURE 4.18. Viscous lidocaine (2% to 2.5%) can be applied to the deeper mucosal surfaces by means of a long Q-Tip swab.

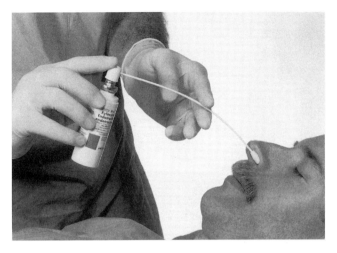

FIGURE 4.19. More concentrated anesthetics (lidocaine 10%, benzocaine 20%) can be sprayed into the nose and applied to deeper mucosal surfaces with long Q-tip swabs soaked with the anesthetic solutions.

Excess local anesthetic may cause gagging or nausea and vomiting if swallowed. This can be prevented by holding a Yankauer suction catheter to the patient's lips between gargles or sprays as recommended by Benumof.[59]

Authors' Method

The authors' method to apply topical anesthetics to the airway is one of many that is efficacious. It will take about 10 minutes to achieve a good level of anesthesia with the method described. Start by applying more dilute solutions of local anesthetics, as the more concentrated solutions tend to irritate the patient's mucosa. The steps to apply topical anesthesia to the airway for fiberoptic intubation are listed below (Figs. 4.17 to 4.22).

1. Lidocaine 2% dripped onto the nasal and nasopharyngeal mucosa (4 to 6 ml)
2. Viscous lidocaine 2% applied deeper into the nasal passage with long Q-tip swabs
3. Lidocaine 10% (or benzocaine 20%) applied to the nasal and nasopharyngeal mucosa with spray and long Q-tip swabs
4. Lidocaine 10% (or benzocaine 20%) applied to the tongue and oropharyngeal mucosa with sprays
5. Supplement with lidocaine 2% to 2.5% ointment on the tongue and in the nose
6. **Test the level of anesthesia with a tongue blade and a long Q-tip before inserting the fiberoptic scope or the endotracheal tube!**

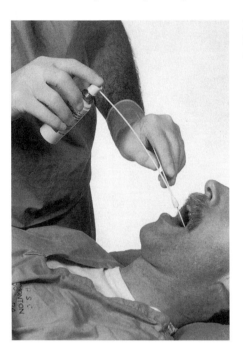

FIGURE 4.20. Concentrated anesthetics can be sprayed on the tongue and into the oropharynx.

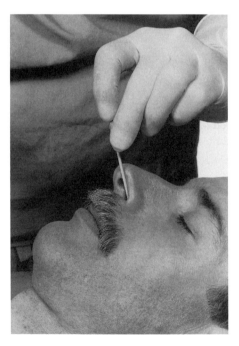

FIGURE 4.21. Test the level of the nasal topical anesthesia by stimulating the nasal and nasopharyngeal surfaces with a long Q-tip. The patient should feel no discomfort.

FIGURE 4.22. Test the level of the oral and oropharyngeal anesthesia by touching the tongue and the pharyngeal wall with a tongue blade. The patient should experience no discomfort or gag reflex.

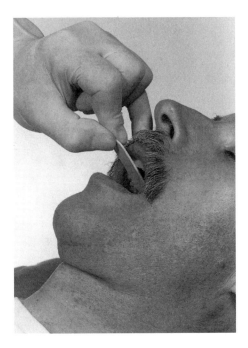

Administer Nerve Block

The internal branch of the superior laryngeal nerve provides sensory innervation to the epiglottis and larynx above the vocal cords. The nerve can be blocked to provide anesthesia to the glottic structures by one of two methods.

The **internal** method involves placing local anesthetic-soaked pledgets in the piriform fossae bilaterally, utilizing a curved Jackson forceps. This method is often not practical because of pathology or secretions.

The **external** method is to inject 2 to 4 ml of lidocaine 1% through a 23-gauge needle to block the superior laryngeal nerve bilaterally as it passes through the thyrohyoid ligament. Do this by palpating the tip of the thyroid cornu and then run a finger medially 1 to 1.5 cm and inject at this point. Direct the needle over the thyroid cartilage and aim it toward the thyrohyoid ligament (below the hyoid bone). Insert the needle 1 to 1.5 cm into the tissue or until it is immediately external to the thyrohyoid ligament (Fig. 4.23). If done correctly, this block will provide sensory anesthesia in 2 to 5 minutes.

Tracheal Anesthesia

The trachea and larynx below the vocal cords can be anesthetized by one of three methods:

1. Aerosol nebulizer: lidocaine 2% to 4% (4 to 6 ml)
2. Transtracheal injection of local anesthetic: lidocaine 2% to 4% (4 to 6 ml)

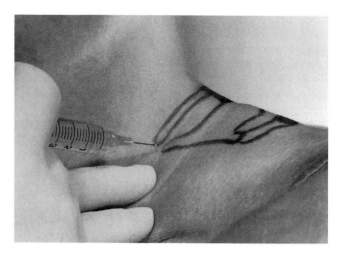

FIGURE 4.23. Superior laryngeal nerve block.

3. Injection of lidocaine onto the vocal cords and into the trachea through the fiberoptic scope: lidocaine 2% to 4% (4 to 6 ml)

Transtracheal Injection

The trachea can be anesthetized by injecting 4 to 6 ml of lidocaine 2% to 4% through the cricothyroid ligament. The ligament is identified by placing one finger on the thyroid cartilage and the other on the cricoid cartilage. Inject the lidocaine through a small (23-gauge) needle, or a 22-gauge intravenous catheter, inserted in the midline. **Aspirate air before injecting.** Remove the needle quickly, as the patient will probably cough as the lidocaine is injected. The trachea will be anesthetized very quickly (Fig. 4.24).

Care should be taken when performing the superior laryngeal nerve block or the transtracheal injection. Intravascular injection could cause a seizure. Misdirected injection of local anesthetic could cause phrenic nerve block or spinal or epidural anesthesia. Surrounding structures such as the esophagus could be damaged. A case of subcutaneous emphysema has been reported after transtracheal injection of local anesthetic.[60] To avoid these complications, **inject local anesthetics through the scope on the vocal cords and into the trachea.**

Awake Intubation Techniques

Whether one performs a nasal or an oral intubation, oxygen should be administered to the patient. Figures 4.25 and 4.26 illustrate two oxygen delivery systems.

Manipulating the Scope

One can stand at the patient's side or at his head to perform fiberoptic intubation. The techniques described refer to an operator standing at the patient's head,

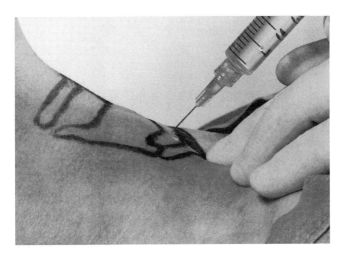

FIGURE 4.24. Transtracheal injection of local anesthetic. Aspirate air before injecting the anesthetic solution.

facing the patient. The controls of the scope are operated by the nondominant hand. The fine movements involved with fiberoptic intubations are made with the dominant hand, moving the scope forward and back and guiding it in right and left turns. The dominant hand may gently contact the patient's face to sense depth of scope insertion and movement of the patient during endoscopy (Fig. 4.27).

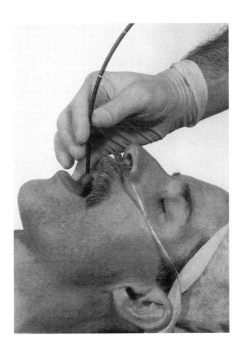

FIGURE 4.25. Nasal prongs can be used to supplement oxygenation during oral fiberoptic intubation.

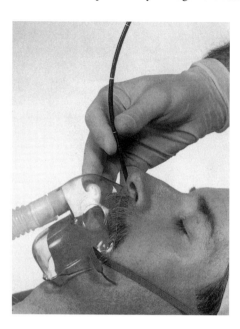

FIGURE 4.26. A modified face mask can be used to supplement oxygenation during nasal fiberoptic intubation.

The handle of the scope should be held so that the black reference marker, seen through the eyepiece, is oriented in the 12 o'clock position. The black reference marker orients the scope anteriorly and in the midline. The tip of the scope can be curved upward or downward with the hand controls. The operator can also activate suctioning with a hand control. The depth that the scope is inserted

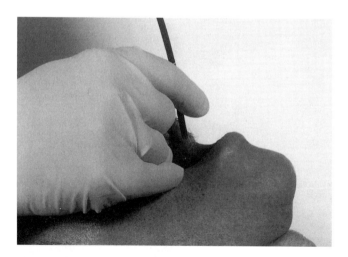

FIGURE 4.27. During intubation, the endoscopist stands at the patient's head and directs the scope's fine movements with his dominant hand, which can come into gentle contact with the patient's face.

into the airway is controlled by the dominant hand. The operator should look through the scope as it is inserted and try to recognize anatomic landmarks as soon as possible. To turn the scope to the right, the operator curves the tip upward, then turns the handle to the right, leaning one's body into the turn. To turn the scope to the left, the operator curves the tip upward, then turns the handle to the left, leaning to the left. **Do not try to turn the scope by twisting the fiberoptic bundle! This maneuver will damage the scope!** Direct the scope with short, controlled movements. Finally, be careful to hold the scope with the fiberoptic bundle fully extended so that the glass fibers are not broken by coiling or angulation.

Prepare the Scope and Endotracheal Tube

One should lubricate both the endoscope and the endotracheal tube to decrease friction and ease insertion. The tube and scope can be lubricated with a water-soluble gel (Fig. 4.28). Lubricate the inside of the tube as well by passing a flexible catheter covered with gel through the tube (Fig. 4.29).

Before lubricating the tube, soften it by placing it in some warm, sterile water or saline (Fig. 4.30). This is especially important if a nasal intubation is planned.

Immediately before starting the intubation, be sure to focus the scope and clean the viewing channel. Warming the scope's tip with warm water or by placing it

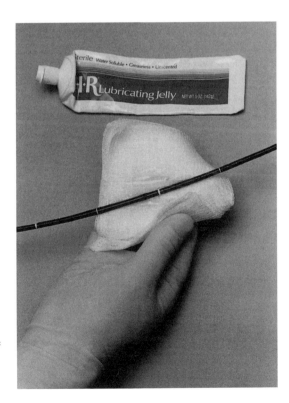

FIGURE 4.28. The endoscope should be well lubricated with KY-Jelly or viscous anesthetic gel.

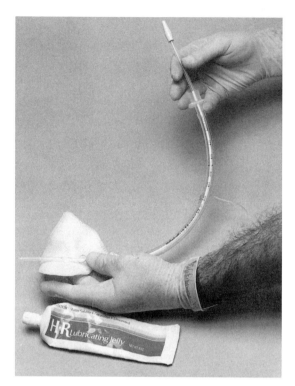

FIGURE 4.29. To facilitate passage of the endoscope, the inside of the endotracheal tube should be lubricated. A flexible suction catheter covered with KY-Jelly or viscous anesthetic gel can be run through the tube to deposit lubricant inside.

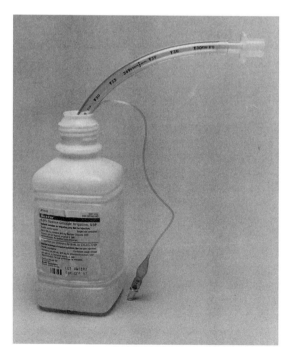

FIGURE 4.30. The endotracheal tube can be softened in warm water or saline. A softer tube will curve more easily and cause less trauma to the nasal passage.

near the outflow of a forced air warming device[61] will help prevent fogging when the scope is placed into the patient's airway.

Awake Nasotracheal Fiberoptic Intubation

With the operator standing at the patient's head, initiate the intubation with the tip of the endotracheal tube in the patient's nasal passage or with the tube pulled proximally onto the endoscope (Fig. 4.31).

If you start with the tip of the tube in the nasal passage, **do not pass the tube as far as the pharynx or the tube will direct the scope toward the esophagus.** One advantage to starting with the tube pulled onto the endoscope is that the tube will not impede the scope's movement or tip deflection, making maneuvering of the scope and tip easier.

With the patient's head in a neutral or slightly extended position (if safe),[62] insert the tip of the scope into the nose. **Begin viewing through the scope immediately.** If the tip of the endotracheal tube is already in the nose, observe the endotracheal tube through the scope and watch the endoscope pass out of the tube. Next, watch the scope move through the nasal passage and enter the pharynx. At this point, deflect the tip of the scope **upward.** The epiglottis and glottic opening should come into view in the midline. If the laryngeal structures are

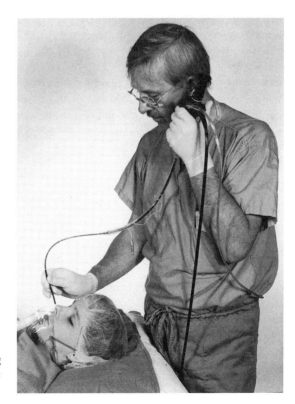

FIGURE 4.31. Performing a nasotracheal fiberoptic intubation.

not seen, move the tip of the scope to the right and left by rotating the handle and leaning into the turn. Ask the patient to take a deep breath or vocalize. Movement of the larynx may make it easier to visualize the epiglottis or glottis. Once the glottis is seen, move the scope toward the opening. You may spray local anesthetic through the working channel of the scope to anesthetize the vocal cords and trachea. Anticipate coughing at this point. Once the patient is calm, pass the endoscope into the trachea and observe the tracheal rings and the carina.

When the scope is in the trachea, slide the tube over the scope into the trachea. This maneuver should be easy. However, one may find that the endotracheal tube does not pass with ease. **Do not force passage of the endotracheal tube.** You may try various rotational maneuvers to help the tip of the tube to pass into the trachea.[63–65] Start by turning the tube $-90°$ to the left, then to $-180°$, then back to the right $+90°$. You may try turning the tube to the right. If the tube still does not pass, consider using a tube with a different tip (as described earlier in the chapter), an anode tube, or a smaller standard endotracheal tube. If you sense that the tube is "stuck" to the endoscope, **do not force the tube off the scope! Doing so can cause an expensive tear to the scope's outer sheath.** Instead, try to inject 4 to 5 ml of saline into the distal end of the tube. This maneuver may lubricate the scope and allow the tube to be passed over the scope.[66] If the tube remains "stuck" to the scope, remove the scope and tube as one unit and start again.

Once the tube has been successfully passed into the trachea, note its depth, verify that the tube is in the trachea by observing the carina, inflate the cuff, and remove the scope. Confirm tube placement.

One common problem encountered by the novice is poor visualization or observing the notorious **"red out"** when looking through the scope. Use the suction liberally. Take the scope out and clean the optic channel as often as is necessary. Do not deflect the tip of the scope onto a mucosal surface. Be careful not to pass the scope quickly into the esophagus. The vocal cords usually come into view when the scope is passed only 5 to 10 cm into the airway.

Awake Orotracheal Fiberoptic Intubation

With the operator standing at the patient's head, have the patient place his head in a neutral or slightly extended position (if safe) and have an assistant lift the mandible.

The mandibular lift maneuver is very important. The epiglottis will be lifted off the pharyngeal wall and the operator will be able to visualize the glottis (Figs. 4.32 and 4.33). Aoyama et al.[67–69] reiterate this recommendation and further describe a mechanical device that they have used to support jaw thrust, both in awake and anesthetized patients (Fig. 4.34).

Next, lubricate and insert an intubating airway. The airway will help direct the scope and prevent the patient from biting the scope. Pass an endotracheal tube onto the scope. If the airway does not have a slit in the intubating channel, be sure to remove the 15-mm adapter from the tube.

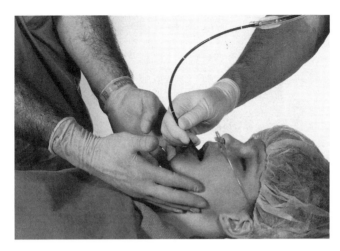

FIGURE 4.32. Performing an orotracheal fiberoptic intubation. An assistant lifts the mandible, a maneuver that raises the epiglottis off of the pharyngeal wall, improving visualization of the glottis.

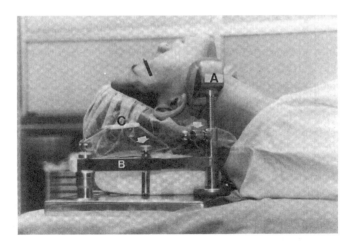

FIGURE 4.33. A new jaw support device supporting the bilateral angle of the jaw. The device maintains jaw thrust and head extension. Bilateral heads (A) attached to the easy-locking poles are adjustable to the desired height and direction by simply pulling up. Bilateral universal arms (B) attached to a stainless board can be fixed only by pushing the levers (C). The device may be additionally secured in place by using two screws (white arrow) on each side. The head is covered with a soft cushion that can support the angle of the jaw without discomfort, even in a conscious patient. (From Aoyama, 2000,[69] with permission.)

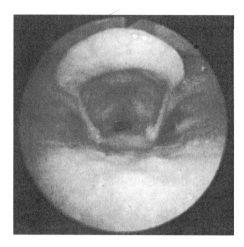

FIGURE 4.34. By applying proper technique, one should obtain a laryngeal view as illustrated in this photograph. (From Ovassapian A. *Fiberoptic Airway Endoscopy in Anesthesia and Critical Care*. New York: Raven Press; 1990:17, with permission.)

Insert the endoscope through the intubating airway's guide channel. **Begin visualization through the scope immediately.** Watch the tip of the scope pass over the airway, the base of the tongue, and into the pharynx. Deflect the tip of the scope upward and proceed as described in the previous section on awake nasotracheal fiberoptic intubation.

After intubation and verification of tube placement, you can remove the intubating airway and replace it with a standard oral airway.

If awake orotracheal fiberoptic intubation proves difficult, you may try various maneuvers to pass the tube as described earlier. You may try to facilitate visualization by having an assistant displace the airway's soft tissue by inserting a Macintosh 3 or 4 laryngoscope blade[70,71] or having an assistant put anterior traction on the tongue.[72]

Verify Tube Placement

The following steps will help verify that the endotracheal tube is positioned in the mid-trachea, below the glottis, and above the carina.

For an awake patient:

1. Observe the carina and tracheal rings before removing the endoscope.
2. Note that the depth of the endotracheal tube is appropriate.
3. After attaching the tube to the breathing circuit, observe whether the chest rises and listen for breath sounds when positive pressure is applied to the system.
4. When the patient breathes spontaneously, watch for the bag to deflate or feel air movement at the tip of the tube.
5. Monitor the end-tidal CO_2.

6. With a fiberoptic scope in the pharynx, observe whether the tube passes into the glottis. Make sure that the cuff is completely below the vocal cords.

7. Obtain a chest X ray.

8. With the tube in place, ask the patient to phonate. He will not be able to do so if the endotracheal tube is between the vocal cords.

For an anesthetized patient:

All of the steps listed above, except step 8, can be used to verify tube placement if the patient is anesthetized.

Fiberoptic Intubation for an Anesthetized Patient

Either nasal or oral fiberoptic intubation can be performed with the patient anesthetized. Oxygen 100% should be administered for a few minutes before starting. The patient may breathe spontaneously, he may have his ventilation controlled, or he may be apneic. If the patient is breathing spontaneously or having his ventilation controlled, an intubating face mask (as described previously) should be employed. Other authors have described various methods to provide ventilation through laryngeal tubes placed in the pharynx during fiberoptic ventilation.[73–75] If fiberoptically guided intubation is conducted through a Portex adapter, tubes up 6.0 mm ID cuffed and 6.5 mm uncuffed may be used. If an intubating mask is not used, fiberoptic intubation can be conducted with the patient asleep, apneic, and thoroughly preoxygenated before the intubation sequence begins. Always monitor the patient with an oxyhemoglobin saturation monitor.

The procedural steps to intubate the anesthetized patient are the same as for the awake patient. **The mandibular lift may markedly facilitate visualization of the glottis.**

Performing a fiberoptic intubation with the patient anesthetized may be harder to perform than if he were awake, for the reasons stated previously. However, the technique is very useful when the patient is combative or very young. If having trouble intubating the patient when he is anesthetized, **consider waking him up and trying other techniques to establish an airway, including awake fiberoptic intubation.**

Success Rate of Fiberoptic Intubation

Ovassapian[1(p98)] reported that the success rate of fiberoptic intubations at his institution was approximately 98%. (About 20% were described as "moderately difficult" and about 5% were described as "difficult.")[1(p99)] This rate of success should be achieved if you are well trained and continue to practice fiberoptic techniques to maintain **proficiency.**

Causes of Failed Fiberoptic Intubation

Table 4.8 lists some of the causes of failed fiberoptic intubation.

TABLE 4.8. Causes of failed fiberoptic intubaton

1. Lack of training or experience
2. Unprepared patient
a. Inadequate instruction/education
b. Insufficient topical anesthesia
c. Insufficient sedation
3. Excessive secretions, blood
4. Distorted airway anatomy
a. Masses
b. Infection
c. Cysts
d. Floppy epiglottis
e. Burns
f. Trauma
5. Inability to pass the endotracheal tube over the scope
6. Inability to withdraw the scope from the endotracheal tube
7. Rushing
8. Equipment failure
9. Fogging
10. Starting with the scope too deep (in the esophagus)

Source: Modified from Ovassapian, 1996,[1] and Reed, 1995,[76] with permission.

Complications of Fiberoptic Intubation

The complications associated with fiberoptic intubation are rare. Table 4.9 lists actual, and possible, complications associated with the technique.

Special Uses of the Fiberoptic Endoscope

The fiberoptic endoscope has many applications other than straightfoward intubation of the trachea. A few of these will be discussed in more detail. They include the following:

1. Endobronchial tube placement
2. Retrograde wire-guided intubation
3. Endotracheal tube change
4. Use in the ICU
5. Pediatric use
6. Use with various "new" airways: Combitube, COPA, LMA
7. Video fiberoptic systems
8. Use of the fiberoptic endoscope as a conduit for jet ventilation
9. Use of the fiberoptic endoscope in the "difficult airway" scenario

Cautionary Note: All of the techniques described above should be practiced on models and mannequins before being attempted on a patient!

TABLE 4.9. Complications of fiberoptic intubation

1. Laryngospasm
2. Bronchospasm
3. Gagging
4. Vomiting (aspiration)
5. Hematoma (at the sight of transtracheal injection of local anesthetic)
6. Nerve block and transtracheal injection–related problems
    a. Seizures
    b. Injury to surrounding structures
    c. Epidural or spinal injection of local anesthetic
    d. Nerve injury
    e. Barotrauma (subcutaneous emphysema)
7. Oversedation
    a. Loss of the airway
    b. Hypoventilation/hypoxemia
8. Barotrauma, gastric distension/rupture, if oxygen is insufflated through the endoscope
9. Cardiovascular problems
    a. Hypertension
    b. Tachycardia
    c. Vagal reflexes
10. Damage to the scope or other equipment
11. Unpleasant recall by the patient

Source: Modified from Ovassapian, 1996,[1(p101)] with permission.

Endobronchial Tube Placement

Once a double-lumen endobronchial tube is placed, the fiberoptic scope can be used to verify that the tube has been placed correctly.

To confirm placement, the operator looks down the **tracheal lumen** of the double-lumen tube and visually verifies the following:

1. That the tip of the endobronchial tube has entered the correct mainstem bronchus.
2. That the cuff on the distal or bronchial end of the tube can **barely** be seen at the carina when the cuff is inflated. This will verify that the distal tip of the tube is not too far into the mainstem bronchus.

Retrograde Wire-Guided Intubation

The fiberoptic endoscope may be used to assist retrograde wire-guided intubation. (See Chapter 10.) The technique has been described by many authors and used to intubate adult[77] and pediatric[78] patients. The steps of the technique follow:

1. Check equipment. Make sure the wire to be passed is at least 6 to 10 inches longer than the fiberoptic endoscope and that it passes through the working port of the scope.
2. Place a lubricated endotracheal tube over the fiberoptic bundle and run it back to the handle of the scope.

3. Pass the retrograde wire through the cricothyroid ligament and direct it out through the mouth or nose as described in Chapter 10.
4. Pass the wire through the distal end of the fiberoptic scope and feed it all the way through the scope so that it comes out the proximal end of the working port. Have an assistant grasp or clamp the wire to keep it from being lost in the scope.
5. Pass the scope along the wire into the airway. View its passage through the airway. Watch as it passes into the trachea.
6. Pass the tube into the trachea, positioning it above the carina. The tube and scope can be moved together. Provide slack in the wire by feeding more wire through the cricothyroid ligament. If the wire kinks or prohibits insertion of the scope and tube, it can be cut off at the skin and pulled back through the scope. Do not cut the wire until the scope is definitely in the trachea.
7. Remove the wire.
8. Inflate the cuff and verify placement of the tube in the trachea.
9. Remove the endoscope.

Endotracheal Tube Change

A patient's endotracheal tube may need to be changed because of cuff failure or tube damage. Executing a tube change with the fiberoptic endoscope requires **expert skill** with the instrument. Equipment for, and personnel competent to perform, an emergency cricothyroidotomy should be standing by if the technique is attempted on a patient with a very tenuous or abnormal airway, **since loss of the airway during tube changing could be a life-threatening event.**

1. Apply appropriate monitors.
2. Allow the patient to continue breathing spontaneously.
3. Denitrogenate the lungs by placing the patient on 100% oxygen for at least 5 minutes.
4. Judiciously consider the appropriateness of sedation, topical anesthesia, and nerve blocks. Apply topical anesthesia to the trachea by injecting 2 to 4 ml of lidocaine 4% into the endotracheal tube.
5. Use the nasal approach unless contraindicated.
6. Pass a lubricated endotracheal tube onto the fiberoptic bundle and slide it back to the handle.
7. Gently insert the endoscope nasally and advance it until the existing tube can be seen passing into the glottis. Carefully examine the anatomy and review contingency plans.
8. At this point, you have two options:
    a. You may pass the fiberoptic scope into the trachea alongside the existing tube before removing the tube. The scope may have to pass **anterior to the existing tube as it enters the anterior commissure of the glottic opening.**[1(pp166–175)] Deflate the cuff of the existing tube to allow passage of the scope. After the scope is in the trachea, remove the existing tube and pass the new tube into the trachea. Confirm tube placement.

b. Sometimes the scope will not pass into the trachea with the existing tube in place. In this case, pass the new tube down to the end of the scope and position the scope close to the glottic opening. Remove the existing tube and insert the scope into the trachea. Advance the new tube over the scope. You can make this option safer by passing a flexible tube changer, a bougie, through the damaged tube before removing it. If the new tube or scope cannot be passed into the trachea, you can attempt to pass a tube over the bougie into the trachea.

Use in the ICU

All of the techniques that have been described can be used in the ICU. In addition, other specific uses in this setting include the following:

1. Endotracheal and endobronchial lavage and suctioning
2. Evaluation of airway anatomy for trauma, foreign bodies, or pathology at any level
3. Verifying the position of other equipment (NG tube)
4. Obtain samples for bacterial/cytological examination

Pediatric Use

Every use described for adults can be applied to pediatric patients. The fiberoptic endoscope has been used to evaluate the airways of very young awake patients[79,80] to intubate pediatric surgical patients who were anesthetized and difficult to intubate with standard instruments,[81] or predicted to be difficult,[82] as well as to manage the airways of pediatric patients with known bronchial pathology.[83] You cannot consider yourself **proficient** in all aspects of fiberoptic endoscopic airway management unless you have mastery of adult **as well as** pediatric techniques.

Fiberoptic Endoscopy and the "New" Airway Devices

Much has been written concerning use of the Combitube, the COPA and the LMA. Following is a review of the use of these devices and the fiberoptic endoscope.

Combitube (Kendall, Mansfield, MA)

Gaitini et al.[84] described a nasal fiberoptically guided intubation in an anesthetized patient who had a Combitube in place. The fiberoptic scope was advanced until the pharyngeal section of the Combitube was seen positioned superolateral to the larynx. The pharyngeal cuff was partially deflated and the bronchoscope was passed into the trachea. The patient was intubated, then the Combitube was removed. The authors state that the technique was adapted to a similar technique described by Ovassapian et al.[85]

Gaitini et al[86] also published a study comparing 20 anesthetized, nonparalyzed, spontaneously breathing patients with 20 anesthetized, paralyzed, and mechanically ventilated patients who had a Combitube placed after induction of anesthesia. The patients were then intubated using a nasotracheal fiberoptic technique. An armored endotracheal tube was used in the study. The pharyngeal cuff was partially deflated during the intubation. The rates of successful intubations were 90% in the spontaneously breathing group of patients and 75% for the paralyzed patients.

Kraft et al[87] described a modified Combitube allowing passage of the fiberoptic scope through the airway. The technique described by Kraft et al. also required use of a guide wire over which the endotracheal tube was placed.

These reports document that fiberoptic intubation directed outside a Combitube, which is already in place, is a reasonable option to consider if one deems it necessary to exchange the Combitube with an endotracheal tube.

COPA (Cuffed Oropharyngeal Airway) (Mallinckrodt Medical Inc., St. Louis)

Hawkins et al[88] described a fiberoptic intubation technique in which a scope, covered with an Aintree intubation catheter, was passed through a COPA airway into the trachea of 20 anesthetized, paralyzed patients. The scope and COPA were then removed, leaving the Aintree catheter in the trachea. A standard endotracheal tube was then "railroaded" over the catheter into the trachea. The authors reported that all patients were successfully intubated. The only difficulty arose when the operator failed to lubricate the Aintree catheter.

Greenberg and Kay[89] reported a study of 40 anesthetized patients who were intubated either nasally or orally with a COPA in situ. The fiberoptic endoscope was passed outside of the COPA and the cuff was not deflated. After the scope was passed into the trachea, the COPA was removed and an endotracheal tube was passed into the trachea over the scope. The authors reported one episode of coughing causing transient hypoxemia, and one patient being withdrawn from the study because of "secretions." The authors concluded that the COPA should be considered as a useful adjunct to fiberoptic intubation, especially since the device allows ventilation during the intubation process to continue.

LMA (Laryngeal Mask Airway) (LMA North America, San Diego)

Fiberoptic intubations have been performed for years through the LMA.[90,91] The LMA has proven to be a useful guide through which to perform neonatal and pediatric laryngoscopy and bronchoscopy.[92] Fiberoptic intubation techniques utililizing the LMA have been described for pediatric surgical patients, some with preexisting difficult airway anatomy.[93,94]

The manufacturers of the LMA now market the **Fastrach-LMA** (LMA North America), which is designed to facilitate "blind" intubations through the mask, and to be used as an intubating LMA with the fiberoptic endoscope. The **Fastrach** is packaged with three reusable **Fastrach Endotracheal Tubes** that have silicone tapered tips. The **Fastrach-LMA** has a modified diaphragm (epiglottic elevator) through which an endoscope and a tube can be passed.

In practice, the LMA is used most often to facilitate fiberoptic intubation in an anesthetized patient. However, an LMA may be placed in an awake patient who is topically anesthetized and/or sedated. To use the **Fastrac** to facilitate fiberoptic intubation, start by placing it into proper pharyngeal position and then inflate the cuff. The patient can be ventilated or he may breathe spontaneously. Next, place an endotracheal tube (without the 15-mm adapter) onto the fiberoptic bundle of the scope. Pass the scope through the **Fastrach** into the trachea. Pass the tube over the scope into the trachea. Remove the scope. Next, place a **"stabilizer bar or device"** on the end of the endotracheal tube. The **"stabilizer device"** holds the endotracheal tube in place as the **Fastrach** is withdrawn from the mouth. Place a standard airway into the patient's mouth, replace the 15-mm adapter on the distal end of the tube, inflate the cuff, and verify tube position. One may not wish to remove the **Fastrach.** If one does not remove the **Fastrach** and the patient wakes up with it in place, he may damage it by biting (Figs. 4.35 to 4.37). (Note the precaution associated with Fastrach used in patients with cervical pathology [see Chapter 15]).

The LMA is a uniquely designed airway that is adaptable to many settings in which it can be used to facilitate fiberoptic intubation as well as evaluation of the laryngeal anatomy and function.

Video Fiberoptic Systems

Both Olympus and Pentax market video fiberoptic systems. These systems are useful teaching aids. With more use by practitioners, they will become as popu-

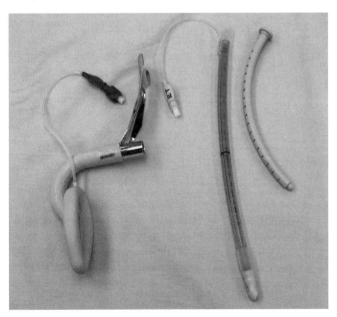

FIGURE 4.35. The Fastrach LMA, Fastrach Endotracheal Tubes, and the "stabilizing device" used to hold an endotracheal tube in place if the Fastrach is removed after fiberoptic intubation. (LMA North America Inc., with permission.)

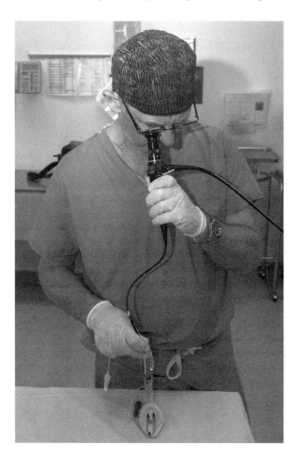

FIGURE 4.36. Fiberoptic intubation through a Fastrach LMA. (LMA North America Inc., with permission.)

lar as traditional fiberoptic endoscopes to perform all of the functions of the traditional scope.

Fiberoptic Endoscope and Jet Ventilation

The fiberoptic endoscope has been used as a conduit to apply jet ventilation. One example describing its use was published by David et al.[95] They applied low-frequency jet ventilation through the suction channel of an endoscope that had been passed through the tracheal anastomosis of a patient who required aggressive pulmonary toilet. The technique, as described, was both simple and efficacious. Many variations of the technique, for many different purposes, could be proposed.

Fiberoptic Endoscopy in the Difficult Airway Scenario

Fiberoptic intubation is offered as one choice in the ASA difficult airway algorithm along the "non-emergency pathway."[17] Controversy exists between those who feel that they are very competent in the application of fiberoptic airway tech-

FIGURE 4.37. Use the "stabilizing device" to hold the endotracheal tube in place as the Fastrach is withdrawn from the mouth. (LMA North America Inc., with permission.)

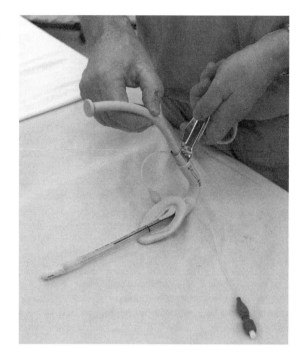

niques, even in the **emergency setting,** and those who do not. A quote from Dr. Ovassapian, commenting on use of the fiberoptic scope in the failed intubation scenario, puts the argument in proper perspective.[96]

> **The only thing hindering the routine use of (the) fibrescope (endoscope) in failed intubation, is lack of experience, skill, and confidence.**

The A.S.A. difficult airway algorithm suggests a way for practitioners to think about their approach to managing the difficult airway. You must weigh your airway management strengths with your weaknesses. Roberts[97] offers many thoughtful observations and suggestions concerning various options to choose from when dealing with the difficult airway. **In the final analysis, you must decide for yourself how aggressively you will apply your fiberoptic airway management skills when faced with a difficult airway.**

Summary

The development of fiberoptic endoscopic techniques and the proliferation of teaching protocols and workshops is testimony to the utility of this revolutionary airway management intervention. To gain **proficiency:**

1. Attend a workshop presented by a recognized authority and teacher in the field of fiberoptic airway management techniques.

2. Develop an organized and efficient training protocol in your institution.
3. Practice as many different fiberoptic airway techniques as possible under the guidance of a competent colleague.
4. Use the fiberoptic endoscope on a **routine** basis.
5. Apply the techniques to pediatric as well as adult patients.

Finally, you must define your **level of competence** with fiberoptic airway techniques. Knowing your level will allow you to apply your skills appropriately when dealing with a difficult airway.

References

1. Ovassapian A. *Fiberoptic Endoscopy and the Difficult Airway.* 2nd ed. Philadelphia: Lippincott-Raven, 1996.
2. Fulling PD, Roberts, JT. Fiberoptic intubation. *Inter Anesth Clin.* 2000;38(3):189–217.
3. Dierdorf SF. The physics of fiberoptic endoscopy. *Mt Sinai J Med.* 1995;62(1):3–9.
4. Dierdorf SF. Use of the flexible fiberoptic laryngoscope. *Mt Sinai J Med.* 1995;62(1): 21–26.
5. Society for Airway Management. PO Box A 3982, Chicago, IL 60690-3982; Tel: (773) 834-3171; http://www.samhq.org.
6. American Society of Anesthesiologists. 520 N. Northwest Highway, Park Ridge, IL 60068-2573; Tel: (847) 825-5586; http://www.asahq.org.
7. Lefebvre DL, Stock MC. Fiberoptic glottic examination to promote safe prolonged tracheal intubation. *Anesthesiology.* 1988;69:A177.
8. Dellinger RP, Bandi V. Fiberoptic bronchoscopy in the intensive care unit. *Crit Care Clin.* 1992;8:755.
9. Clark PT, et al. Removal of proximal and peripheral endobronchial foreign bodies with the flexible fiberoptic bronchoscope. *Anaesth Intensive Care* 1989;17:205–208.
10. Koppel JN. Learning fiberoptic-guided endotracheal intubation. *Mt Sinai J Med.* 1995;62(1):41–46.
11. Colley PS, Freund P. An aid to learning to use the fiberoptic bronchoscope for intubation. *Anesth Analg.* 1997;85:464–465.
12. Naik VN, et al. Fiberoptic orotracheal intubation on anesthetized patients. *Anesthesiology.* 2001;95(2):343–348.
13. Mallios C, et al. Fiberoptic cart for intubation and teaching. *Can J Anaesth.* 1998; 45(12):1220–1221.
14. Schaefer HG, et al. Teaching fiberoptic intubation in anaesthetised patients. *Anaesthesia.* 1994;49:331–334.
15. Erb T, et al. Teaching the use of fiberoptic intubation in anesthetized, spontaneously breathing patients. *Anesth Analg.* 1999;89:1292–1295.
16. Erb T, et al. Teaching the use of fiberoptic intubation for children older than two years of age. *Anesth Analg.* 1997;85:1037–1041.
17. ASA Difficult Airway Algorithm. 2001. Available at: http://www.asahq.org.
18. Chung D. A modified Williams airway intubator to assist fiberoptic intubation. *Can J Anaesth.* 1998;45(1):95.
19. Aoyama K, et al. Simple modification of the Ovassapian fiberoptic intubating airway. *Anesthesiology.* 1999;91(3):897.
20. Ravindran RS. Another advantage of marking Ovassapian fiber-optic intubating airway. *Anesthesiology.* 2000;92(6):1843.

21. Goskowicz R, et al. Fiberoptic tracheal intubation using a nipple guide. *Anesthesiology.* 1996;85(5):1210.
22. Krensavage TJ. Oral obturator a useful adjunct for fiberoptic tracheal intubation. *Anesthesiology.* 1996;85(4):942.
23. Higgins MS, Marco AP. An aid in oral fiberoptic intubation. *Anesthesiology.* 1992; 77:1236.
24. Frei FJ, Ummenhofer W. A special mask for teaching fiber-optic intubation in pediatric patients. *Anesth Analg.* 1993;76:458.
25. Okuda M, et al. A new device for fiberoptic endotracheal intubation under general anesthesia. *Anesthesiology.* 1988;69:637.
26. Magaro T, et al. Ventilation via a mouth mask facilitates fiberoptic nasal tracheal intubation in anesthetized patients. *Anesthesiology.* 1993;78:603.
27. Waring PH, Vinik HR. A potential complication of the Patil-Syracuse endoscopy mask. *Anesth Analg.* 1991;73:668.
28. Williams L, et al. Foreign body from a Patil-Syracuse mask for fiberoptic intubation. *Anesth Analg.* 1991;73:359.
29. Davis K. Alterations to the Patil-Syracuse mask for fiberoptic intubation. *Anesth Analg.* 1992;74:472.
30. Barker KF, et al. Ease of laryngeal passage during fiberoptic intubation: a comparison of three endotracheal tubes. *Acta Anaesthesiol Scand.* 2001;45:624–626.
31. Greer JR, et al. A comparison of tracheal tube tip design on the passage of an endotracheal tube during oral fiberoptic intubation. *Anesthesiology.* 2001;94(5):729–731.
32. Greer R, et al. Comparison of two tracheal tube tip designs for oral fiberoptic intubation. *Br J Anaesth.* 2000;84(2):281.
33. Jones HE, et al. Fiberoptic intubation: influence of tracheal tube tip design. *Anaesthesia.* 1993;48:672–674.
34. Rosenblatt WH. Overcoming obstruction during bronchoscope-guided intubation of the trachea with the double setup endotracheal tube. *Anesth Analg.* 1996;83:175–177.
35. Marsh NJ. Easier fiberoptic intubations. *Anesthesiology.* 1992;76:860–861.
36. Brull SJ, et al. Facilitation of fiberoptic orotracheal intubation with a flexible tracheal tube. *Anesth Analg.* 1994;78:746–748.
37. Hakala P, et al. Comparison between tracheal tubes for orotracheal fiberoptic intubation. *Br J Anaesth.* 1999;82(1):135–136.
38. Olympus America, Inc. 2001.
39. Pentax. Orangeburg, NY: 2001.
40. Guzman JL. Use of a short flexible fiberoptic endoscope for difficult intubations. *Anesthesiology.* 1997;87(6):1563–1564.
41. Saruki N, et al. Swift conversion from laryngoscopic to fiberoptic intubation with a new, handy fiberoptic stylet. *Anesth Analg.* 1999;89:526–528.
42. Morris IR. Fibreoptic intubation. *Can J Anaesth.* 1994;41(10):996–1008.
43. Cole AR, et al. Fibreoptic intubation. *Can J Anaesth.* 1995;42(9):840.
44. Hershey MD, Hannenberg AA. Gastric distention and rupture from oxygen insufflation during fiberoptic intubation. *Anesthesiology.* 1996;85(6):1479–1480.
45. Ovassapian A, Mesnick PS. Oxygen insufflation through the fiberscope to assist intubation is not recommended. *Anesthesiology.* 1997;87(1):183.
46. Brookman CA, et al. Anticholinergics improve fiberoptic intubating conditions during general anaesthesia. *Can J Anaesth.* 1997;44(2):165–167.
47. Ezri T, et al. Central anticholinergic syndrome complicating management of a difficult airway. *Can J Anaesth.* 1996;43(10):1079.

48. Smith JE, Reid AP. Selecting the safest nostril for nasotracheal intubation with the fibreoptic laryngoscope. *Br J Anaesthesia.* 1999;82(suppl 1):26.
49. Balatbat JT, et al. Controlled intermittent aerosolization of lidocaine for airway anesthesia. *Anesthesiology.* 1999;91(2):596.
50. Smith T. Jetting lidocaine through the atomizer. *Anesthesiology.* 1999;90(2):634.
51. Barclay PM, O'Sullivan E. Systemic absorption of cocaine during fibreoptic bronchoscopy. *Br J Anaesth.* 1999;83:518P–519P.
52. Khorasani A, et al. Canister tip orientation and residual volume have significant impact on the dose of benzocaine delivered by Hurricane spray. *Anesth Analg.* 2001;92:379–383.
53. Ellis FD, et al. Methemoglobinemia: a complication after fiberoptic orotracheal intubation with benzocaine spray. *J Bone Joint Surg.* 1995;77-A(6):937–939.
54. Chung DC, et al. Anesthesia of the airway by aspiration of lidocaine. *Can J Anaesth.* 1999;46(3):215–219.
55. Drummond JC, et al. Airway anesthesia: the toothpaste method. *Can J Anaesth.* 2000;47(1):94.
56. Jones JM, Bramhall J. Airway anaesthesia during fibreoptic endoscopy. *Can J Anaesth.* 1997;44(7):785.
57. Vloka J, et al. A simple adaptation to the Olympus LF1 and LF2 flexible fiberoptic bronchoscopes for instillation of local anesthetic. *Anesthesiology.* 1995;82(3):792.
58. Bacon GS, et al. Dyclonine hydrochloride for airway anesthesia: awake endotracheal intubation in a patient with suspected local anesthetic allergy. *Anesthesiology.* 1997;86(5):1206–1207.
59. Benumof JL, et al. Upper airway obstruction. *Can J Anaesth.* 1999;46(9):906.
60. Wong D, McGuire GP. Subcutaneous emphysema following trans-cricothyroid membrane injection of local anesthetic. *Can J Anaesth.* 2000;47(2):165–168.
61. Dunn SM, Pulai I. Forced air warming can facilitate fiberoptic intubations. *Anesthesiology.* 1998;88(1):282.
62. Roberts JT, et al. Why cervical flexion facilitates laryngoscopy with a Macintosh laryngoscope, but hinders it with a flexible fiberscope. *Anesthesiology.* 1990;73:A1012.
63. Katsnelson T, et al. When the endotracheal tube will not pass over the flexible fiberoptic bronchoscope. *Anesthesiology.* 1992;76:151.
64. Cossham PS. Fibreoptic orotracheal intubation. *Br J Anaesth.* 1999;83(4):683–684.
65. Randell T. Response to Cossham. *Br J Anaesth.* 1999;83(4):683–684.
66. Krensavage TJ. Saline solution as lubrication to manipulate a stuck fiberoptic bronchoscope. *Anesth Analg.* 1999;88:965.
67. Aoyama K, et al. Jaw thrust maneuver for endotracheal intubation using a fiberoptic stylet. *Anesth Analg.* 2000;90:1457–1458.
68. Aoyama K, et al. The jaw support device facilitates laryngeal exposure and ventilation during fiberoptic intubation. *Anesth Analg.* 1998;86:432–434.
69. Aoyama K, et al. New jaw support device and awake fiberoptic intubation. *Anesth Analg.* 2000;91:1309–1310.
70. Johnson C, et al. Fiberoptic intubation facilitated by a rigid laryngoscope. *Anesth Analg.* 1991;72:714.
71. Dennehy KC, Dupuis JY. Fibreoptic intubation in the anaesthetized patient. *Can J Anaesth.* 1996;43(2):197.
72. Archdeacon J, Brimacombe J. Anterior traction of the tongue—a forgotten aid to awake fiberoptic intubation. *Anaesth Intens Care.* 1995;23(6):750–757.
73. Slots P, Reinstrup P. One way to ventilate patients during fibreoptic intubation. *Acta Anaesthesiol Scand.* 2001;45:507–509.

74. Chen L, et al. Continuous ventilation during transnasal fiberoptic bronchoscope-aided tracheal intubation. *Anesth Analg.* 1996;82(3):674.

75. Cavdarski A. Continuous ventilation during transnasal fiberoptic intubation. *Anesth Analg.* 1996;83:1133.

76. Reed AP. Predictable problems with flexible fiberoptic laryngoscopy. *Mt Sinai J Med.* 1995;62(1):31–35.

77. Gupta B, et al. Oral fiberoptic intubation over retrograde guidewire. *Anesth Analg.* 1989;68:517.

78. Audenaert SM, et al. Retrograde-assisted fiberoptic tracheal intubation in children with difficult airways. *Anesth Analg.* 1991;73:660.

79. Downing GJ, Kibride HW. Evaluation of airway complications in high-risk preterm infants: application of flexible fiberoptic airway endoscopy. *Pediatrics.* 1995;95(4):567–572.

80. Berkowitz RG. Neonatal upper airway assessment by awake flexible laryngoscopy. *Ann Otol Rhinol Laryngol.* 1998;107:75–80.

81. Blanco G, et al. Fibreoptic nasal intubation in children with anticipated and unanticipated difficult intubation. *Paediatric Anaesthesia.* 2000;111:49–53.

82. Hakala P, et al. Orotracheal fibreoptic intubation in children under general anaesthesia. *Paediatric Anaesthesia.* 1997;7:371–374.

83. Monrigal JP, Granry JC. Excision of bronchogenic cysts in children using an ultrathin fibreoptic bronchoscope. *Can J Anaesth.* 1996;43(7):694–696.

84. Gaitini LA, et al. Replacing the combitube by an endotracheal tube using a fibre-optic bronchoscope during spontaneous ventilation. *J Laryngol Otol.* 1998;112:786–787.

85. Ovassapian A, et al. Fiberoptic tracheal intubation with combitube in place. *Anesth Analg.* 1993;76:S315.

86. Gaitini LA, et al. Fiberoptic-guided airway exchange of the esophageal-tracheal combitube in spontaneously breathing versus mechanically ventilated patients. *Anesth Analg.* 1999;88:193–196.

87. Kraft P, et al. Bronchoscopy via a redesigned combitube in the esophageal position: a clinical evaluation. *Anesthesiology.* 1997;86:1041–1045.

88. Hawkins M, et al. Fiberoptic intubation using the cuffed oropharyngeal airway and Aintree intubation catheter. *Anaesthesia.* 1998;53:891–894.

89. Greenberg RS, Kay NH. Cuffed oropharyngeal airway (COPA) as an adjunct to fiberoptic tracheal intubation. *Br J Anaesth.* 1999;82:395–398.

90. Chen L. Continuous ventilation during trans-laryngeal mask airway fiberoptic bronchoscope-aided tracheal intubation. *Anesth Analg.* 1996;82:891–892.

91. Barnett RA, Ochroch EA. Augmented fiberoptic intubation. *Crit Care Clinics.* 2000;16(3):453–462.

92. Hinton AE, et al. Neonatal and paediatric fibre-optic laryngoscopy and bronchoscopy using the LMA. *J Laryngol Otol.* 1997;111:349–353.

93. Holmstrom A, Akeson J. Fibreoptic laryngotracheoscopy via the LMA in children. *Acta Anaesth Scand.* 1997;41:239–241.

94. Walker RWM, et al. A fibreoptic intubation technique for children with mucopolysaccharidoses using the LMA. *Paediatric Anaesth.* 1997;7:421–426.

95. David I, et al. Jet ventilation for fiberoptic bronchoscopy. *Anesthesiology.* 2001;94(5):930–932.

96. Ovassapian A, et al. Fibreoptic bronchoscope and unexpected failed intubation. *Can J Anaesth.* 1999;46:806–807.

97. Roberts J. Fiberoptic intubation and alternative techniques for managing the difficult airway. *ASA Refresher Course.* 1999:136.

5
Evaluation of the Airway

It has been estimated that as many as 600 patients die each year from complications related to airway management.[1] A recent report from France[2] indicated that among 198,000 patients, 162 either died from or sustained permanent brain damage following airway intervention.

Three mechanisms of injury account for most serious airway complications: esophageal intubation, failure to ventilate, and difficult intubation—with difficult intubation playing a role in all three.[3] The vast majority of difficult intubations (98%) may be anticipated by performing a thorough evaluation of the airway in advance.[4] Nevertheless, many clinicians pay little attention to this important task and confine their examination to a cursory observation of the mouth and teeth.

The information in this chapter will allow you to anticipate with a reasonable degree of accuracy when airway management may be difficult.

The technique of endotracheal intubation depends heavily on the ability to manipulate the cervical spine, the atlantooccipital joint, the mandible, oral soft tissues, neck, and hyoid bone. Therefore, any disease, congenital or acquired, that interferes with the mobility of these structures can create difficulties that prevent you from seeing the larynx during direct laryngoscopy. The same factors apply to successful nasal intubation, but in addition, patency of the nasal passages is required. It should also be remembered that the ability to see the larynx does not always ensure a successful intubation. Occasionally, abnormal dentition or obstruction by other, more proximal structures may impair your ability to place an endotracheal tube between the vocal cords. Unrecognized pathology in the vicinity of the larynx may impede the passage of an endotracheal tube large enough to allow adequate ventilation. This background information should be kept in mind when evaluating patients for intubation.

The Normal/Abnormal Airway

There are a number of wide-ranging characteristics and measurements in adults that constitute a "normal airway" (Box 5.1). When patients with these features present for airway management, problems do not usually occur. There are also a number of features that make up the "difficult airway" (Box 5.2), and when patients with these characteristics present for airway management, problems frequently occur.

Predictive Tests for Difficult Intubation

Anesthesiologists are constantly seeking ways to develop a foolproof system for predicting difficult intubation. The Mallampati test has undeserved status as a reliable predictor of difficult intubation. In reality a Mallampati score of 3 only has a positive predictive value of 21% for laryngoscopy grades 3 and 4 combined and only 4.7% for laryngoscopy grade 4 alone. Therefore, if we relied solely on this test to predict difficult intubation we would be performing a considerable number of unnecessary awake intubations. It may seem unreasonable to single out this one test; however, in reality anesthesiologists have given great credence. The truth, of course, is that most of the other tests we use for this purpose are equally disappointing when positive predictive value is measured, with the exception of a history of difficult intubation.

Box 5.1. Factors Characterizing the Normal Airway in Adolescents and Adults

1. History of one or more easy intubations without sequelae
2. Normal appearing face with "regular" features
3. Normal clear voice
4. Absence of scars, burns, swelling, infection, tumor, or hematoma; no history of radiation therapy to head or neck
5. Ability to lie supine asymptomatically; no history of snoring or sleep apnea
6. Patent nares
7. Ability to open mouth widely with TMJ rotation and subluxation (3 to 4 cm or two to three finger-breadths)
8. Mallampati/Samsoon Class I (i.e., with patient sitting up straight, opening mouth as wide as possible, with protruding tongue; the uvula, posterior pharyngeal wall, entire tonsillar pillars, and fauces can be seen)
9. At least 6.5 cm (three finger-breadths) from tip of mandible to thyroid notch with neck extended
10. At least 9 cm from symphysis of mandible to mandibular angle
11. Slender supple neck without masses; full range of neck motion
12. Larynx movable with swallowing and manually movable laterally (about 1.5 cm on each side)
13. Slender to moderate body build
14. Ability to extend atlantooccipital joint (normal extension is 35°)

Source: Compiled from Smith DE. In: Miller RD, ed. *Anesthesia.* 2nd ed. New York: Churchill-Livingstone; 1986:233–234; Gordon RA. *Int Anesthesiol Clin.* 1972;10:37; and Liu PL. *Principles and Procedures.* Philadelphia: JB Lippincott; 1992.

How reliable is our predictability if we use a combination of tests? Common sense tells us that if we use more than one test to predict difficult intubation, our chances of predicting difficulty increase. However, one of the problems noted is that there is very poor interobservational reliability for many of the tests that we commonly use to predict difficult intubation. A recent paper by El-Ganzouri et al[5] demonstrated increased accuracy predicting difficult intubation when one used objective airway risk criteria. They prospectively studied 10,507 patients presenting for intubation under general anesthesia.

Risk factors for difficult intubation include the following:

• Mouth opening less than 4 cm
• Thyromental distance less than 6 cm
• Mallampati 3
• Neck movement less than 80%

Box 5.2. Signs Indicative of a Difficult Intubation

1. Trauma, deformity; burns, radiation therapy, infection, swelling; hematoma of the face, mouth, pharynx, larynx, and/or neck
2. Stridor or "air hunger"
3. Intolerance of the supine position
4. Hoarseness or abnormal voice
5. Mandibular abnormality
   a. Decreased mobility or inability to open the mouth at least three finger-breadths
   b. Micrognathia, receding chin
      i. Treacher Collins, Pierre Robin, other syndromes
      ii. Less than 6 cm (three finger-breadths) from tip of the mandible to thyroid notch with neck in full extension (adolescents and adults)
   c. Less than 9 cm from angle of the jaw to symphysis
   d. Increased anterior or posterior mandibular depth
6. Laryngeal abnormalities: fixation of the larynx to other structures of neck, hyoid, or floor of mouth
7. Macroglossia
8. Deep, narrow, high-arched oropharynx
9. Protruding teeth
10. Mallampati/Samsoon Classes 3 and 4 (see Figs. 5.6 and 5.7); inability to visualize the posterior oropharyngeal structures (tonsillar fossae, pillars, uvula) on voluntary protrusion of the tongue with mouth wide open and the patient seated
11. Neck abnormalities
    a. Short and thick
    b. Decreased range of motion (arthritis, spondylitis, disk disease)
    c. Fracture (possibility of subluxation)
    d. Obvious trauma
12. Thoracoabdominal abnormalities
    a. Kyphoscoliosis
    b. Prominent chest or large breasts
    c. Morbid obesity
    d. Term or near-term pregnancy
13. Age between 40 and 59 years
14. Gender (male)

Source: Modified from Smith DE. In: Miller RD, ed. *Anesthesia.* 2nd ed. New York: Churchill-Livingstone; 1986:233–234; Gordon RA. *Int Anesthesiol Clin.* 1972;10:37; and Liu PL. *Principles and Procedures,* Philadelphia: JB Lippincott; 1992.

Table 5.1. Accuracy of risk factors in predicting difficulty with tracheal intubation

Risk factor	Laryngoscopy grade[a]	True positives	True negatives	False positives	False negatives	Sensitivity (%)	Specificity (%)	Positive predictive value (%)	Negative predictive value (%)
Mouth opening <4 cm	≥III	169	9359	506	473	26.3	94.8	25.0	95.2
	IV	50	9775	625	57	46.7	93.9	7.4	99.4
Thyromental distance <6.0 cm	≥III	45	9793	72	597	7.0	99.2	38.5	94.3
	IV	18	10301	99	89	16.8	99.0	15.4	99.1
Mallampati Class III	≥III	287	8785	1080	355	44.7	89.0	21.0	96.1
	IV	64	9097	1303	43	59.8	87.4	4.7	99.5
Neck movement <80°	≥III	67	9705	160	575	10.4	98.4	29.5	94.4
	IV	18	10191	209	89	16.8	97.9	7.9	99.1
Inability to prognath	≥III	106	9456	409	536	16.5	95.8	20.6	94.6
	IV	28	9913	487	79	26.2	95.3	5.4	99.2
Body weight >110 kg	≥III	71	9333	532	571	11.1	94.6	11.8	94.2
	IV	14	9811	589	93	13.1	94.3	2.3	99.1
Positive history of difficult intubation	≥III	29	9852	13	613	4.5	99.8	69.0	94.1
	IV	10	10368	32	97	9.3	99.7	23.8	99.1

[a]Laryngoscopy grade categorized as either IV alone or III and IV combined. (From El-Ganzouri,[5] with permission.)

- Inability to advance the mandible (prognathism)
- Body weight greater than 110 kg
- Positive history of difficult intubation

Following induction of anesthesia the laryngeal view at laryngoscopy was graded. Poor intubating conditions were noted in 107 cases (1%). Logistic regression identified all 7 criteria as independent predictors of difficulty. A composite airway risk index as well as a simplified risk weighting system revealed a higher predictive value for grade 4 laryngoscopy (Table 5.1). While it may be impractical to perform these calculations on all cases, they certainly have potential for the future. The real message here is that multiple abnormal tests predicting difficult intubation are better than a single test.

Elective Intubation

Most elective intubations are performed by anesthetists or anesthesiologists on patients presenting for elective surgery. Occasionally, patients will be intubated on an elective basis on the ward. In all elective intubations, a brief assessment of the patient's medical status is advised.

History

Evaluation of the airway is a very important component of the overall evaluation of a patient for anesthesia. Patients should be specifically questioned about:

Previous intubations (review old records whenever possible)
Dental problems (bridges, caps, fillings, appliances, loose teeth)
Respiratory disease (sleep apnea syndrome, smoking, sputum production, wheezing)
Arthritis (temporomandibular joint [TMJ] disease, ankylosing spondylitis, rheumatoid arthritis)
Clotting abnormalities (especially before nasal intubation)
Congenital abnormalities and syndromes
Type I diabetes mellitus

Diabetes Mellitus

It has been estimated[6] the incidence of difficult intubation is about 10 times higher in patients suffering from long-term diabetes mellitus than in normal healthy patients. The limited joint mobility syndrome occurs in 30% to 40% of insulin-dependent diabetics and is thought to be due to glycosylation of tissue proteins that occurs in patients with chronic hyperglycemia.[7]

Limited joint mobility is best seen when a diabetic patient's hands assume the "prayer sign" position (Fig. 5.1). The patient typically is unable to straighten the interphalangeal joints of the fourth and fifth fingers. Another way of demonstrating this deficiency is to obtain palm print scores on patients with diabetes.

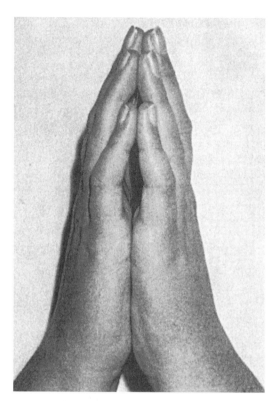

FIGURE 5.1. Hands of a 31-year-old diabetic woman in the "prayer sign" position. Her palm print score appears in Figure 5.2, D. Conditions for laryngoscopy in this individual were very poor. (From Reissell, et al,[6] with permission.)

The palm of the hand is stained with black ink and an imprint is made on white paper. This problem is well illustrated by Reissell et al, who compared palm prints in a normal patient with those from patients with varying degrees of joint mobility limitation (Fig. 5.2). It has been postulated that the same process affects the cervical spine, TMJ, and larynx. Nadal et al[8] recently tested the validity of the palm print test in 83 adult diabetics scheduled for surgery under general anesthesia. They evaluated the airway using the Mallampati test, the thyromental distance, head extension, and the palm print. The sensitivity, specificity, and the positive predictive value were calculated for each test. The palm print test had the highest sensitivity (100%). The other three tests failed to detect 9 out of 13 difficult airways.

NPO Status

Elective intubation of the trachea frequently involves the administration of potent intravenous anesthetic agents and neuromuscular blocking drugs, and patients who have recently ingested solid food and liquids are at considerable risk when airway intervention is performed in the presence of a full stomach. Therefore, it is incumbent upon you to ascertain the NPO status of the patient in ad-

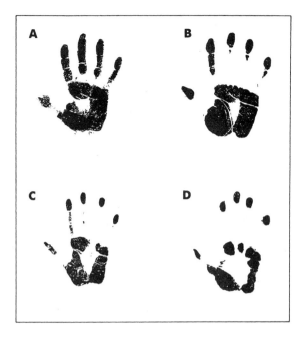

FIGURE 5.2. **A.** Complete palm print (score, 0) of a patient in whom laryngoscopy was easy (score, 0). **B.** Palm print (score, 1) of a patient in whom there is deficiency in the interphalangeal areas of the fourth and fifth digits. Laryngoscopy conditions were scored 1 in this individual. **C.** Palm print (score, 2) in which changes have spread into the interphalangeal areas of the second and third digits. Laryngoscopy in this patient was found to be difficult (score, 2). **D.** Palm print showing only the fingertips (score, 3). Several attempts were needed, and the introducer was used for laryngoscopy in this case (score, 3). (From Reissell, et al,[6] with permission.)

vance. Elective intubation should not be performed if an adult patient has ingested food within the last 6 hours.[9]

Physical Examination

General

On first approaching patients presenting for elective intubation, it is advisable to make a general assessment—i.e., the level of consciousness, the facies and body habitus, the presence or absence of cyanosis, the posture, and pregnancy. Rose and Cohen[4] have shown that the incidence of difficult intubation increases in males, persons aged 40 to 59, and the obese.

Facies

Particular attention should be paid to the facial appearance of the patient. A number of syndromes and disease states can make intubation difficult, many of which are associated with abnormal facial features, (e.g., Pierre-Robin, Treacher Collins, Klippel-Feil, Apert's, fetal alcohol). (See appendix at the end of this chapter.) Thus, when you encounter a patient with abnormal facial features, inquire as to specific syndromes or consult a pediatrician. Schmitt et al recently described a high incidence of difficult intubation in acromegalic patients. They studied 128 patients and reported difficulty in 26% of cases.[10]

Nose

The nose should be carefully examined when nasotracheal intubation is planned, observing the position of the nasal septum and whether the patient has any polyps. Nasal intubation should be avoided in the presence of a clotting abnormality, CSF leakage, nasal polyps, a history of epistaxis, or a basal skull fracture. The patency of each nostril can be tested by having the patient breathe forcefully through the unoccluded nostril. In many cases, one nostril will be more patent than the other.

Temporomandibular Joint (TMJ)

The patient's ability to open his mouth may be limited by disease of the TMJ or by masseter spasm, or a combination of both.

The function of the TMJ is complex, involving articulation and movement between the mandible and cranium. The mandible may be depressed, elevated, or manipulated anteriorly, posteriorly, or laterally. There are two distinct components to this action, each contributing about 50% to the total. The first is a hinge-like movement of the condyle through the synovial cavity, accounting for the first 20 mm or so of opening, and the second is the forward displacement of the disc and condyle, accounting for an additional 25 mm or so[11] (Fig. 5.3A, Fig. 5.3B).

A number of conditions can affect temporomandibular joint function, prominent among them are the arthritides, including rheumatoid arthritis, ankylosing spondylitis, psoriatic arthritis, and, most commonly, degenerative joint disease. TMJ function should be assessed in all patients presenting for endotracheal intubation. With the middle finger of each hand posterior and inferior to the patient's earlobes, place your index fingers just anterior to the tragus (Fig. 5.4) and instruct the patient to open widely. Two distinct movements should be felt[12]: the first is rotational, and the second involves advancement of the condylar head (Fig. 5.5). Listen and palpate for clicks and crepitus, both of which indicate joint dysfunction.

TMJ function may also be assessed by inserting, or asking the adult patient to insert, two or three extended fingers held vertically in the oral cavity along the midline. Normal adults are capable of inserting three fingers, which corresponds to a maximum mandibular opening of 50 to 60 mm.[13] Patients capable of inserting only two or fewer are considered to have some limitation and may be more difficult to intubate. If the maximal mandibular opening is less than 30 mm

FIGURE 5.3. Temporomandibular joint in closed **A** and open positions **B**. Note the rotation and translation of the condyle. (From Aiello and Metcalf,[11] with permission.)

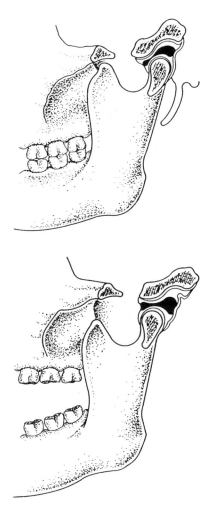

in the adult, oral surgeons feel that significant TMJ dysfunction is present. If less than 25 mm, it is unlikely that the larynx will be visible by conventional laryngoscopy, since exposure of the larynx depends to a great extent upon the ability to move the mandible and soft tissues forward. If 20 mm or less, a Macintosh 3 blade will not fit in the mouth and fiberoptically assisted intubation is recommended.

It is important to be able to distinguish between limited mouth opening due to muscle spasm and restriction due to joint disease. The former will respond to muscle relaxation, the latter will not. Patients with mandibular fractures have severely limited mouth opening because of trismus. If the fracture does not involve TMJ, it is safe to induce general anesthesia with muscle relaxation in these patients in preparation for intubation. If there is some doubt, an intravenous or inhalational

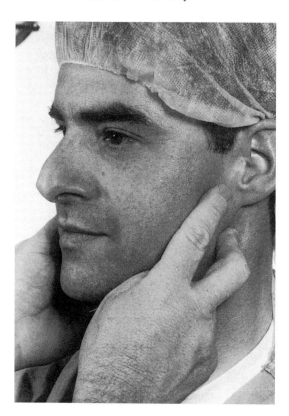

FIGURE 5.4. Assessment of temporomandibular joint function.

anesthetic should be administered first, without a muscle relaxant, and the ability to open tested in this fashion before committing to the use of muscle relaxants.

Also caution should be used when performing laryngoscopy in patients with TMJ disease. Additional damage can occur in the presence of profound muscle relaxation. If an alternative method of anesthesia is available, intubation should be avoided in any patient with significant TMJ disease.

The **mandibular protrusion test** can be performed when assessing temporo-mandibular function. This test is performed by asking the patient to advance the mandible as far as possible and the classification is as follows:

Class A: the lower incisors can be protruded beyond the upper incisors.
Class B: the lower incisors can be advanced only to the level of the upper incisors.
Class C: the lower incisors cannot reach the level of the upper incisors.

Impaired mandibular protrusion is associated with difficult laryngoscopy and difficult mask ventilation.[14,15]

Lips

A cleft lip deformity can present problems during instrumentation of the airway, in that the laryngoscope blade tends to enter the cleft. Absence of the philtrum

FIGURE 5.5. Palpating an advanced condylar head.

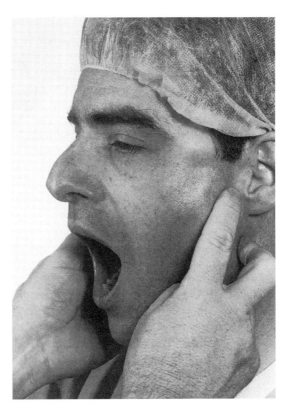

should alert you to the fetal alcohol syndrome,[16] which is associated with difficult intubation.

Oral Cavity

Before intubation, the state of oral hygiene should be assessed. Occasionally, foreign bodies such as a piece of candy or chewing gum may be hidden in the recesses of the oral cavity, especially in children.

Teeth

After examining the oral cavity, inspect the teeth. Long, protruding teeth (buck teeth) can restrict the amount of access. During direct laryngoscopy, damage is usually caused by excessive pressure on teeth that are already loose or repaired (e.g., fillings, caps, bridges, or other attachments). The incisors and canines are usually at greater risk, because the laryngoscope is generally inserted in close proximity to the teeth.

Your experience will be a major factor in the frequency of damage to the teeth. Experienced intubationists exert little if any pressure on the upper teeth, unless they are protruding. Teeth can be injured by vigorous manipulation of oral airways. Dental damage occurring in association with anesthesiology procedures accounted for 24.8% of all litigations against St. Paul Fire and Marine Insurance Company between the years 1973 and 1978.[17] More recent data from a New Zealand study[18] confirm earlier observations that dental damage is still one of the most common reasons for complaints against anesthesiologists. A review of files from the Accident Compensation Corporation in New Zealand covering a 2-year period revealed 76 claims. Interestingly, the number of claims made by women was twice that by men. Most injuries occurred to teeth that had already been restored (60%) and, as expected, the upper central incisors were usually involved. The most common injury was fracture or displacement of a filling or crown during intubation. However, a significant number occurred during emergence from anesthesia, and many of these involved oral airways. A separate survey of dental damage associated with anesthesia in New Zealand revealed an incidence of 10.4 injuries per 1,000 cases, which was much greater than that reported to the Accident Compensation Corporation.

If the patient is properly informed of potential dental problems, and reasonable care is taken during the procedure, the clinician is not considered liable if damage occurs. Davies[19] emphasized the importance of careful scrutiny of the dentition and recommended including a schematic diagram of the dentition on the evaluation sheet (Table 5.2).

Patients presenting with loose or exfoliating teeth are at increased risk for aspiration or ingestion of teeth. Consequently, it is advisable to discuss the potential risks with the patient and seek permission to remove the tooth or teeth prior to intubation. Most patients are agreeable to this approach. Children frequently present for surgery with loose deciduous teeth, and the parents are usually quite willing to consent to a minor dental procedure while the child is anesthetized; also, an unheralded visit from the "tooth fairy" tends to lessen the tension that may attend the perioperative assessment of the patient.

Having discussed the implications of the teeth with reference to intubation, it is appropriate to mention that the edentulous state is rarely associated with difficulty visualizing the airway. On the other hand, airway management using bag/mask/valve ventilation is usually more difficult under these circumstances because the normal contour of the face is distorted and collapsed and it is difficult to maintain a mask seal. There is a suggestion that bag/valve/mask ventila-

TABLE 5.2. Dental Chart

Right	Left
7,6,5,4,3,2,1	1,2,3,4,5,6,7
7,6,5,4,3,2,1	1,2,3,4,5,6,7

Schematic representation of anterior view of dentition with teeth numbered sequentially from midline. Indicate abnormalities as: A = Appliance; B = Bridge; C = Caps; L = Loose; M = Missing.
Source: Modified with permission from Davies, 1991,[19] with permission.

tion may be facilitated in the presence of dentures. However, most patients are required to remove dentures before entering the operating suite. Perhaps the logic of that convention should be revisited. The insertion of an oral airway usually allows more effective ventilation in the edentulous state.

Tongue

Two features of the tongue may interfere with your ability to visualize the larynx. One is its size in relation to the oral cavity, and the other is mobility. The tongue may be abnormally large and therefore occupy a greater proportion of the oropharynx or, conversely, be of normal size in an unusually small oropharynx. Mallampati[20] and Mallampati et al[21] have studied the correlation between the ability to observe intraoral structures and the incidence of subsequent difficult intubation. The patient is instructed to sit erect with the head in neutral position, to open as widely as possible, and to protrude the tongue maximally. Samsoon and Young[22] modified the Mallampati classification as follows: the examiner sits opposite the patient at eye level and observes various intraoral structures using a flashlight—Class I: soft palate, tonsillar fauces, tonsillar pillars, and uvula visualized; Class II: soft palate, tonsillar fauces, and uvula visualized; Class III: soft palate and base of uvula visualized; Class IV: soft palate not visualized (Fig. 5.6). In general, exposure of the airway is easy in Class I and II with a Macintosh blade but Class III or IV are difficult to intubate. It should be remembered, however, that this classification is only a guideline and cannot be relied upon to be the sole predictor of difficult intubations. Cohen et al,[23] using Cormack and Lehane's[24] grading system for ease or difficulty of intubation (Fig. 5.7), compared the Mallampati classification with the actual grade observed during attempted laryngoscopy and found a high correlation at the extremes. Pilkington et al showed that the Mallampati grade increased during pregnancy. They studied 242 pregnant patients. They performed the Mallampati test at 12 weeks and 38 weeks gestation and showed that the number of grade 4 cases had increased by 34%. This observation may explain why the incidence of difficult intubation occurs more frequently in obstetric patients (1.7%) compared to general surgical patients (1.3%). They speculated that the reason for the change in Mallampati grade was most likely fluid retention.[25]

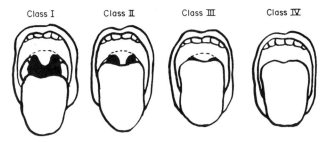

FIGURE 5.6. Classification of pharyngeal structures. Note that in Class III the soft palate is visible but in Class IV it is not. (From Samsoon and Young,[22] with permission.)

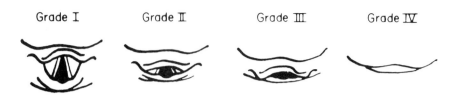

FIGURE 5.7. These are the best views obtainable at laryngoscopy, assuming correct technique. The frequencies apply to patients without neck pathology. Severe disease of the neck may produce a Grade IV view, but this rarely if ever occurs. The approximate frequencies are as follows: Grade I, 99%; Grade II, 1%; Grade III, 1/2000; Grade IV, $< 1/10^5$. (Courtesy of Circon Corporation.)

The diseased tongue may also prevent you from visualizing the larynx—e.g., tumors tend to limit lingular mobility and thus your ability to expose the larynx. The presence of lingual tonsillar tissue can also create unexpected difficulty with intubation, resulting in catastrophic airway obstruction.[26]

Ectopic thyroid tissue can be found at the base of the tongue and may bleed following laryngoscopy, leading to difficulties with the airway. This anomaly is rare, occurring in 1:100,000 cases.[27]

Tongue piercing has become popular among the younger generation. This new trend may pose problems for those performing any form of airway management. Metal or plastic objects in the tongue may become detached and aspirated or ingested or plainly lost in the course of an anesthetic. Pressure of the laryngoscope, oropharyngeal airway, or endotracheal tube on the object may cause pressure necrosis and there is also a risk of electrocautery burns. For all of these reasons it is advisable to remove tongue rings before inducing anesthesia. Patients should be informed of the risks and encouraged to remove these objects before arrival in the operating room. Patients express concerns that the opening in the tongue closes in quickly when the tongue ring is removed. It is our understanding that a pierced tongue remains patent for several hours following removal. Epidural catheters have been threaded through the opening in the tongue to maintain patency. In summary, patients should be encouraged to remove tongue rings before arrival in the operating room.[28,29]

Mandible and Floor of Mouth

The optimal position for exposure of the larynx when using a Macintosh laryngoscope is attained by flexing the neck and extending the atlantooccipital joint.[30] In individuals with normal anatomy this aligns the axes of the larynx, pharynx, and mouth so they are almost parallel (Fig. 5.8). A number of factors can interfere with the ability to align these axes, however, such as a large or tethered tongue, a short mandible, protruding upper incisors, pathology in the floor of the mouth, or reduced size of intra- and submandibular space. Some of these limitations are nicely illustrated in Fig. 5.9.

Two well-known congenital anomalies associated with mandibular shortening

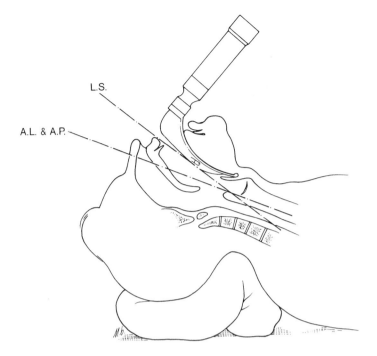

FIGURE 5.8. Final exposure.

are the Treacher Collins and Pierre Robin syndromes. In these conditions mandibular shortening is obvious and extreme. A number of individuals, however, will present with less obvious shortening of the mandible. Two very simple measurements that can be made at the bedside are the **thyromental distance,** which should exceed 6.5 cm in adults when the atlantooccipital is fully extended[31] (Fig. 5.10), and the **mandibular angle-mental symphysis distances,** which should be at least 9 cm in adults (Fig. 5.11). Ramadhani et al. recently published

FIGURE 5.9. Anatomical factors relevant to a difficult intubation. At laryngoscopy the line of vision to the cords must be clear. Difficulty can arise if the tongue (*3*), upper teeth (*2*), or cords (*1*) are displaced in the direction of the *arrows*. Even with no pathology, however, difficulty can occur because of variations in the normal anatomy. (From Cormack and Lehane,[24] with permission.)

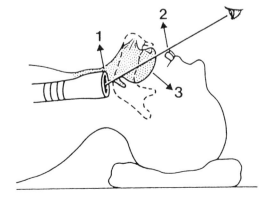

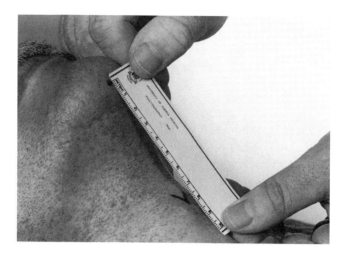

FIGURE 5.10. Thyromental distance.

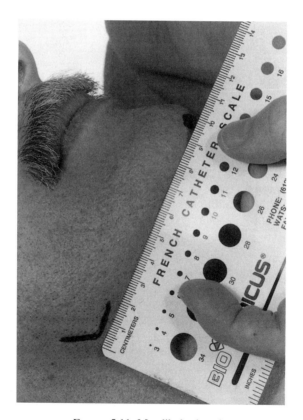

FIGURE 5.11. Mandibular length.

a report suggesting that the **sternomental distance** was a useful, sole predictor of difficult intubation in obstetric patients. A **sternomental distance** of less than 13.5 cm was a predictor of difficult laryngoscopy in obstetric patients. To our knowledge, this claim has never been validated.[32]

When these measurements are reduced, you can expect to have difficulty exposing the larynx with a Macintosh laryngoscope. Few clinicians use a ruler; rather, they estimate the anterior mandibular space by placing the fingers horizontally beneath the patient's chin. In normal adults the distance from the hyoid bone to the mandibular symphysis is about three finger-breadths (Fig. 5.12). If it is two finger-breadths or less, the mandible is considered hypoplastic. A number of other measurements may be used but they are of little practical value.

Neck, Cervical Spine, and Hyoid Bone

The neck and cervical spine should be carefully examined before intubation; the general neck contour should be inspected first.

Obese patients with short, muscular, thick necks (which have a limited range of motion) are more difficult to intubate than patients with normal, supple, or elongated necks. Patients with Klippel-Feil syndrome (characterized by a reduced number of cervical vertebrae) present problems at intubation, since the neck is shorter and thus has impaired mobility.

During examination of the neck, the skin color should be noted. Pigmentation changes may indicate that a patient has had previous radiotherapy, which could have caused acute inflammatory changes with later scarring and fibrosis in the neck region. Particular attention should be paid to scars or masses in the neck. Though almost all of these warrant some concern, any due to vascular injuries are particularly ominous because the airway could become occluded without

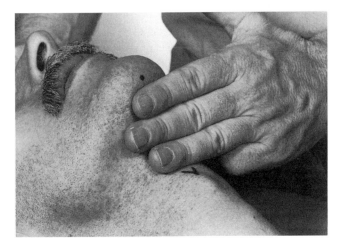

FIGURE 5.12. Assessing the mandibular space.

warning when bleeding occurs. Previous tracheostomy scars should lead you to suspect tracheal stenosis. Always check for deviation of the trachea and evaluate the degree of tracheal mobility. Relative immobility of the trachea has been associated with difficult intubation.

What role does the hyoid bone play in facilitating laryngoscopy? A significant number of patients in the general population develop calcification of the stylohyoid ligament, which may interfere with your ability to elevate the epiglottis during laryngoscopy using a Macintosh laryngoscope. There are a limited number of case reports in the literature on this topic.[33-35] The clinical sign that should lead you to suspect this problem is relative immobility of the hyoid bone or larynx. Laryngeal mobility should be routinely checked in any patient presenting for endotracheal intubation.

In palpating the neck, you should assess the degree of mobility of the cervical spine and note any limitation in flexion or extension. The optimal position for endotracheal intubation is flexion of the cervical spine and extension of the head at the atlantooccipital joint. Consequently, flexion or extension deformities of the cervical spine associated with the arthritides may make direct laryngoscopy difficult or impossible. Recently, Keenan et al[36] have reported that problems intubating patients with flexion and extension deformities of the cervical spine are not entirely due to failure to align the axes of the larynx, pharynx, and oral cavity. Rather, an additional factor is present, shortening of the cervical spine, which can cause laryngeal and tracheal deviation or forward buckling of the trachea, and this tends to force the larynx into an anterior position.

Under normal circumstances, 35° of cervical extension is possible at the atlantooccipital joint.[37] (Fig. 5.13). This angle can be readily estimated at the bedside by asking the patient to sit straight up, with the head erect and the line of sight parallel to the ground. Then ask the patient to open wide. In this position the occlusal surfaces of the upper teeth are horizontal to the ground. On extending the atlantooccipital joint, the angle created by moving the occlusal surfaces is estimated. Goniometry may be used to estimate the angle more accurately, but in practice the angle is estimated visually.

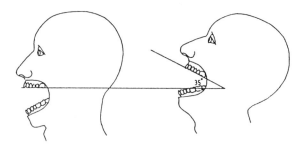

FIGURE 5.13. An assessment of atlantooccipital translation can be made by estimating the angle traversed by the maxillary teeth when the neck is extended. (From Bellhouse and Doré,[1] with permission.)

Vocal Quality

In listening for vocal quality, try to assess whether stridor is present and, if so, in which phase(s) of respiration it occurs. Lesions that are predominantly supraglottic are usually associated with inspiratory stridor, whereas subglottic lesions tend to cause both inspiratory and expiratory stridor.

Cardiorespiratory System

An examination of the airway is incomplete without a review of the cardiac and respiratory systems. This will give some measure of the patient's cardiorespiratory reserve. The minimum information required, even in emergencies, are the vital signs. Time permitting, all patients undergoing endotracheal intubation should have a thorough cardiorespiratory examination that includes a history and physical examination.

History

Every patient should be questioned about coughs and colds and whether they are acute or chronic. A patient presenting with recent cold symptoms is not a good candidate for general anesthesia because inhalation agents tend to irritate the already inflamed mucosa of the larynx, trachea, and bronchi and this can lead to laryngospasm, bronchospasm, and hypoxemia both intraoperatively and postoperatively.

If sputum is produced, its color and amount should be estimated. Greenish or yellowish sputum or an increased production of sputum suggests acute infection, and elective procedures should be delayed until it has cleared. Each patient should be questioned about smoking, and the number of pack-years recorded. Patients should be questioned about dyspnea, orthopnea, or paroxysmal nocturnal dyspnea that has occurred, and an effort should be made to determine if it is of cardiac or respiratory origin.

The patient should then be questioned about asthma; the severity of asthma can be estimated by the number of hospital admissions and the medications required. An asthmatic individual presenting for surgery and requiring steroid therapy has advanced disease and will need supplementation. Patients can usually apprise you of the current status of their asthma and can subjectively rate their chest tightness. Endotracheal intubation in the presence of wheezing often aggravates the situation and elective surgery should be delayed whenever possible. On the other hand, emergency intubation may be required in a patient suffering an acute asthmatic episode. In this case, if the patient presents with a clear history of asthma, you should pretreat with aerosolized bronchodilators and beta-2 agonists whenever possible.

Information needs to be obtained about the patient's past medical and surgical history pertaining to the respiratory system (e.g., previous thoracotomy, pulmonary aspiration, pneumothorax).

Physical Examination

It is necessary to determine if the patient is cyanotic and, if so, whether the cyanosis is central or peripheral. The degree of cyanosis can be determined by performing pulse oximetry. Does the patient appear dyspneic? Record the respiratory rate and whether retractions are present. The normal adult will breathe 16 to 20 times per minute. Does the chest expand symmetrically? Is the patient wheezing? Look for scars indicating previous surgery or chest tubes. A patient with a history of chronic bronchitis and emphysema will often have an increased anterior–posterior (AP) diameter (barrel chest).

When palpating the chest, feel the larynx and trachea and determine if they are in the midline, deviated, or mobile. Check for lymph nodes in the supraclavicular fossae and axillae. Feel the apical beat and determine its position. Does the chest expand symmetrically?

Percussion may help determine if atelectasis, pneumothorax, consolidation, or pleural effusion is present.

Listen carefully to the breath sounds over both lung fields. Are they normal? Are they equal on both sides? Are there any additional sounds? If rhonchi are present, are they coarse or high pitched, occasional or diffuse, unilateral or bilateral? Crepitations or rales are moist sounds that usually indicate pulmonary edema. They are often present in older patients but usually clear on coughing. Tubular sounds or bronchial breathing may indicate pulmonary consolidation. Diminished or absent breath sounds may indicate pneumothorax, atelectasis, or pleural effusion but are frequently due to obesity and emphysema.

Cardiovascular System

Endotracheal intubation may have a profound effect on the cardiovascular system, so a thorough history and physical examination is necessary in elective situations.

History

Ask the patient about chest pain. If present, determine its exact site and radiation. Also try to determine its quality. You may suggest adjectives that best describe it to the patient (e.g., gripping, stabbing, burning, dull ache, or heartburn). Is it continuous or intermittent? Is it associated with respiration? What relieves the pain? Does it radiate? If so, where? Is it associated with exercise? If so, what is the exercise tolerance? What brings it on and what relieves it? Are any medications being taken? Time spent eliciting details about chest pain is most important and should never be rushed.

If dyspnea is present, try to evaluate if it is of cardiac or respiratory origin. Does the patient have orthopnea or paroxysmal nocturnal dyspnea? Does he suffer from palpitations, fainting spells, or ankle edema? Patients with cardiac failure often complain of tiredness and weakness. Pertinent history includes questions about hypertension, previous myocardial infarction (MI), and rheumatic fever. Find out what cardiac medications the patient is taking. Record details about smoking and alcohol intake, both of which can cause serious cardiac disease.

Physical Examination

The physical will entail inspection, palpation auscultation, and electrocardiography.

Observe the patient for cyanosis. Look at the neck veins. Jugular venous distention may be an indication of cardiac dysfunction.

Palpate the apical beat and determine its exact location. In normal adults it is in the fifth left intercostal space $3^1/_2$ inches from the midline. Determine blood pressure and pulse rate.

Listen for heart sounds. The first heart sound is best heard at the apex, and the second at the base in the aortic area. Also listen for additional sounds. An S_3 gallop indicates left ventricular dysfunction, and an S_4 may be indicative of an atrial abnormality. Mitral murmurs are best heard at the apex, and aortic at the base. If murmurs are present, where are they best heard and do they radiate? Listen for carotid bruits.

A cardiac examination is incomplete unless the ECG is evaluated. Routine ECGs are usually required in patients with a history of cardiac disease or in patients who are 50 years of age or older.

Structured Approach

In 1991 Davies designed a systematic approach to airway evaluation using the acronym MOUTHS (Table 5.3). It is a quite useful approach and may encourage clinicians to pay more attention to this component of patient evaluation.

Bag/Valve/Mask Ventilation

In the process of evaluating the airway, we focus perhaps too much on anticipating difficult intubation and not enough on anticipating difficult mask ventilation. When confronted with difficult intubation, we rely heavily on our ability to perform effective mask ventilation. We must always keep this issue in mind when evaluating the airway. Bag/valve/mask ventilation can be difficult under certain circumstances—for instance, in bearded individuals, the edentulous, and very obese. However, not only may finding a suitable mask fit be difficult but, more important, the force required to ventilate the lungs may necessitate using two

TABLE 5.3. MOUTHS

Components	Descriptors	Assessment activities
Mandible	Length and subluxation	Measure hyomental distance and anterior displacement of mandible
Opening	Base, symmetry, range	Assess and measure mouth opening in centimeters
Uvula	Visibility	Assess pharyngeal structures and classify
Teeth	Dentition	Assess for presence of loose teeth and dental appliances
Head	Flexion, extension, rotation of head/neck and cervical spine	Assess all ranges of movement
Silhouette	Upper body abnormalities, both anterior and posterior	Identify potential impact on control of airway of large breasts, buffalo hump, kyphosis, etc.

Source: Modified from Davies, 1991,[19] with permission.

TABLE 5.4. Difficult mask ventilation

Variable	Odds ratio (95% C I)	P value
Beard	3.18 (1.39–7.27)	0.006
BMI >26	2.75 (1.64–4.62)	<0.001
Edentulous	2.28 (1.26–4.10)	0.006
Age >55 years	2.26 (1.34–3.81)	0.002
History of snoring	1.84 (1.09–3.10)	0.002

hands and will require an assistant. The mouth and nose may be distorted following trauma, preventing maintenance of an adequate seal. Bag/valve/mask ventilation may be impossible when penetrating objects are lodged in the vicinity of the mouth and nose. Patients with mandibular deformities are sometimes more difficult to manage using bag/valve/mask ventilation. Similarly, patients with serious flexion deformities of the cervical spine may not only be impossible to intubate but also difficult to ventilate using bag/valve/mask ventilation. Tracheostomy may also be very difficult under these circumstances.

Langeron et al[15] recently published a study on the topic of difficult mask ventilation (DMV). They studied 1,502 patients and reported a 5% incidence of difficult mask ventilation. Using a univariate analysis, risk factors for DMV included: increased body mass index (BMI), age, macroglossia, the presence of a beard, the edentulous state, a history of snoring, increased Mallampati grade, and a short thyromental distance. They identified 5 independent factors for DMV in a multivariate analysis (Table 5.4). The presence of two of these criteria was an accurate predictor of DMV (sensitivity and specificity greater than 70%). The authors also showed that DMV was the harbinger of difficult intubation in 30% of cases.

The introduction of the laryngeal mask airway (LMA) has lessened our anxiety about DMV. In a "cannot intubate, cannot ventilate" situation, you should not hesitate to insert an LMA.

Additional Information

Arterial Blood Gases

The decision to perform endotracheal intubation often depends upon arterial blood gas results, and so this information is usually readily available. Arterial blood gas specimens are not required in healthy patients undergoing intubation for elective surgery. However, if these data are available, record them and use them to assess the success or failure of your subsequent intervention.

ENT Consultation

An ENT consultation is warranted if you suspect pathology in the vicinity of the airway. Indirect laryngoscopy, which is usually performed by an ENT surgeon, involves examination of the larynx by observing its reflection via a laryngeal mirror or fiberoptic laryngoscope. Thus, the airway can be visualized and the nature and extent of any disease assessed before the patient is anesthetized for direct laryngoscopy and intubation. Yamamoto et al[38] evaluated indirect laryngoscopy as a predictor of difficult intubation in more than 6,000 patients. This test had a specificity of 98.4%, a sensitivity of 69.2%, and a positive predictive value of 31%. The test could not be performed in 15% of patients because of an excessively active gag reflex.

Radiologic Studies

Most patients presenting for emergency intubation will probably have had a recent chest X-ray examination. The chest X ray is worth reviewing because in addition to being a useful screening test, it can reveal pathology not evident clinically—pathology that could later be attributed to your intervention. AP and lateral neck films should always be obtained whenever there is encroachment on the airway, regardless of the etiology. Norton et al[37] recommend dynamic fluoroscopy primarily to assess soft tissue position and motion. If these initial radiologic studies yield insufficient information, it is worthwhile to request a radiology consultation for recommendations on which additional studies to perform. Appropriate selection is important, since unnecessary studies are time-consuming and costly, and needlessly expose patients to radiation. Recent technological advances in radiology (e.g., computed tomography [CT] and magnetic resonance imaging [MRI]) have greatly improved our ability to diagnose complex airway disorders.

The "Awake Look"

The "awake look" is a procedure used when airway difficulties are anticipated but have not been definitively diagnosed. After the patient has been sedated and topical anesthesia applied to the supraglottic structures, direct laryngoscopy is attempted. If the epiglottis can be readily elevated and vocal cords can be easily seen, there is no reason to perform an awake intubation. Generally, intubation under anesthesia, with the aid of muscle relaxants, is a far more pleasant experience for the patient than awake intubation. Although the "awake look" may also be an unpleasant experience, it in no way compares with a poorly performed awake intubation. It should always be considered before attempting intubation in a patient with suspected airway difficulty if the problem has not been well defined. The "awake look" has never been validated as a useful test to predict difficult intubation.

Flow-Volume Loops

A flow-volume loop is a pulmonary function study in which the forced expiratory volume (FEV) and forced inspiratory volume (FIV) are recorded in succession on a spirogram. Flow is plotted on the vertical axis, and volume on the horizontal. Flow-volume loops help distinguish between small and large airway obstructions. They also may help pinpoint the site of large airway obstruction and whether the obstruction is fixed or variable and whether the obstruction is intrathoracic or extrathoracic. A series of flow-volume loops is depicted in Figure 5.14.

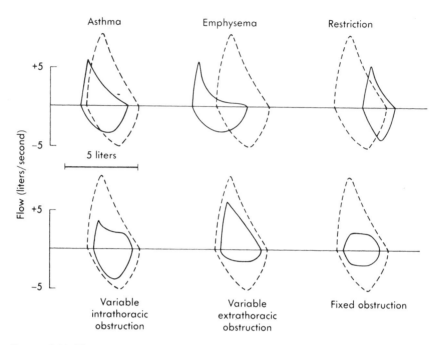

FIGURE 5.14. Flow-volume loops depicting obstruction of the airways. The upper series shows small airways, the lower series large airways. Dashed curves are normal. (From Ruppel G. *Manual of Pulmonary Function Testing.* 6th ed. St Louis: Mosby; 1994:56, with permission.)

Difficult Airway Clinic

In 1987 Norton et al[37] established a "difficult airway" clinic at the University of Michigan. Patients with potential airway difficulties are referred to the clinic by anesthesiologists and surgeons. In this setting, a formal evaluation of the airway is carried out and a plan of action is formulated.

Summary

It is important to conduct a thorough evaluation of the airway before intubation—bearing in mind, of course, that this will not always be possible under emergency circumstances. Whereas a thorough airway evaluation may not allow you to predict the ease or difficulty with which intubation can be performed in every case, it will in about 98% of cases. An unanticipated difficult intubation is a medical emergency that, if not dealt with quickly and appropriately, can lead to serious morbidity or even death. Therefore, every effort must be made, in advance, to detect an airway problem, and the best way this can be done is to conduct a thorough airway evaluation.

References

1. Bellhouse CP, Doré C. Criteria for estimating likelihood of difficulty of endotracheal intubation with Macintosh laryngoscope. *Anaesth Intensive Care.* 1988;16:329–337.
2. Tiret L, et al. Complications associated with anaesthesia—a prospective survey in France. *Can J Anaesth.* 1986;33:336–344.
3. Caplan RA, et al. Adverse respiratory events in anesthesia: a closed claims analysis. *Anesthesiology.* 1990;72:828–833.
4. Rose DK, Cohen MM. The airway: problems and predictions in 18,500 patients. *Can J Anaesth.* 1994;41:5,372–383.
5. El-Ganzouri AR, McCarthy RJ, Tuman KJ, et al. Preoperative airway assessment: predictive value of a multivariate risk index. *Anesth Analg.* 1996;82:1197–1204.
6. Reissell E, et al. Predictability of difficult laryngoscopy in patients with long term diabetes mellitus. *Anaesthesia.* 1990;45:1024–1027.
7. Salazarulo HH, Taylor LA. Diabetic Stiff Joint Syndrome as a cause of difficult endotracheal intubation. *Anesthesiology.* 1986;64:366–368.
8. Nadal JLY, Fernandez BG, Escobar IC, et al. The palm print as a sensitive predictor of difficult laryngoscopy. *Acta Anaesthesiol Scand.* 1998;42:199–203.
9. The Canadian Anaesthetists' Society Inc. Guidelines for the basic standards of practice of anaesthesia. 1981:6.
10. Schmitt H, Buchfelder M, Radespiel-Troger, et al. Difficult intubation in acromegalic patients. *Anesthesiology.* 2000;93:110–114.
11. Aiello G, Metcalf I. Anaesthetic implications of TMJ disease. *Can J Anaesth.* 1992; 39:610–616.
12. Block C, Brechner VL. Unusual problems in airway management: the influence of the temporomandibular joint, the mandible and associated structures and endotracheal intubation. *Anesth Analg.* 1971;50:114.
13. Posselt U. *Physiology of Occlusion and Rehabilitation.* 2nd ed. Oxford: Blackwell; 1968.
14. Calder I, Calder J, Crockard HA. Difficult direct laryngoscopy in patients with cervical spine disease. *Anaesthesia.* 1995;50:756–763.
15. Langeron O, Masso E, Huraux C, et al. Prediction of difficult mask ventilation. *Anesthesiology.* 2000;92:1229–1236.
16. Finucane BT. Difficult intubation associated with the foetal alcohol syndrome. *Can Anaesth Soc J.* 1980;27:6,574–575.
17. St. Paul Fire and Marine Insurance Co. Physician and Surgeon Professional Liability Countrywide Summary Report by Allegation. 1978.
18. Burton JF, Baker AB. Dental damage during anaesthesia and surgery. *Anaesth Intensive Care.* 1987;15:262–268.
19. Davies J. MOUTHS. *Can J Anaesth.* 1991;38:687–688.
20. Mallampati SR. Clinical signs to predict difficult tracheal intubation [hypothesis]. *Can Anaesth Soc J.* 1983;30:316–317.
21. Mallampati SR, et al. A clinical sign to predict difficult tracheal intubation: a prospective study. *Can Anaesth Soc J.* 1985;82:429.
22. Samsoon GLT, Young JRB. Difficult tracheal intubation: a retrospective study. *Anaesthesia.* 1987;42:487–490.
23. Cohen SM, et al. Oral exam to predict difficult intubation: a large prospective study. *Anesthesiology.* 1989;71:A937.
24. Cormack RS, Lehane J. Difficult tracheal intubation in obstetrics. *Anaesthesia.* 1984;39:1105–1111.

25. Pilkington S, Carli F, Dakin MJ, et al. Increase in Mallamapati score during pregnancy. *Br J Anaesth.* 1995;74:638–642.
26. Jones DH, Cohle SD. Unanticipated difficult airway secondary to lingual tonsillar hyperplasia. *Anesth Analg.* 1993;77:1285–1288.
27. Buckland RW, Pedley J. Lingual thyroid—a threat to the airway. *Anesthesia.* 2000; 55:1103–1105.
28. Rosenberg AD, Young M, Bernstein RL, et al. Tongue rings: just say no. *Anesthesiology.* 1998;89:1279.
29. Brown DC. Anesthetic considerations of a patient with a tongue piercing and a safe solution. *Anesthesiology.* 2000;93:307.
30. Bannister FB, MacBeth RG. Direct laryngoscopy and tracheal intubation. *Lancet.* 1944;1:651.
31. Patil V, et al. *Fiberoptic Endoscopy in Anesthesia.* 1st ed. Chicago: Year Book; 1983.
32. Ramadhani SAL, Mohamed LA, Rocke DA, et al. Sternomental distances a sole predictor of difficult laryngoscopy in obstetric anesthesia. *Br J Anaesth.* 1996;77:312–316.
33. Walls RD, et al. Difficult intubation associated with calcified stylohyoid ligament. *Anaesth Intens Care.* 1990;18:110–126.
34. Sherwood-Smith GH. Difficulty in intubation: calcified stylohyoid ligament. *Anaesthesia.* 1976;31:508–510.
35. Akinyemi OO, Elegbe EO. Difficult laryngoscopy and tracheal intubation due to calcified stylohyoid ligaments. *Can Anaesth Soc J.* 1981;28:80–81.
36. Keenan MA, Stiles CM, Kaulman RL. Acquired laryngeal deviation associated with cervical spine disease in erosive polyarticular arthritis. *Anesthesiology.* 1983;58:441.
37. Norton ML, Wilton N, Brown ACD. The difficult airway. *Anesthesiology Review.* 1988;15:25–28.
38. Yamamoto K, Tsubokawa T, Shibita K, et al. Predicting difficult intubation with indirect laryngoscopy. *Anesthesiology.* 1997;86:316–321.
39. Steward DJ. *Manual of Pediatric Anesthesia.* New York: Churchill-Livingstone; 1985: 289–343.

Suggested Readings

Bainton, Cedric R. Difficult intubation—what's the best test? *Can J Anaesth.* 1996;43: 541–543.
Charters P. Analysis of mathematical model for osseous factors in difficult intubation—report of investigation. *Can J Anesth.* 1994;41:594–602.
Jacobson J, et al. Preoperative evaluation conditions in patients scheduled for elective surgery. *Acta Anaesthesiol Scand.* 1996;40:421–424.
Jimson C, Tse, et al. Predicting difficult endotracheal intubation in surgical patients scheduled for general anesthesia: a prospective blind study. *Anesth Analg.* 1995;81:254–258.
Kanaya N, et al. The utility of three-dimensional computed tomography in unanticipated difficult endotracheal intubation. *Anesth Analg.* 2000;91:752–754.
Karkouti K, et al. Predicting difficult intubation: a multivariable analysis. *Can J Anesth.* 2000;47:730–739.
Naguib M, et al. Predictive models for difficult laryngoscopy and intubation: a clinical, radiologic and three-dimensional computer imaging study. *Can J Anesth.* 1999;46:748–759.
Nath G, Sekar M. Predicting difficult intubation—a comprehensive scoring system. *Anaesthesia and Intensive Care.* 1997;25:482–486.
Sawwa D. Prediction of difficult tracheal intubation. *Br J Anesth.* 1994;73:149–153.

Appendix

Syndrome	Description	Airway Implications
Anderson syndrome	Severe midfacial hypoplasia, relative mandibular prognathism, abnormal structure and angle of mandible (triangular facies), kyphoscoliosis	Possible airway problems; intubation may be difficult; assess respiratory status
Angioedema (angioneurotic edema), hereditary	Episodic edema of extremities, face, trunk, airway, and abdominal viscera, usually for 24 to 72 hr (4 hr to 1 wk; onset in childhood differentiates this from idiopathic form; etiology: abnormal levels of C1 and C4 esterase inhibitor, leading to accumulation of vasoactive substances, then to increased vascular permeability, and then to edema; usually painless but may be accompanied by prodromal focal tingling or "tightness"; often induced by trauma or vibration; may also be accompanied by bouts of abdominal pain, diarrhea; hemoconcentration leading to hypotension, shock, pharyngeal edema (usually develops slowly); most deaths from laryngeal edema; mortality rate up to 33%; long-term treatment is with antifibrinolytic and hormonal agents; may be adverse side effects of long-term epsilon-aminocaproic acid therapy	Check results of complement assay, hematocrit, fluid status, treatment history, previous drug reactions; observe for voice change or dysphasia; prophylaxis (especially for dental or oropharyngeal manipulation): epsilon-aminocaproic acid for 2 to 3 days and/or fresh frozen plasma for 1 day preoperatively; continue epsilon-aminocaproic acid IV pre- and postoperatively; danazol (androgen) may be useful; acute attack: give epinephrine, steroids, antihistamine, possibly fresh frozen plasma; if pharyngeal edema is imminent or develops: endotracheal or nasotracheal intubation (leave in place for 24 to 72 hr); if this is not possible perform tracheostomy; anesthesia: regional when possible; otherwise, extreme care when instrumenting airway
Apert syndrome (acrocephalo-syndactyly)	Hypoplastic maxilla and exophthalmos; craniosynostosis, possibly with increased intracranial pressure; mental retardation and syndactyly; congenital heart disease may be present	If congenital heart disease present: antibiotic prophylaxis preoperatively; intubation may be difficult
Arthrogryposis multiplex	Multiple congenital contractures; congenital heart disease in about 10% of cases	If congenital heart disease present: antibiotic prophylaxis preoperatively; minimal thiopental required—muscles replaced by fat; possible airway problem from limitation of mandibular movement

(continued)

Appendix (*Continued*)

Syndrome	Description	Airway Implications
Beckwith syndrome (Beckwith-Wiedemann syndrome, "infantile gigantism")	Birth weight > 4,000 g; macroglossia, exophthalmos, visceromegaly, umbilical hernia	Airway problems caused by large tongue; monitor blood glucose carefully and and treat hypoglycemia
Behçet syndrome	Gross ulceration of mouth (usually first sign, may extend to esophagus) and genital area; uveitis, iritis, conjunctivitis, skin lesions, nonerosive arthritis; may also be vasculitis, myocardial, and CNS involvement; risk of sepsis at sites of skin puncture, etc.	Use sterile technique; may have history of steroid therapy; nutritional status often poor; intubation may be difficult because of scarring in pharynx
Binder syndrome	Maxillonasal dysplasia; if severe, may be corrected surgically	Advancement of maxilla with with wiring of maxilla and and mandible may cause airway problems pre- and postoperatively
Carpenter syndrome (acrocephalo-polysyndactyly)	Mental retardation, oxycephaly, peculiar facies, syndactyly, deformed extremities, congenital heart disease, hypogenitalism	If congenital heart disease present: antibiotic prophylaxis preoperatively; hypoplastic mandible may may make intubation difficult; problems associated with heart disease
Cherubism	Fibrous dysplasia of mandible	Intubation may be extremely difficult
Chotzen syndrome	Craniosynostosis, associated renal anomalies	Intubation may be difficult, renal excretion of drugs impaired
Christ-Siemens-Touraine syndrome (anhidrotic ecto-dermal dysplasia)	Absence of sweating and tearing, heat intolerance due to inability to control temperature by sweating, poor mucus formation leading to persistent respiratory infections	Hypoplastic mandible may make intubation difficult; monitor body temperature carefully and be prepared to institute cooling; tape eyes closed; chest physiotherapy pre- and postoperatively
Chubby puffer syndrome	Obesity, upper airway obstruction, daytime somnolence, respiratory distress when sleeping; patient may be hyperactive and aggressive; blood gases may show hypoxemia and hypercapnia; cor pulmonale may develop	Patient may present for tonsillectomy; avoid pre-operative sedation; monitor carefully postoperatively for airway obstruction; avoid narcotic analgesics; patient with severe obstruction may require tracheostomy

Appendix (*Continued*)

Syndrome	Description	Airway Implications
Collagen disease: dermatomyositis, polyarteritis nodosa, rheumatoid arthritis, systemic lupus erythematosus	Systemic connective tissue diseases with variable systemic involvement: osteoporosis, fatty infiltration of muscle, anemia, pulmonary infiltration or fibrosis	TMJ or cricoarytenoid arthritis may create airway and intubation difficulties; risk of fat embolism after osteotomy, fracture, or minor trauma; supplemental steroid therapy
Cretinism (congenital hypothyroidism)	Goiter, hypothyroidism secondary to defective synthesis of thyroxine, large tongue	Correct hypothyroidism and anemia preoperatively if possible; airway problems due to large tongue
Cri-du-chat syndrome	Mental retardation, abnormal (cat-like) cry, microcephaly, round face, hypertelorism; in some, ears abnormal, micrognathia, epiglottis and larynx small; congenital heart disease may be present	If congenital heart disease present: antibiotic prophylaxis preoperatively; airway problems; stridor, laryngomalacia; intubation may be difficult
Crouzon disease	Craniosynostosis, hypertelorism, parrot beak nose, hypoplastic maxilla	Intubation may be difficult
Down syndrome (mongolism, trisomy 21)	Mental retardation, small nasopharynx, hypotonia; high incidence of congenital heart disease; duodenal atresia in some	If congenital heart disease present: antibiotic prophylaxis preoperatively; do not use barbiturate premedication but give usual doses of atropine; airway problems: large tongue, small mouth; risk of laryngospasm, especially on extubation; problems of cardiac anomalies; patients tolerate extensive surgery quite well
Ellis-van Creveld syndrome (chondroectodermal mesoectodermal dysplasia)	Ectodermal defects and skeletal anomalies; 50% have congenital heart disease, usually septal defects; chest wall anomalies cause poor lung function; may have abnormal maxilla, cleft lip, cleft palate, hepatosplenomegaly; many die before 6 mo	If congenital heart disease present; antibiotic prophylaxis properatively; problems of associated heart disease: assess cardiorespiratory function carefully; airway problems: intubation may be difficult
Farber disease	Sphingomyelin deposition	Assess cardiorespiratory and renal function
Fetal alcohol syndrome	Abnormalities of infant from maternal heavy alcohol consumption: growth retardation, intellectual impairment, craniofacial abnormalities (microcephaly, microphthalmia, hypoplastic upper lip, flat maxilla), cardiac defects (especially ventricular septal defect), renal abnormalities, inguinal hernia	If congenital heart disease present: antibiotic prophylaxis preoperatively; difficult intubation; problems of associated cardiac disease

(*continued*)

Appendix (*Continued*)

Syndrome	Description	Airway Implications
Focal dermal hypoplasia (Goltz syndrome)	Multifarious features, including multiple papillomas of mucous membranes, skin	Airway may contain papillomas
Goldenhar syndrome (oculoauriculo-vertebral syndrome)	Unilateral hypoplasia with mandibular hypoplasia; congenital heart disease in 20%	If congenital heart disease present: antibiotic prophylaxis preoperatively; airway problems and intubation may be difficult; problems of associated cardiac disease
Gorlin-Chaudhry-Moss syndrome	Craniofacial dysostosis, patent ductus arteriosus, hypertrichosis, hypoplasia of labia majora, dental and eye anomalies, normal intelligence	If congenital heart disease present: antibiotic prophylaxis preoperatively; asymmetry of head—difficult airway; problems associated with patent ductus arteriosus
Gorlin-Goltz syndrome (basal cell nevus syndrome)	Multiple nevoid basal cell carci-nomas, hypertelorism, mandibular prognathism, multiple jaw cysts and fibrosarcomas, kyphoscoliosis, incomplete segmentation of cervical and thoracic vertebrae, congenital hydrocephalus, mental retardation, etc.	Extreme care in positioning and intubating—cervical movement may be limited; increased cranial pressure may be unrecognized
Hallervorden-Spatz disease	Autosomal recessive disorder of basal ganglia: dementia and dystonia with torticollis, scoliosis, and trismus	Assess pulmonary status carefully; induction of inhalational anesthesia leads to relaxation of abnormal posturing and trismus, and facilitates intubation; succinylcholine may induce hyperkalemic response
Herlitz syndrome (epidermolysis bullosa)	Skin cleavage at dermalepidermal junction, resulting in erosions and blisters from minor trauma to skin or mucous membrane; possibility of confusion with prophyria (similar skin lesions)	Antibiotic prophylaxis preoperatively; use sterile technique (reverse isolation); airway difficulty: oral lesions, adhesion of tongue; check for history of steroid therapy; avoid trauma to skin or mucous membranes; avoid instrumentation of airway if possible; use only well-padded mask for inhalational anesthesia or use Ketamine; **do not use** adhesive tape
Histiocytosis X (eosinophilic granuloma, Hand-Schuller-	Lesions in bones and viscera (larynx, lungs, liver, and spleen); clinical course similar to acute leukemia; hypersplenism,	Correct anemia and coagulation defects; assess cardio-respiratory status carefully (and, if indicated, fluid

Appendix (*Continued*)

Syndrome	Description	Airway Implications
Christian disease, Letterer-Siwe disease)	pancytopenia, anemia, purpura, hemorrhage; hepatic involvement; pulmonary (diffuse hilar infiltration); respiratory failure, cor pulmonale; gingival inflammation and necrosis, with loss of teeth; diabetes insipidus if sella turcica involved; many die in first year of life	balance); may have history of steroid therapy; laryngeal fibrosis may make intubation difficult
Hurler syndrome (mucopoly-saccharosis Type IH)	Mental retardation, gargoyle facies, deafness, stiff joints, dwarfism	Antibiotic prophylaxis
I-cell disease (mucolipidoses)	Mental retardation, Hurler-type bone changes, severe joint limitation, chronic pulmonary disease; valvular insufficiency common; death in early childhood (most by 1 yr)	Intubation and airway maintenance difficult; limited jaw movement, stiffness of neck and rib cage
Klippel-Feil syndrome	Congenital fusion of two or more cervical vertebrae, causing neck rigidity	Intubation may be very difficult; should be done awake if possible; otherwise inhalational induction without muscle relaxant; do not extubate until fully awake
Larsen syndrome	Multiple congenital dislocations, hydrocephalus, cleft palate, connective tissue defect (poor cartilage in rib cage, epiglottis, arytenoids), chronic respiratory problems	Intubation may be difficult, intracranial pressure increased
Leopard syndrome	Multiple large freckles, hypertelorism, eyelid ptosis, etc., congenital heart disease (pulmonary stenosis in 95%); ECG anomalies include aberrant conduction; growth retardation common; pectus carinatum, hyphosis, etc. in some; genitourinary anomalies (hypospadias)	If congenital heart disease present: antibiotic prophylaxis preoperatively; assess cardiac status, lung function; intubation may be difficult; problems of associated cardiac disease
Meckel syndrome (dysencephalia splanchnocystica)	Microcephaly, micrognathia, cleft epiglottis, congestive heart disease, renal dysplasia; most die in infancy	Antibiotic prophylaxis preoperatively; assess cardiac status; intubation may be difficult; care with drugs excreted by kidneys
Median cleft face syndrome	Various degrees of cleft face; lipomas and dermoids over frontal bone	Cleft nose, lip, and palate may cause intubation difficulties

(*continued*)

Appendix (*Continued*)

Syndrome	Description	Airway Implications
Moebius syndrome (congenital oculofacial paralysis)	Congenital paralysis of cranial nerves VI and VII, limb deformities, micrognathia; feeding difficulties and aspiration may cause chronic pulmonary problems	Assess respiratory status carefully; intubation may be difficult
Myositis ossificans (fibrodysplasia ossificans progressiva)	Bony infiltration of tendons, fascia, aponeuroses, and muscle; thoracic involvement greatly reduces thoracic compliance; progressive respiratory failure	Check respiratory function, history of steroid therapy; airway and intubation problems if neck rigid and mouth fixed
Myotonia dystrophica	Weakness and myotonia, eyelid ptosis, cataracts, frontal baldness, cardiac conduction defects and arrhythmias, impaired ventilation	Check respiratory function; do not use succinylcholine (which causes myotonia in 50%)
Noack syndrome	Craniosynostosis and digital anomalies, obesity	Intubation may be difficult because of skull deformity
Orofaciodigital syndrome	Cleft lip and palate, lobed tongue, hypoplastic mandible and maxilla, digital anomalies, hydrocephalus, polycystic kidneys	Airway problems and intubation may be difficult; possible renal impairment—do not use drugs excreted by kidneys
Osteogenesis imperfecta (fragilitas ossium)	I—Congenita: usually stillbirth or rapidly fatal; II—Tarda: pathological fractures, blue sclerae, deafness; osteoporosis causes kyphoscoliosis and lung pathology; fragility of vessels results in subcutaneous hemorrhage; dentinal deficiency leads to carious and fragile teeth	Use extreme care in positioning and intubating; teeth easily broken
Patau syndrome (trisomy 13)	Mental retardation, microcephaly, micrognathia, cleft lip or palate, congestive heart disease, (usually ventricular septal defect and/or dextrocardia); most die by 3 yr	If congestive heart disease present, antibiotic prophylaxis preoperatively; intubation may be difficult; problems associated with heart disease
Pierre Robin syndrome	Cleft palate, micrognathia, glossoptosis, congestive heart disease in some; neonates have respiratory obstruction that can lead to cor pulmonale; maintain airway by nursing prone on a frame; may require tongue suture, intubation, or tracheostomy	If congestive heart disease present: antibiotic preoperatively; intubation may be very difficult; use awake technique; patient should be fully awake before extubation
Pompe disease (glycogen storage disease Type II)	Deposits of glycogen in muscles, severe hypotonicity, large tongue, massive cardiomegaly; death from cardiorespiratory failure before 2 yr of age	**Extreme care:** do not use respiratory or cardiac depressant or muscle relaxants; large tongue may cause airway problem

Appendix (*Continued*)

Syndrome	Description	Airway Implications
Pyle disease (metaphyseal dysplasia)	Craniofacial abnormalities, enlarged mandible, cranial nerve paralyses	Assess airway carefully
Rieger syndrome	Hypodontia, malformations of anterior chamber of eye, myotonic dystrophy; may be other developmental abnormalities, including maxillary hypoplasia	Anesthetic requirements dictated by muscle disease; *see also* Myotonia dystriphica; congenital
Silver-Russel dwarfism	Short stature, skeletal asymmetry, micrognathia, low birth weight; may also have anomalous sexual development	Intubation may be difficult
Sleep apnea syndromes (*see also* Chubby puffer syndrome)	Disorders of breathing during sleep, including: I. Central sleep apnea, due to CNS immaturity (? sudden infant death syndrome), trauma, infections or neoplasms, and primary central alveolar hypoventilation (Ondine's curse); apnea occurs without evidence of respiratory muscle activity II. Obstructive sleep apnea due to obesity, adenoid hypertrophy, Pierre Robin syndrome, or any other condition causing chronic airway obstruction; apnea occurs because of obstruction and is accompanied by increased respiratory muscle activity III. Mixed forms; medical history may include daytime somnolence, loud snoring, restless sleep, insomnia, fatigue; children may be hyperactive and aggressive	Assess airway carefully; avoid preoperative sedation; intubate and ventilate during anesthesia; beware of acute obstruction during induction of anesthesia; intubation may be difficult; avoid narcotic analgesics during and after anesthesia; awaken patient completely during transfer to postoperative recovery; monitor closely for apnea postoperatively
Smith-Lemil-Opitz syndrome	Microcephaly, mental retardation, genital and skeletal anomalies (including micrognathia), thymic hypoplasia, hypotonia; may have increased susceptibility to infection	Use sterile technique; airway and intubation problems; care with muscle relaxants; assisted or controlled ventilation may be necessary pre- and postoperatively
Soto syndrome (cerebral gigantism)	Acromegalic features, dilated cerebral ventricles but normal intracranial pressure; nonprogressive	Possible airway problems due due to acromegalic skull; no other problems reported
Stevens-Johnson syndrome (erythema multiforme)	Urticarial lesions and erosions of mouth, eyes, genitalia; possible hypersensitivity to exogenous agents (drugs, infections, etc.); if pleural blebs, pneumothorax	Antibiotic prophylaxis preoperatively; check cardiac and fluid status and pulmonary function; use sterile technique (reverse

(*continued*)

Appendix (*Continued*)

Syndrome	Description	Airway Implications
	may occur; dehydration and malnutrition common; may include myocarditis/pericarditis	isolation); oral lesions: avoid intubation and insertion of esophageal stethoscope; **monitoring is difficult** (because of skin lesions) **but essential;** danger of ventricular fibrillation; temperature control: febrile episodes; IV infusion essential but do not use cut-down (possibility of infection); Ketamine is probably best anesthetic agent
Tangier disease (an alpha lipoproteinemia)	Low plasma cholesterol, large orange tonsils, anemia and thrombocytopenia because of hypersplenism, peripheral neuropathy and abnormal electromyogram, premature coronary disease	Check hemoglobin and platelet count preoperatively; do not use muscle relaxants; be alert for premature ischemic heart disease
Treacher Collins syndrome (mandibulofacial dysostosis)	Micrognathia, aplastic zygomatic arches, microstomia, choanal atresia; congenital heart disease may be present	If congenital heart disease present: antibiotic prophylaxis preoperatively; possible airway and intubation difficulties (less severe than with Pierre Robin deformity)
Turner syndrome (gonadal dysgenesis)	XO females; short stature, infantile genitalia, webbed neck, possible micrognathia, coarctation, dissecting aneurysm of aorta or pulmonary stenosis; renal anomalies in more than 50%	If congenital heart disease present: antibiotic prophylaxis preoperatively; intubation may be difficult; assess cardiovascular status; care with drugs excreted by kidneys
Urbach-Wiethe disease (cutaneous mucosal hyalinosis)	Hoarseness or aphonia (hyaline deposits in larynx and pharynx), skin eruptions	Establishing and maintaining airway may be difficult
Velocardiofacial syndrome	Speech difficulties because of velopharyngeal anomalies, learning disability (mild), congenital heart disease (especially ventricular septal defect), and characteristic facies: large nose with broad nasal bridge, vertically long face, narrow palpebral fissures, retruded mandible	May present for pharyngoplasty, considerations of congenital heart disease; obstructive sleep apnea may occur after pharyngoplasty and can cause death

Appendix (*Continued*)

Syndrome	Description	Airway Implications
Welander muscular atrophy (late distal hereditary myopathy)	Initially involves distal muscles; prognosis: for life good, for ambulation poor; *see also* Werdnig-Hoffman disease	May require spinal fusion; use extreme care with thiopental and muscle relaxants; do not use respiratory depressant drugs
Werdnig-Hoffman disease (infantile muscular atrophy)	Earlier onset and more severe than Welander muscular atrophy; feeding difficulties, aspiration of stomach contents, chronic respiratory problems; most die before puberty	Minimal anesthesia required; do not use muscle relaxants or respiratory depressant drugs; ventilatory support may be needed and weaning from this can be difficult

Source: Modified from Steward DJ, 1985.[39]

6

Indications and Preparation of the Patient for Intubation

NEUROMUSCULAR BLOCKING DRUGS
  Depolarizing drug—succinylcholine
  Nondepolarizing drugs
  Methods of administering a neuromuscular blocking drug
  Reversal of neuromuscular blockade
SUMMARY

Endotracheal intubation has been an established technique in anesthesia for more than 50 years. It was first performed in 1880 by MacEwan[1] in Glasgow, who blindly introduced a metal tube into the trachea using the oral route. Over the years, as the technique and equipment became more refined, endotracheal intubation evolved into a routine procedure for adults and children undergoing general anesthesia, resuscitation, and respiratory care. Nevertheless, the decision to intubate should not be made lightly. You must always weigh the risks of the procedure against those of nonintervention. If intubation is necessary, select the most appropriate route as well as the type of sedation and anesthesia required.

General Indications for Intubation

As a technique, endotracheal intubation is one of the most common lifesaving procedures performed today. However, the decision whether to intubate or not is not always clear-cut and ethical issues surrounding the initiation of advanced life support are being raised more frequently. The indications for intubation are outlined in Box 6.1 and will be discussed in detail in this chapter.

Ventilatory Support

Respiratory failure requiring mechanical ventilation and/or oxygen therapy is a common indication for endotracheal intubation. The tube provides a conduit through which you can apply various modalities of ventilatory support—intermittent mandatory ventilation (IMV), control mode ventilation (CMV), and in certain cases, high frequency ventilation (HFV). Furthermore, you can institute various end-expiratory

---

Box 6.1. Indications for Intubation

Ventilatory support (assisted or mechanical)
Protection of the airway
Ensuring airway patency
Anesthesia and surgery
Suctioning

Box 6.2. Objectives in Ventilatory Support

1. Make the correct etiological diagnosis
2. Institute therapy to treat pathology
   a. Pneumonia: antibiotics
   b. Cardiogenic pulmonary edema: cardiac support and diuretics
   c. Status asthmaticus: bronchodilators
3. Oxygenation goals
   a. Wean $FiO_2 \leq 50\%$
   b. Oxyhemoglobin saturation $\geq 90\%$
   c. $PaO_2 \geq 60$ mm Hg
   d. Pulmonary shunt fraction $\leq 18\%$
4. Ventilation goals
   a. Adjust the minute ventilation to achieve pH homeostasis (provided there is no profound metabolic acidosis) $7.35 \leq pH \leq 7.45$
5. Be prepared to react to complications and problems

---

maneuvers (e.g., positive end-expiratory pressure [PEEP] or continuous positive airway pressure [CPAP]) to enhance oxygenation, increase the functional residual capacity (FRC), improve lung compliance, and decrease the work of breathing in selected patients. (See Chapter 11 for further details on ventilatory support.)

Once you have determined the etiology of the pulmonary pathology, you can determine whether ventilatory support should be directed toward treating primarily an oxygenation problem, a ventilation problem, or both (as commonly occurs). When treating ventilated patients, it helps to direct your efforts toward specific goals (Box 6.2). The remainder of this section discusses the various conditions that necessitate ventilatory support, most of which fall under the heading hypoxia.

Hypoxia

Hypoxia, as an inadequate supply of oxygen to meet physiologic demands of the tissues,[2] can be arbitrarily subdivided into six categories (Box 6.3). The most common cause, requiring ventilatory support or oxygen supplementation, is **hypoxic hypoxia;** thus, in this chapter, considerable emphasis will be placed on this category. The term *hypoxic hypoxia* is synonymous with **hypoxemia.**

Hypoxemia

Hypoxemia is defined as a reduced partial pressure of oxygen in arterial blood (P_aO_2). The normal P_aO_2 varies with age and can be estimated using the following formula:

$$P_aO_2 \text{ (mm Hg)} = 102 - 0.33 \text{ Age (in years)}$$

Box 6.3. Classification of Hypoxia

1. Hypoxic
   $\downarrow PaO_2$, hypoxemia
2. Anemic
   $\downarrow O_2$ carrying capacity, anemia
3. Histotoxic
   Impaired O_2 utilization (e.g., cyanide poisoning)
4. Stagnant
   Inadequate tissue perfusion (e.g., shock, cardiac failure, pulmonary embolus)
5. Hypermetabolic
   $\uparrow O_2$ demand (e.g., shock, cardiac failure, pulmonary embolus)
6. Interference with O_2 transport mechanisms (e.g., carbon monoxide poisoning, methemoglobin, hemoglobinopathies)

Hypoxemia per se is not an indication for intubation and ventilation. Supplemental oxygen can be administered to patients via a face mask or nasal prongs. However, intubation should be considered if:

1. The patient cannot maintain an oxyhemoglobin saturation of at least 90% or a P_aO_2 of at least 60 mm Hg on a concentration of inspired oxygen less than 50%.
2. The disease causing the hypoxemia is expected to persist and signs of exhaustion are observed.

During this observation period you need to assess the patient carefully for signs of further deterioration and be ready to intubate immediately if necessary.

The ensuing discussion covers the five general causes of hypoxemia (Box 6.4): decreased inspired oxygen concentration, hypoventilation, ventilation/perfusion inequality, decreased diffusion capacity, and anatomical shunt.

Box 6.4. Common Causes of Hypoxemia

1. Decreased inspired oxygen concentration
2. Hypoventilation
3. Decreased diffusion capacity
4. Ventilation/perfusion inequality
5. True or anatomical shunt

Decreased Oxygen Content of Inspired Air

Atmospheric pressure at sea level is about 760 mm Hg. Thus, the partial pressure of inspired oxygen at sea level is about 150 mm Hg:

$$P_IO_2 = (P_b - P_{H_2O}) \times F_IO_2$$
$$= (760 - 47) \times 0.21$$
$$= 149.72 \text{ mm Hg}$$

where P_IO_2 is the partial pressure of inspired oxygen, P_b the barometric pressure (760 mm Hg at sea level), P_{H_2O} the water vapor pressure (47 mm Hg at 37°C) and

$$F_IO_2 \text{ the concentration of inspired oxygen in room air (0.21).}$$

On ascending to high altitudes, the partial pressure of oxygen in inspired air decreases; at 30,000 feet, for example, it is only about 40 mm Hg. Low oxygen content may occur during the administration of anesthesia (e.g., selection of hypoxic gas mixtures, plumbing accidents involving oxygen delivery systems, or faulty equipment). Oxygen analyzers are a valuable means of detecting the delivery of hypoxic gas mixtures to patients.

Hypoventilation

Respiration is rigorously regulated by a complex feedback system in the CNS. The rhythmic movements of the diaphragm and other respiratory muscles are controlled by impulses originating in the brain stem that reach the motor units peripherally through the phrenic, vagus, and intercostal nerves. Central chemoreceptors in the medulla are exquisitely sensitive to even small changes in carbon dioxide tension in the arterial blood. Likewise, peripheral chemoreceptors (in the carotid and aortic bodies) are very sensitive to falling oxygen tensions, especially when the P_aO_2 falls below 60 mm Hg. Numerous disease processes and medications may interfere with normal respiratory function, leading to respiratory pump failure or hypoventilation.

Hypoventilation occurs when the movement of air in and out of the lungs in a given period is insufficient to meet the oxygen demands and carbon dioxide excretory requirements of the organism. Its causes are legion, but they may be broadly divided into two main categories: central and peripheral.

The hallmark of hypoventilation is an elevation in the alveolar carbon dioxide tension (P_ACO_2). The relationship between P_ACO_2 and alveolar ventilation is best expressed by the alveolar ventilation equation[3]:

$$\dot{V}_A = \dot{V}_{CO_2}/P_ACO_2 \times K$$

Therefore:

$$P_ACO_2 = \dot{V}_{CO_2}/\dot{V}_A \times K$$

where $\dot{V}_A$ is alveolar ventilation (liters/min), $\dot{V}_{CO_2}$ is CO_2 production (L/min), P_ACO_2 is alveolar CO_2 tension (mm Hg) (note that this is nearly identical to the arterial CO_2 tension [P_aCO_2] in normal subjects, and K is 0.863 (conversion factor relating $\dot{V}_A$ at BTPS and V_{CO_2} STPD and correcting for alveolar P_{H2O}). $\dot{V}_A$ and $\dot{V}_{CO_2}$ are the only determinants of P_ACO_2, and ultimately of P_aCO_2.

If an individual hypoventilates while breathing room air, the space occupied by carbon dioxide in the alveoli expands, to the detriment of the space available for the other respiratory gases (including oxygen). This is a simple way of explaining why hypoxemia occurs when patients hypoventilate. This phenomenon may be clarified by studying the clinically useful alveolar air equation:

$$P_AO_2 = F_IO_2 (P_B - P_{H2O}) - P_ACO_2/R$$

where P_AO_2 is the alveolar oxygen tension (mm Hg), F_IO_2 the concentration of inspired oxygen, P_ACO_2 the alveolar carbon dioxide tension (mm Hg), and R the respiration quotient (usually assumed to be 0.8). For example, if F_IO_2 is 0.2, P_b 760 mm Hg, P_{H2O} 47 mm Hg, P_ACO_2 40, and R 0.8, then the $P_AO_2 = 100$.

Hypoventilation is a common cause of hypoxemia usually seen in patients with chronic obstructive lung disease and in persons who have received excessive doses of narcotics and other respiratory-depressant drugs. In addition to causing hypoxemia, it can seriously interfere with acid/base balance. Hypoventilation caused by respiratory depressant drugs may require only supplemental oxygen therapy. However, hypoventilation caused by respiratory pump failure (e.g., Guillain-Barre syndrome) may require urgent and prolonged mechanical ventilatory support.

Decreased Diffusion Capacity

There are two major causes of decreased diffusion capacity: **loss of lung tissue** following surgery or disease that decreases the surface area available for gas exchange, and **failure of equilibrium** between the alveolar oxygen tension (P_AO_2) and the alveolar carbon dioxide tension (P_ACO_2). Diffusion impairment also occurs if equilibrium is not reached between the alveolar oxygen tension (P_AO_2) and the arterial oxygen tension (P_aO_2). Diseases that cause a change in the thickness of the respiratory membrane fall into this category. Hypoxemia may not manifest itself unless the patient is exercised. Hypoxemia caused by diffusion impairment may be corrected by administering a high F_IO_2 to the patient.

Ventilation/Perfusion Inequality

Ventilation/perfusion inequality occurs when the normal relationships of ventilation and perfusion in the lung are mismatched as a result of various disease processes. A simple description of ventilation/perfusion ratios in Riley's in a three-compartment model of the lung consists of three zones:

1. Ventilated but unperfused alveoli (dead space)
2. Perfused but unventilated alveoli (shunt or venous admixture)
3. Ideally ventilated and perfused alveoli

The institution of an end-expiratory maneuver (e.g., PEEP or CPAP) may improve oxygenation in patients with diseases that cause venous admixture: atelectasis, acute respiratory distress syndrome (ARDS), and pneumonia.

True or Anatomic Shunt

A shunt is produced when blood passes through an unventilated portion of the lung or bypasses the lung altogether. A physiologic shunt may be the result of any disease that causes a venous admixture. However, there are other causes. In patients with congenital heart disease, blood may bypass the lungs through an atrial or ventricular defect or a patent ductus arteriosis. One form of intrapulmonary shunt may result from an arteriovenous fistula in a tumor. In contrast to the other causes of hypoxemia, increasing the F_IO_2 in these patients will not increase the P_aO_2 to levels seen in normal subjects. Once the etiology of the hypoxemic condition is determined, the underlying defect must be corrected as soon as possible. The moment hypoxemia is detected, patients must receive immediate supplemental oxygen, preferably 100% until the exact quantification of the hypoxemia has been established.

Protection of the Airway in a Patient with Impaired Laryngeal Reflexes

One of the most important indications for intubation is protection of the airway in patients who have depressed laryngeal reflexes. These reflexes may be impaired because of stupor and coma (e.g., anesthesia, encephalopathy, cerebrovascular accident (CVA), drug overdose, ethanol intoxication, cardiac arrest, seizures, postictal state, airway burns, tracheoesophageal fistula, partial paralysis of the laryngeal musculature). Such patients are at great risk for aspiration of gastric contents, which can result in aspiration pneumonitis. In most instances, endotracheal intubation with a cuffed endotracheal tube prevents regurgitated material from entering the trachea.

Ensuring Airway Patency in a Patient with Abnormal Pathology or Depressed Level of Consciousness

Comatose patients may not be able to breathe adequately because of airway obstruction by the tongue or by any encroachment on the airway from without or within. Tumors of the larynx are among the most common cause, but other diseases and conditions can also interfere—acute epiglottitis, croup, airway burns, foreign-body aspiration, vascular trauma to the neck, anaphylaxis. The passage of an endotracheal tube in these persons may be lifesaving.

Anesthesia and Surgery

Endotracheal intubation is required during surgery whenever the site of the operation will interfere with the ability to safely administer an anesthetic. Most operations on the head, neck, and face fall into this category, for without an endotracheal tube the surgeon simply does not have sufficient access to the operative site. In addition, there is a risk of aspiration of blood or other materials during surgery. Furthermore, contamination of the surgical field may occur because of proximity of the anesthesiologist and equipment to the surgical site. If a patient is at risk from aspiration of gastric contents, a cuffed endotracheal tube should be inserted during general anesthesia (e.g., emergency surgery).

Endotracheal intubation should be performed whenever neuromuscular blocking drugs are used (with some exceptions), because the protective reflexes are significantly impaired during paralysis. It is called for also when elective surgical procedures are likely to last more than two hours, to facilitate the delivery of oxygen and anesthetic gases and reduce the risk of aspiration. Intubation is also indicated when the patient is in an operative position that will interfere with ventilation (e.g., prone, sitting, lateral, head down, or extreme lithotomy).

Positive-pressure ventilation is usually required during thoracic surgical procedures and it is best achieved with an endotracheal tube in place. Occasionally mask anesthesia can fail because of the inability to maintain an adequate mask seal, especially if the patient is edentulous, obese, large, or bearded.

Specific Indications

The following specific circumstances call for endotracheal intubation during the administration of anesthesia:

Surgery on the head, face, or neck
Emergency surgery
Muscle paralysis
Lengthy surgery
Thoracic surgery
Failure of mask anesthesia
Abnormal positions
Limited access

Suctioning

An endotracheal tube allows access to the tracheobronchial tree to suction secretions. Occasionally a patient will produce large quantities of secretions during surgery, especially surgery in the vicinity of the airway. This can be prevented by the administration of anticholinergic drugs preoperatively, such as atropine, scopolamine, or glycopyrolate. The administration of succinylcholine, however, is often associated with excessive secretions, especially if anticholinergic drugs are not used. Any surgical patient who has recently had a cold will produce an excessive quantity of secretions, which may necessitate intubation. If secretions cannot be readily handled through an endotracheal tube, the patient undergoing prolonged ventilation may require a tracheostomy.

Selecting the Route of Intubation

Once the decision has been made to intubate a patient, you need to select the appropriate route—orotracheal, nasotracheal, or transtracheal. Although orotracheal is by far the most common, the other routes are preferable in selected circumstances.

Orotracheal Intubation

Except in the specific clinical situations, the oral route is routinely selected for intubation. General indications are listed in Box 6-1. Orotracheal intubation is used in most surgical patients undergoing general anesthesia. It is especially necessary for avoiding contamination of the surgical field. This latter issue is important from a historical perspective. Formerly, surgeons were limited in their ability to operate on lesions in the mouth or in the vicinity of the airway while the patient was receiving anesthesia by mask. It was this particular problem that motivated MacEwan in 1880 to introduce the technique of endotracheal intubation, and today surgical field avoidance remains one of the most common indications for oral intubation.

Contraindications

There are very few absolute contraindications to oral intubation. And, quite simply, these are the usual indications for nasotracheal intubation:

Surgical field avoidance
Poor oral access
Prolonged ventilation

Nasotracheal Intubation

In selected circumstances, the nasotracheal route is preferred to orotracheal. Its indications include surgical field avoidance, poor oral access, and prolonged ventilation.

Surgical Field Avoidance

Otolaryngologists, oral surgeons, plastic surgeons, and dentists often require access to the mouth and occasionally wire the maxilla and mandible together. Although an oral endotracheal tube may suffice in most situations, occasionally it will obscure the operative site. Accordingly, nasotracheal intubation is selected. When dealing with specialists in this area, it is best to discuss their preferences before proceeding.

Poor Oral Access

Gaining access to the mouth may be difficult in patients with trismus, status epilepticus, fractured mandible, or arthritis of the TMJ or cervical spine. In these situations, nasotracheal intubation is the method of choice. Also, if you are unable to elevate the epiglottis when attempting oral intubation, the nasal route is often successful because the tube, upon emerging from the nasopharynx, tends to point beneath the epiglottis toward the vocal cords.

Prolonged Ventilation

Specialists generally agree that the nasal route is more comfortable than the oral route for patients requiring prolonged intubation. Nasal tubes are also easier to stabilize. In addition, patients tend to salivate less, and there is no danger of damage to the tube from dental occlusion.

Contraindications

Nasotracheal intubation is contraindicated in the following circumstances:

Bleeding disturbances
Nasal pathology (epistaxis, polyps, septal deviation, infections)
Basal skull fracture
CSF leakage
Chronic sinusitis
Nasal stenosis

Transtracheal Intubation

An endotracheal tube can be readily inserted into the trachea via an existing tracheostomy stoma.

Endobronchial Intubation

Endobronchial intubation is employed when ventilation of only one lung is desired. The indications are listed in Box 6.5.

Box 6.5. Indications for Endobronchial Intubation

Absolute

1. Isolation of one lung
    a. Unilateral infection
    b. Massive hemorrhage
2. Control of the distribution of ventilation
    a. Bronchopleural fistula
    b. Bronchopleural cutaneous fistula
    c. Giant unilateral lung cyst
3. Unilateral bronchopulmonary lavage

Relative

1. Surgical exposure
2. Upper lobectomy
3. Aortic aneurysm resection

Preparation of the Patient for Intubation Outside the Operating Room

Anesthesiologists are occasionally called upon to assist in airway problems that occur outside the operating room. Although general anesthesia is not usually required in these situations because the patient is already obtunded or even comatose, many patients are far from comatose and require airway intervention because of respiratory failure. The following preparatory measures are recommended in these cases:

Patient interview
Sedation
Topical anesthesia
Nerve block
General anesthesia

Patient Interview

When possible, it is strongly recommended that a few moments be spent with the patient before awake intubation to explain the reasons for the intervention and what to expect vis-à-vis pain and discomfort. All too often clinicians, eager to solve a life-threatening problem, forge ahead with intubation and fail to pay attention to these all-important and humane aspects of medical care.

Sedation

When It Is Needed

Most conscious patients presenting for intubation benefit from sedation; they are anxious about the procedure, and the application of topical anesthesia and nerve blocks can cause discomfort. In an emergency there may not be time, but in elective situations you should take the time to provide adequate sedation. Effective sedation requires patience and a good knowledge of the pharmacology of sedative and hypnotic drugs. Sedation is associated with impaired reflex activity, and therefore patients who have recently eaten are at increased risk from aspiration. Adults presenting for elective surgery should refrain from food for 6 hours and clear liquids for at least 3 hours before the operation. Regurgitation and pulmonary aspiration is a real risk during attempts at intubation in sedated patients because they are supine, somewhat restrained, and partially obtunded.

How It Is Done

The best way to sedate a patient is first to obtain reliable venous access (plastic cannulae are better for this than metal ones), and to select an appropriate combination of agents (a benzodiazepine and a narcotic are optimal). Of the benzo-

TABLE 6.1. Sedation/topical anesthesia

Indications	Medication	Dose*
Sedation/Analgesia	Midazolam (Versed)	0.5 to 1 mg increments IV
	Fentanyl (Sublimaze)	25 to 50 μg increments IV
	Morphine	1 to 3 mg increments IV
	Demerol	20 to 25 mg increments IV
	Propofol	20 mg increments IV
Topical anesthesia	Lidocaine 4 to 10%	3.5 to 7 mg/kg
	Cocaine 4%	2 mg/kg
Topical vasoconstriction	Phenylephrine (Dristan 0.5%)	Up to 3 sprays per nostril
	Oxymetazoline (Afrin 0.05%)	Up to 3 sprays per nostril

*Suggested doses, when drugs are used alone; may be modified at the discretion of the clinician. Doses should be titrated carefully to desired effect. All doses should be reduced when combined with other centrally active drugs. These are the recommended doses for adults only.

diazepines, one of the most popular is midazolam.[4] This water-soluble compound appears to have all the benefits of diazepam without the problems (Table 6.1). It also has a much shorter half-life (2 to 4 hours) than other benzodiazepines, and the incidence of venous thrombosis with it appears to be insignificant. It is 2 to 4 times more potent than diazepam on a milligram-for-milligram basis, and thus no more than 1.0 mg increments should be used.

In preparing a patient for intubation, opiates such as fentanyl and morphine or demerol are often injected with a benzodiazepine. They not only provide analgesia but also suppress the cough reflex, enabling the patient to better tolerate the intubation procedure. Morphine is administered in a dose of 1 to 3 mg intravenously, and its effects may persist for 1 to 2 hours. In contrast, fentanyl, which is administered in a dose of 25 to 50 μg intravenously, has a much shorter duration of action, 30 to 60 minutes. The most serious side effect of opiates is respiratory depression. Additional side effects include hypotension, bradycardia, nausea, vomiting, and pruritis. The effects of narcotic overdose can be reversed by the opiate antagonist naloxone, 0.1 to 0.4 mg intravenously. Since naloxone has a short duration of action (30 to 60 minutes), however, repeated doses may be necessary. Propofol is a very effective sedative/hypnotic when given in small increments (20mg); however, it is associated with pain on injection. This pain can be alleviated by adding small doses of lidocaine (20 to 40 mg IV).

The combination of a benzodiazepine and a narcotic is synergistic; therefore, caution must be used because of the enhanced respiratory-depressant effects. They also shift the CO_2 response curve to the right (increasing the ventilatory rate in response to increasing arterial PCO_2) and alter the slope of the curve in an adverse (downward) direction. Benzodiazepine/morphine and benzodiazepine/fentanyl are combinations commonly used. Intravenous increments are as follows: midazolam, 0.5 mg; morphine, 2 mg; fentanyl, 25 μg. However, these drugs should be used only if the person administering them is fully familiar with their properties, side effects, and dosage.

How the Patient Should Be Monitored

Vital signs (blood pressure [BP], pulse, respirations) should be monitored at regular intervals (at least every 5 minutes) while you are sedating a patient. A precordial stethoscope facilitates monitoring heart and respiratory rates simultaneously. Electrocardiogram monitoring, pulse oximetry, and arterial blood gases, if available, provide the clinician with additional information that may help assess the effects of sedation.

When It Is Adequate

Small increments of sedative drugs are injected, and sufficient time is allowed to assess their effects. Some patients require large quantities; others very little. Sedation is adequate when the patient appears to be sleeping quietly yet is responsive to oral commands. Other indicators include slurred speech, decreased respiratory rate (<12 breaths per minute), and a lowered blood pressure. Snoring, retractions, and unresponsiveness are signs of oversedation and may indicate impending airway obstruction.

Local Anesthetic Techniques

If, upon using these end points, you feel that the patient is adequately sedated, a topical anesthetic should be applied to the nose or oropharynx, depending upon the route of intubation. If the patient appears disturbed by this intervention, more sedation may be necessary. It must be clearly understood, however, that sedation of patients for intubation can result in significant cardiovascular and respiratory depression, and therefore, life-sustaining equipment must always be immediately available. Local anesthetic techniques have been described in detail in Chapter 4.

General Anesthesia

Few patients require general anesthesia for intubation outside the operating room. If a patient must be restrained to the degree that a general anesthetic is required for intubation, you should seriously question the indication for intubation. However, situations do exist in which general anesthesia is necessary—for example, in patients with cerebral injury or acute epiglottitis and when the patient is totally uncooperative.

Cerebral Injury

Occasionally a patient who is quite responsive will present in the emergency room with serious cerebral damage requiring hyperventilation to reduce intracranial pressure. In this situation a poorly performed awake intubation can aggravate the intracranial injury. However, general anesthesia administered by a competent anesthesiologist allows the intubation to be performed with skill and alacrity. Furthermore, the intravenous barbiturates often used during induction of anesthesia help to reduce intracranial pressure and cerebral oxygen consumption.

Acute Epiglottitis

When a child presents with acute epiglottitis, no attempt should be made to confirm the diagnosis by examining the airway. Instrumentation of these children in the awake state is strictly contraindicated. Time permitting, they should be brought to the operating room, where general anesthesia can be induced. Premature intubation of a child in the awake or semianesthetized state may lead to laryngospasm and complete airway obstruction. Occasionally, however, time does not permit the luxury of general anesthesia. If bag/valve/mask ventilation fails under these circumstances, awake intubation or a tracheostomy may be the only option.

Uncooperative Patient

On occasion, patients present in the emergency room with life-threatening airway compromise that requires urgent intervention but he (or she) is uncooperative. Rarely, general anesthesia may be the only option for safe intubation. Hypoxia, alcohol ingestion, and the use of mind-altering substances all can cause a person to behave abnormally or erratically, forcing you to employ a general anesthetic. The new inhalation anesthetic Sevoflurane can be used to suppress an otherwise agitated patient and may be an alternative to intravenous anesthesia in a patient with an abnormal airway.

However, once this course of action is decided upon, remember: You are responsible for sustaining the patient's life; if difficulty is anticipated in securing the airway, it may be preferable to restrain the patient physically and attempt an awake intubation.

Neuromuscular Blocking Drugs

Neuromuscular blocking drugs, introduced into anesthesia practice by Griffith and Johnson[5] in 1941, have revolutionized the practice of anesthesia and surgery. Up to that time, muscle relaxation was achieved by deepening the level of inhalation anesthesia, with the consequent prolongation of recovery. Following the introduction of neuromuscular blocking drugs, the concept of balanced anesthesia—consisting of hypnosis, analgesia, and muscle relaxation—was developed and it was no longer necessary to expose patients to deep levels of inhalation agents for long periods in order to achieve adequate muscle relaxation. Furthermore, the technique of endotracheal intubation was greatly facilitated by the muscle relaxants.

These drugs may be divided into two classes depending upon their mechanism of action. **Depolarizing** agents (mainly succinylcholine) act as acetylcholine receptor agonists and depolarize the motor end plate; since they are not hydrolyzed by acetylcholinesterase, they remain at the neuromuscular junction, preventing repolarization (and mimicking the effects of excessive acetylcholine). The **nondepolarizing,** competitive agents (e.g., pancuronium, atracurium, vecuronium) act as antagonists and compete with acetylcholine for receptor sites on the motor end plate. All striated muscle groups, including respiratory muscles, are affected; smooth muscle is not. When using any neuromuscular blocking agent, therefore, it is advisable to monitor the degree of muscle paralysis with a nerve stimulator.

Since these drugs cause respiratory paralysis, the implications of their use are enormous. They should never be prescribed for patients outside the operating room without consulting an anesthesiologist or another physician who is fully familiar with their pharmacology. Also, they are rarely administered unless intubation and mechanical ventilation are anticipated. (*Note:* Use of the term *muscle relaxant* can be deceptive. Physicians not fully familiar with these drugs might construe *relaxant* to mean relaxer or sedative, which would be disastrous!)

It should be clearly understood that neuromuscular blocking drugs have no inherent sedative effects. Although the lack of movement gives the impression that a patient is resting quietly, he or she may actually be quite anxious. It is inhumane to paralyze and mechanically ventilate an alert patient without providing an adequate level of sedation.

Depolarizing Drug—Succinylcholine

Unless there are contraindications to its use, succinylcholine is the drug of choice when rapid intubation is required. Its neuromuscular blocking effects (first described by Bovet et al[6] in 1949) are widely utilized, and the compound has been the "gold standard" since Foldes et al[7] reported using it in 1952 for muscular relaxation in patients undergoing surgery.

The drug has a rapid onset of action (about 30 seconds) and a relatively short duration. In the average adult a 1 mg/kg dose lasts 5 to 20 minutes. Within about 30 seconds of injection, there is a marked muscle fasciculation of varying intensity followed by a profound flaccid paralysis lasting 5 to 20 minutes, depending upon the dose and the patient. Succinylcholine is rapidly hydrolyzed by plasma pseudocholinesterase.

One serious side effect (Box 6.6), however, is life-threatening hyperkalemia—which can occur following an injection in patients with burns, muscle injury, upper or lower motor neuron disease, or a number of other conditions—owing to the massive potassium efflux during prolonged muscle depolarization. In a few susceptible individuals, succinylcholine can trigger malignant hyperthermia. Bradycardia often follows a repeat dose, especially in children, and can be prevented by administering atropine.

The duration of action of succinylcholine is determined by the degree of pseudocholinesterase activity in the plasma, which may be influenced by hereditary factors, disease states, pregnancy, or medications. Hereditary factors are

Box 6.6. Disadvantages of Succinylcholine (Classified by Mechanism of Action)

Depolarization (end plate and muscle)
  Fasciculation and increased abdominal pressure
  Contracture
    Denervated, extraocular, and jaw muscles
  Potassium efflux and cardiac consequences
  Muscle pain
  Changing nature of block
    Tachyphylaxis and slow recovery
Other agonist actions
  Tachycardia and hypertension, other dysrhythmias
  Sinus bradycardia and arrest
Idiosyncratic responses
  Failure to metabolize succinylcholine
    Atypical plasma cholinesterase
  Exaggerated multisystem reactions
  Malignant hyperthermia
  Muscular dystrophies
Active metabolites
Drug interactions and complicating medical conditions
  Cardiac dysrhythmias
    Hyperkalemia in burns, renal failure, etc.
    Other electrolyte imbalances
    Cardiac glycosides
  Contractures and cardiac dysrhythmias
    Major neurological lesions
    Muscular dystrophies
  Reduced metabolism of succinylcholine
    Physiological (e.g., pregnancy, obesity, age extremes)
    Cholinesterase inhibition
  Increased metabolism of succinylcholine
  Increased neuromuscular sensitivity (e.g., magnesium, myasthenia gravis [nondepolarizing agents])
  Reduced neuromuscular sensitivity (e.g., myasthenia gravis [depolarizing agent])

most often responsible for delayed recovery.[8] In these cases the deficiency is due not so much to the quantity of the enzyme present as to the atypical nature of the enzyme. Patients with this hereditary defect may remain apneic and paralyzed for up to 8 hours. Atypical homozygous pseudocholinesterase deficiency occurs in approximately 1 out of every 2,500 patients. Deficient quantities of the enzyme are most commonly found in patients receiving echothiophate eyedrops and cyclophosphamide (Cytoxan) therapy, but there may also be deficiencies in patients who are suffering from severe liver disease or have recently undergone plasmapheresis and in women who are pregnant. One of the major advantages of succinylcholine is its rapid onset and short duration of action. It is ideal when profound relaxation is required for a short time, as for intubation. The usual intravenous dose in adults is 1 mg/kg, and in children, 2 mg/kg. In children, it should be preceded by atropine or another suitable anticholinergic drug that blocks the undesirable muscarinic effects of acetylcholine (e.g., salivation, bronchial secretions, bradycardia). (*Note:* Anticholinesterase agents do not reverse, but rather **potentiate,** the effects of succinylcholine.) The use of succinylcholine has been restricted in children to emergency use only because of potential risks associated with its use in children.

Nondepolarizing Drugs

In contrast to depolarizing neuromuscular drugs, which are few (and, practically speaking, there is just one), there are several nondepolarizing drugs to choose from.[9–11] A number of new neuromuscular blocking drugs have been introduced in the past 10 years, but it is not necessary for you to be familiar with all of them. Nondepolarizing drugs are most frequently used in anesthesia to provide muscle relaxation during surgery. They are also used to facilitate mechanical ventilation in some cases. Table 6.2 shows a classification of nondepolarizing drugs.

Nondepolarizing neuromuscular blocking drugs are predominantly used by anesthesiologists and critical care specialists in patients who require neuromuscular blockade during surgery or to facilitate mechanical ventilation in critical care units. Curare is now considered obsolete and the only long-acting agent in frequent use is pancuronium. Side effects of pancuronium include tachycardia and hypertension, which are dose dependent and may be undesirable in patients with limited cardiac reserve. Neuromuscular blocking effects of pancuronium tend to persist long after reversal. Doxacurium is even longer-acting than pancuronium and is used infrequently in clinical practice today.

Vecuronium has minimal effects on the cardiovascular system and is devoid

TABLE 6.2. Classification of nondepolarizing drugs

Long-acting	Intermediate	Short-acting
d-tubocurarine	Vecuronium	Mivacurium
Pancuronium	Atracurium	Rocuronium
Doxicurium	Cisatracurium	Rapacuronium

of histamine-releasing properties, but it is metabolized in the liver and excreted in the urine; thus, prolonged effects occur in patients with liver or renal disease.

Atracurium is a benzylisoquinolium nondepolarizing neuromuscular blocking drug. It is metabolized by ester hydrolysis ($^2/_3$) and Hofman elimination (nonenzymatic degradation at body temperature and pH). Hypotension and tachycardia occur with high doses and it causes histamine release.

Cisatracurium is a more potent version of atracurium and is devoid of histamine-releasing properties and accompanying cardiovascular effects.

Mivacurium is a short-acting, nondepolarizing drug that is metabolized by pseudocholinesterase, just like succinylcholine, and should be avoided in patients with pseudocholinesterase deficiency. Cardiovascular side effects secondary to histamine release are minimal unless given in large doses. Rocuronium is now one of the most frequently used neuromuscular blocking drugs in North America. It is an aminosteroid and has a very rapid onset of action (60 seconds following 1 mg/kg IV) and an intermediate duration (30 to 45 min, depending upon the dose and other conditions).

Rapacuronium is also an aminosteroid with an equally rapid onset to rocuronium, but in contrast to rocuronium it also has a very rapid recovery. Rapacuronium has recently been withdrawn from clinical use because of severe bronchospasm in children.

Methods of Administering a Neuromuscular Blocking Drug

Neuromuscular blocking drugs may be administered by **bolus injection** with intermittent supplementation or by **continuous infusion.** There is considerable individual variation in patients' reactions to a given dose (Table 6.3),[12] so neuromuscular function should be monitored using a nerve stimulator.

Reversal of Neuromuscular Blockade

Neuromuscular blocking drugs such as succinylcholine and mivacurium are hydrolyzed quite rapidly; thus, recovery is spontaneous and does not require an-

TABLE 6.3. Comparative clinical pharmacology of commonly used neuromuscular blocking drugs

Drug	ED 95 (mg/kg)	Tracheal intubation (mg/kg)	Onset to maximum effect (min)	Recovery index (25%–75%) (min)
Mivacurium	0.08	0.15 to 0.25	2 to 3	10 to 15
Rocuronium	0.3	0.60 to 1.0	2 to 3	10 to 15
Atracurium	0.2	0.5 to 0.75	5 to 6	10 to 15
Cisatracurium	0.05	0.125 to 0.175	5 to 6	10 to 15
Pancuronium	0.06	0.075 to 0.125	4 to 5	25
Vecuronium	0.05	0.075 to 0.125	5 to 6	10 to 15

(Modified from Marash et al 2001,[12] with permission of the authors and publisher.)

TABLE 6.4. Reversal of neuromuscular blockade, anticholinesterase anticholinergic

Drugs	Dose (mg/kg)	For a 70 kg individual
Neostigmine	0.03 to 0.08	3 mg
Atropine*	0.015 to 0.04	1.2 mg
Edrophonium	0.5 to 1.0	70 mg

*The dose of glycopyrrolate is about half that of atropine.

tagonists. The effects of nondepolarizing drugs, however, are longer-acting and usually require reversal, although they do wear off in time. Two medications that reverse neuromuscular function are (1) an anticholinesterase (e.g., neostigmine, edrophonium), which increases the amount of acetylcholine at the neuromuscular junction, and (2) an anticholinergic (atropine), which reduces the side effects of the anticholinesterase (Table 6.4). An anticholinergic medication should always be administered in advance of or simultaneously with anticholinesterase.

Numerous factors can interfere with the reversal of neuromuscular blocking drugs: neuromuscular disease, hypothermia, certain antibiotics, inhalation anesthesia, electrolyte disturbances, hypermagnesemia, drug interactions, and prolonged use of neuromuscular drugs. The recommended doses of established neuromuscular blocking drugs are presented in Table 6.3, and doses of reversal drugs in Table 6.4.

Summary

It must not always be assumed that endotracheal intubation is indicated; time permitting, a careful assessment should be made of each patient. General indications include ventilatory support that may be required because of hypoxemia and/or tissue hypoxia, prevention of aspiration, maintenance of airway patency, anesthesia and surgery, and suctioning.

Once the need for intubation is established, you will need to select the preferred route. Orotracheal intubation is used most often; however, nasotracheal and transtracheal (or endobronchial) intubation may be indicated under certain circumstances. Sometimes awake intubation is required.

In these circumstances proper preparation of the patient facilitates intubation and minimizes discomfort. Sedating patients with a benzodiazepine in conjunction with an opiate for analgesia alleviates the anxiety and pain associated with the procedure. Unfortunately, few clinicians seem to wait long enough for the sedative drugs to take effect; yet a few extra minutes seem to make all the difference to the patient. Topical anesthesia and/or nerve blocks are usually required for awake intubation. Should general anesthesia be required, an anesthesiologist should always be consulted.

Neuromuscular blocking drugs greatly facilitate the ease with which endotracheal intubation can be performed. A large number of new medications have been introduced within the past 10 years, each with its own subtle advantages. Succinylcholine, however, still has the most rapid onset and is the drug of choice when rapid intubation is required in emergency settings (unless there are contraindications to its use.) Nondepolarizing medications are not indicated for intubation in an emergency unless succinylcholine is contraindicated. Nondepolarizing drugs can be used to facilitate mechanical ventilation in some cases. Patients receiving neuromuscular blocking drugs are paralyzed and unable to breathe; they therefore need to be sedated with careful surveillance, preferably in an intensive care unit.

References

1. MacEwan W. Clinical observations on the introduction of tracheal tube, by the mouth instead of performing tracheostomy or laryngotomy. *Br Med J.* 1880;1:122, 163. Reprinted in *Survey of Anesthesiology.* 1969;13:105.
2. Ganong WF. *Review of Medical Physiology.* 11th ed. Palo Alto, CA: Lange Medical Publications; 1983:551.
3. West JB. *Respiratory Physiology: The Essentials.* 3rd ed. Baltimore: Williams & Wilkins; 1985:17.
4. Reves JG, et al. Midazolam: pharmacology and uses. *Anesthesiology.* 1985;62:310.
5. Griffith HR, Johnson GE. The use of curare in general anesthesia. *Anesthesiology.* 1942;3:418.
6. Bovet D, et al. *R.C. Sanit.* 1949;12(suppl):106.
7. Foldes FE, McNall PG, Borrego-Hinojosa JM. Succinylcholine: a new approach to muscular relaxation in anesthesiology. *N Engl J Med.* 1952;247:596.
8. Whittaker M. Plasma cholinesterase variants and the anaesthetist. *Anaesthesia.* 1980; 35:174.
9. Savarese JJ. Review of new and currently available muscle relaxants. ASA Refresher Lectures. 1992.
10. Payne JP, Utting JE. Symposium on atracurium. *Br J Anaesth.* 1983;55(suppl 1):1–39.
11. Longnecker DE, Murphy FL. *Introduction to Anesthesiology.* 8th ed. Philadephia: WB Saunders; 1992.
12. Marash PG, Cullen BF, Stoelting RK. *Handbook of Clinical Anesthesia.* 3rd ed. Philadelphia: Lippincott Williams & Wilkins; 2001:207.

Suggested Readings

Goldman SA. *Muscle Relaxants.* 2nd ed. Philadelphia: WB Saunders; 1979.
Nunn JF. *Applied Respiratory Physiology.* 3rd ed. London: Butterworths; 1987:270–271.
Katz RL. *Muscle Relaxants: Basic and Clinical Aspects.* New York: Grune & Stratton; 1986.
Savarese JJ. Newer muscle relaxants. ASA Refresher Lectures. 1986;142.
West JB. *Pulmonary Pathophysiology—The Essentials.* 3rd ed. Baltimore: Williams & Wilkins; 1987:22–25.

7
Techniques of Intubation

This chapter provides the necessary information to successfully perform intubation. Individuals who are proficient at intubation can usually complete the procedure in less than 30 seconds.

In learning intubation, some hands-on experience is vital. Patients scheduled for elective surgery, under general anesthesia, and requiring intubation are ideal for teaching clinicians the technique. Allowing the clinician to get his or her feet wet can be stressful for everyone involved. The teacher must allow for the novice's lack of expertise and speed and must, simultaneously, protect the patient from trauma and hypoxia. Also, there is a (small) risk of aspiration of gastric contents. Patients should be preoxygenated before intubation. The traditional method of preoxygenation is 3 minutes of tidal volume breathing at 5 L/min using 100% oxygen.[1] Alternatively, Baraka et al[2] have shown equally good results when breathing 8 deep breaths within 60 seconds at 10 L/min. Nimmagadda et al[3] concurred with Baraka's approach and suggested that maximal preoxygenation was achieved when deep breathing at high flows (10 L/min) was extended for 1.5 to 2 minutes.

Current technology allows the continuous monitoring of a patient's oxygenation during intubation by use of a pulse oximeter. This noninvasive monitoring device—attached to a digit, an earlobe, or the nasal septum—relays information about the patient's oxygen saturation and pulse rate to a receiver that electronically displays this information on a screen. Falling oxygen saturations are signaled by a warning sound. Pulse oximetry has revolutionized the teaching of intubation because it provides an excellent intervention end point. Previously, clinical methods or simply timed intervention was used, but neither was entirely satisfactory.

When teaching medical and other students airway skills, it is more important to teach them how to competently perform bag/valve/mask ventilation as opposed to intubation. However, bag/valve/mask ventilation is more difficult to learn. How quickly do students learn to perform these tasks? There is some information on medical students learning endotracheal intubation. Following didactic lectures and practice on a mannequin, 30 medical students performed intubation on 90 patients. One third of the students correctly intubated patients on their first attempt. However, 47% of these students incorrectly identified the position of the endotracheal tube. Ninety-three percent of the students correctly intubated patients after the third attempt, but of these, 20% failed to recognize incorrect tube placement. It seems unlikely that students obtain sufficient training in airway management in a 1- to 2-week rotation in anesthesia.[4]

Although there are no good yardsticks for determining when a clinician is competent to perform intubation, in simplest terms an individual is probably competent if he or she can place a tube within the trachea in 30 seconds or less and complete all the preliminary and follow-up steps required within 1 minute. We estimate that it may take as many as 70 consecutive intubations (oral and nasal) for a clinician to be exposed to most of the common problems that can occur. Safar[5] suggests using a checklist to measure competence (Fig. 7.1).

Student's name	Date	Evaluator's name

☐ Passed
☐ Failed

Measures	Technique	Time
	☑ Check if correct performance	☑ Check if within correct time lapse

Tracheal intubation of *adult* manikin	☐ Checked laryngoscope light before use	sec.
	☐ Checked tube patency before use	
	☐ Held laryngoscope correctly	
	☐ Used no grossly traumatic manoeuvre during intubation attempt	
	☐ Inserted tube into trachea rapidly . . . . . .☐ < 30	
	☐ Gave first lung inflation rapidly via tube by bag-valve or mouth . . . .☐ < 60	
	☐ Inflated cuff of tube correctly (with helper)	
	☐ Used bite-block, secured tube and connected ventilation device correctly	
	☐ Checked to rule out bronchial intubation	
Tracheal intubation of *infant* manikin	☐ Checked laryngoscope light before use	
	☐ Checked tube patency before use	
	☐ Held laryngoscope correctly	
	☐ Used no grossly traumatic manoeuvre during intubation attempt	
	☐ Inserted tube into trachea rapidly . . . . . .☐ < 30	
	☐ Gave first lung inflation rapidly via tube (by mouth) . . . .☐ < 60	
	☐ Used bite-block, secured tube and connected ventilation device correctly	
	☐ Checked to rule out bronchial intubation	
Tracheal suctioning (curved-tipped catheter)	☐ Used correct technique to suction each lung separately . . . .☐ < 60	

FIGURE 7.1. Checklist for testing intubation competence. (From Safar,[5] with permission.)

Intubation Methods

The vast majority of intubations are performed using direct vision; however, there are also indirect or blind methods, which may be used in specific situations.

Orotracheal Intubation by Direct Vision in an Adult (Macintosh Blade)

Direct vision is the most common method employed in the performance of oral endotracheal intubation in adult patients.

Preparation

The first task is to perform an equipment check. It is essential that one be able to deliver 100% oxygen at high flows (up to 10 liters per minute) using a bag and mask. Other mandatory equipment includes (1) a suction apparatus connected via a clear plastic tubing to a rigid tonsil sucker capable of drawing a negative pressure of 25 cm H_2O, and (2) an intubation tray containing the following items (Fig. 7.2):

Two laryngoscope handles and a variety of straight and curved blades
Tongue depressor
Oral and nasal airways
Variety of endotracheal tubes
Needles and syringes
Stylet
K-Y Jelly
Tonsil sucker (Yankauer) and flexible suction catheter
Magill forceps
Tape
Towels
Local anesthetic solution
Laryngeal mask airways

Both laryngoscopes should be functioning, and the endotracheal tube cuff should be checked for leaks. The tube should be well lubricated and some specialists also recommend lubricating the blade up to the bulb with K-Y Jelly.

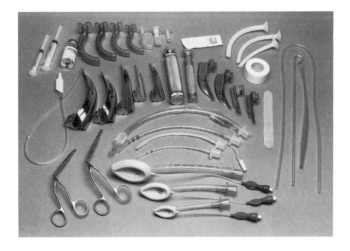

FIGURE 7.2. An intubation tray.

Positioning

In 1944 Bannister and MacBeth[6] suggested that the optimal position of the head
and neck during direct laryngoscopy was flexion of the neck and extension of
the atlantooccipital joint, otherwise known as the *sniffing position*. Failure to flex
the cervical spine and extend the atlantooccipital joint prevents alignment of the
axes of the larynx, pharynx, and mouth (Fig. 7.3). Flexion of the neck or cervical spine is readily achieved by placing a folded towel beneath the occiput
(Fig. 7.4). Atlantooccipital extension is readily achieved by tilting the head backward manually (Fig. 7.5) or by pulling up on the mandible.

What is the optimal positioning of the head and neck for laryngoscopy and
intubation? For years we have been taught that the optimal position of the head
and neck for laryngoscopy was the sniffing position. The *sniffing position* is a
phrase coined by Sir Ivan Magill many years ago and resembles the position
of the head and neck of an individual sniffing the morning air.[7] Anatomically
the *sniffing position* is achieved by flexing the cervical spine and extending the
atlantooccipital joint. Kirstein,[8] an ENT surgeon (otolaryngologist), was among
the first to suggest that the sniffing position was the ideal position for laryngoscopy. Chevalier Jackson,[9] another ENT surgeon, published a study about
optimal position of the head and neck during laryngoscopy for orotracheal intubation, and like Kirstein, he emphasized the importance of neck flexion and
extension of the atlantooccipital joint. Bannister and MacBeth in a landmark
article in the *Lancet* firmly established the sniffing position to be optimal for
laryngoscopy and intubation. They proposed the three axes alignment theory
and demonstrated radiologically that the *sniffing position* aligned the axes of
the larynx, pharynx, and mouth in such a way that the airway was visible
at laryngoscopy. This theory is best illustrated diagrammatically. In Figure 7.3
the head is in the neutral position and the axes of the larynx (AL), pharynx

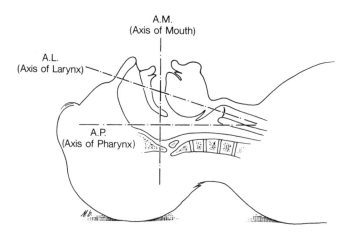

FIGURE 7.3. Poor alignment of the axes of the larynx, pharynx, and mouth.

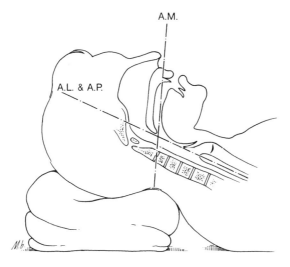

FIGURE 7.4. Cervical flexion.

(AP), and mouth (AM) are poorly aligned. By flexion of the cervical spine the axes of the larynx and pharynx are brought into unison (Fig. 7.4). By extension of the atlantooccipital joint the axis of the mouth is aligned close to the axes of the larynx and pharynx (Fig. 7.5). With proper positioning, all three axes are close to unison with laryngoscopy (Fig. 7.6A). The three axes alignment theory went unchallenged for close to 60 years. Adnet[10] et al recently

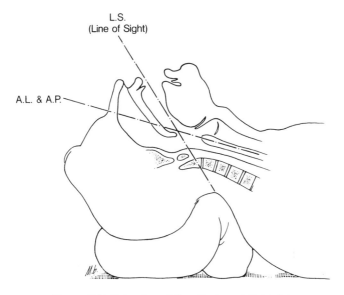

FIGURE 7.5. Extension of the atlantooccipital joint.

demonstrated using MRI that it was not possible to align the three axes into one by adopting the sniffing position (Figs. 7.6B, C, and D). However, they did demonstrate that the sniffing position significantly improved the angle associated with the best laryngoscopic view (Fig. 7.6D). They also showed an improved laryngoscopic view by just extending the atlantooccipital joint (Figure 7.6C), and there was no significant difference in the angles observed when these two maneuvers were compared.

Chou[11] recently contributed to the discussion challenging the time-honored three-axis theory by suggesting that Bannister and MacBeth failed to indicate start and finish points for these axes and only mentioned the direction of the axes. Chou proposed a modified theory. He suggested that direct laryngoscopy involved two axes, the pharynx, and the mouth and tongue. Before the laryngoscope is introduced, the angle between the incisors and the pharynx and glottis is approximately 90°. Head extension converts this angle to approximately 125° and then the advancement of the tongue with the laryngoscope makes this angle approach 180°. However, there are other elements that do not always make it possible to achieve 180° line of sight. These elements are the mobility of the soft tissues and bony structures and the size of the

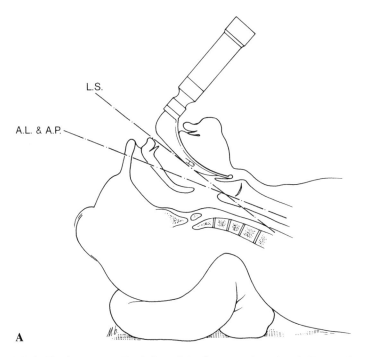

A

FIGURE 7.6. **A.** Final exposure. Evolution of the four axes (mouth axis [MA], pharyngeal axis [PA], laryngeal axis [LA], line of vision [LV]) and the α, β, and δ angles in the three head positions. The magnetic resonance images are shown for patient no. 5. **B.** Neutral position; **C.** simple head extension; **D.** "sniffing position." Continued.

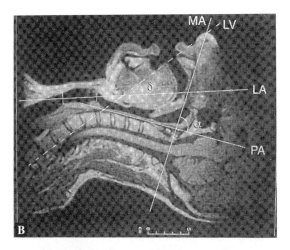

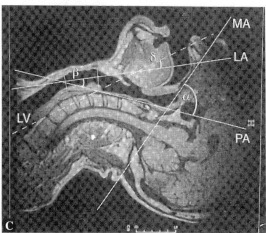

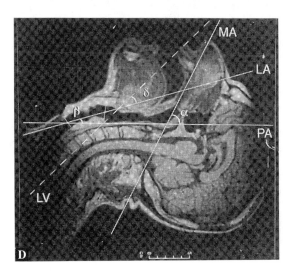

FIGURE 7.6. *Continued.*

oropharyngeal space. The cervical spine cannot be readily extended in arthritic conditions, thereby limiting one's ability to open the 90° angle between the mouth and glottis. Temporomandibular joint disease limits one's ability to move the tongue forward, and those with a hypoplastic mandible or large tongue have a reduced oropharyngeal space. It is with some reluctance that we debunk the theories of old masters. However, it is difficult to refute what Adnet et al and Chou and others have observed. However, although the three-axis theory has been challenged, there is still general agreement that the sniffing position helps facilitate exposure of the glottis.

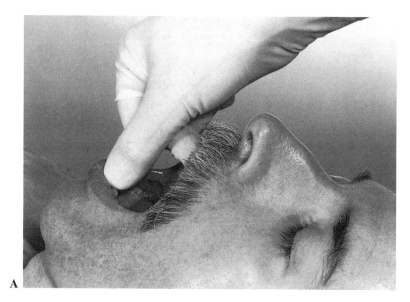

A

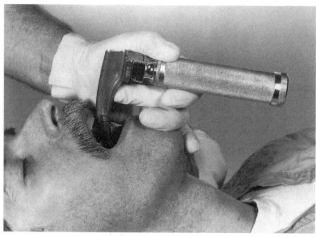

B

FIGURE 7.7. **A.** The scissors maneuver. **B.** The no-touch technique.

Exposure

The final exposure is achieved by opening the mouth and anteriorly displacing the mandible and soft tissues of the oral cavity and neck with the laryngoscope blade (Fig. 7.6A).

To perform the final exposure, stand directly behind the patient's head and take the laryngoscope handle in the left hand (right-handed laryngoscopes are available for left-handed people) as you would a paddle. With the right hand, open the mouth using the **scissors maneuver** (Fig. 7.7A), depressing the lower teeth with the thumb and elevating the upper teeth with the index or middle finger or both. Pressing upon the upper teeth will automatically extend the atlantooccipital joint. Alternatively, you may introduce the laryngoscope using the **no-touch technique,** which involves tilting the head into the sniffing position (Fig. 7.7B). In paralyzed patients the mandible usually descends, allowing room for insertion of the laryngoscope blade without inserting a finger into the mouth (Fig. 7.8). These maneuvers should allow good exposure of the airway. (To reduce the risk of transmitting infectious diseases, gloves are recommended when performing any airway maneuver.)

Visualization

At this stage, the laryngoscope blade is introduced into the mouth with the concave portion arching over the tongue in the midline (Fig. 7.8). If the blade is introduced at the side, it is more likely to tear the mucous membrane near the tonsillar folds on the right.

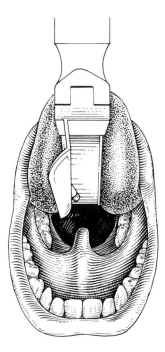

FIGURE 7.8. Introducing the laryngoscope blade.

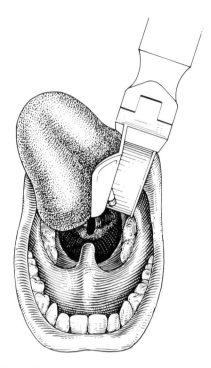

FIGURE 7.9. Displacing the tongue to the left with the laryngoscope.

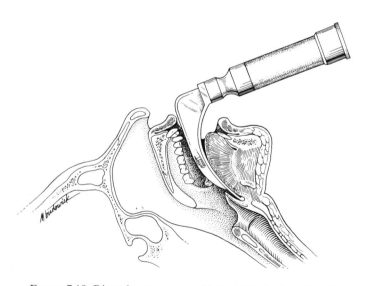

FIGURE 7.10. Direct laryngoscopy with the blade in the vallecula.

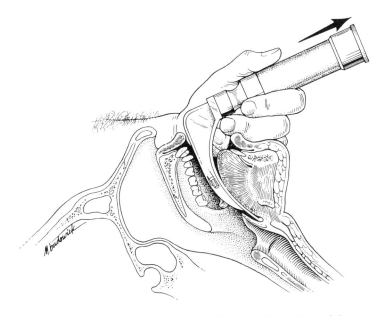

FIGURE 7.11. Forward-upward lift. The wrist should be straight.

Advance the blade over the tongue until the uvula and the tonsillar folds are seen. Then move it to the right side of the mouth so it lies between the aryepiglottic folds and the tongue. This maneuver displaces the tongue to the left (Fig. 7.9). Advance the blade further until its tip lies in the vallecula (Fig. 7.10) and then pull it forward and upward using firm but steady pressure without rotating the wrist (Fig. 7.11). If possible, avoid leaning on the upper teeth with the blade, since damage to the teeth may occur. In most situations the vocal cords should become visible at this stage (Fig. 7.12). If not, exert gentle pressure over the cricoid area to help bring them into view.

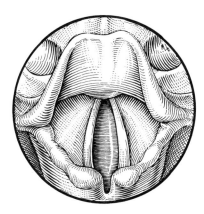

FIGURE 7.12. Direct exposure of the larynx.

Insertion

The endotracheal tube is usually inserted at the right corner of the mouth, below and to the right of the laryngoscope blade, with its concave portion facing toward the ceiling. Occasionally, it is necessary to rotate the tube 90° to the right or left before insertion.

Once the cuff has passed beyond the vocal cords, advance the tube another 3 cm. However, remember that there is a tendency to advance the tube further than necessary when learning this technique. To facilitate placement, have the assistant retract the right corner of the mouth. Occasionally, teeth may damage the cuff of the tube en route to the trachea.

Cuff Inflation

When reasonably satisfied that the endotracheal tube is correctly placed, inflate the cuff with the required amount of air. This is best determined by connecting the tube to the oxygen source and manually applying pressure to the reservoir bag until 20 cm H_2O registers on the airway pressure monitor. Then listen for a leak at the patient's mouth and inflate the cuff until none is audible at 20 cm H_2O. Remember: Overinflation of the cuff can lead to ischemia of the tracheal mucosa adjacent to the cuff.

If the cuff continues to leak despite large quantities of injected air, two possibilities exist: (1) the cuff may have been damaged during intubation, or (2) the tube may not be far enough down (i.e., the tip of the tube may be below the level of the vocal cords but a large portion of the cuff lies above it). This problem can be verified by looking into the patient's mouth with a laryngoscope and identifying the inflated cuff.

Confirmation

Endotracheal intubation is a technique readily learned by physicians and other healthcare personnel. Laryngoscopy and insertion of the tube are usually considered to be the most interesting part of the task, but confirmation of correct tube placement, though perhaps less interesting, is even more important and can never be taken for granted.

Not only must you confirm that the endotracheal tube is in the trachea, you must also ascertain that it is correctly placed within the trachea and not in a mainstem bronchus. Furthermore, since there is no guarantee that once the tube is correctly placed within the trachea it will remain there, you must continue to monitor end tidal CO_2 while the tube remains in place.

Auscultatory methods alone can no longer be relied upon to confirm placement of the tube in the trachea. The anesthesia literature is replete with reports of deaths and serious injuries resulting from undetected esophageal intubation. It is even more sobering to note[12] that "even a conscientious, careful anesthesiologist may be unable to differentiate between tracheal and esophageal intubation by the commonly employed methods." In a review of 29 cases of esophageal intubation by the American Society of Anesthesiologists' Committee on Profes-

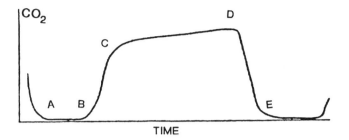

FIGURE 7.13. The normal capnogram. Point D marks the end-tidal CO_2, which is the best reflection of alveolar CO_2 tension. (From Barash, Cullen, and Stoelting,[14] with permission.)

sional Liability,[13] confirmation of correct endotracheal tube placement was entered in the anesthesia record in 18 of these cases.

During the past 10 years continuous carbon dioxide monitoring of exhaled gases, or capnometry, has become a standard of care in many developed countries in the world and is considered the most reliable method of detecting extratracheal tube placement. Capnometry (the measurement of CO_2 concentrations during a respiratory cycle) is different from capnography (the display of wave forms on a screen or a printout)[14] (Fig. 7.13).

Several devices are now available to detect CO_2 in exhaled gases. They range in price from less than $100 to over $10,000. The more expensive are more sophisticated units that provide a visual image of wave forms and numerical values. The end-tidal carbon dioxide detector (Fenem) is a simple, cheap, disposable device that changes color when exposed to carbon dioxide (purple to yellow)[15] (Fig. 7.14).

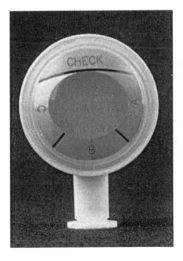
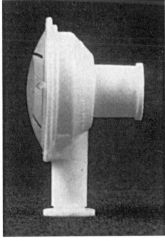

FIGURE 7.14. The Fenam carbon dioxide detector device. (From Denman, Hayes, and Higgins,[15] with permission).

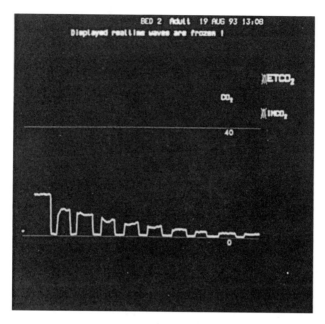

FIGURE 7.15. Simulated capnograph after esophageal intubation and washout of carbon dioxide from the stomach. (From Clyburn and Rosen,[24] with permission.)

It is important to recognize that CO_2 may be detected in the esophagus when exhaled gases enter the esophagus during mask ventilation.[16] Furthermore, CO_2 can be released from the stomach, in varying quantities, from carbonated beverages and antacids.[17] However, the wave forms do not follow the usual patterns (Fig. 7.15). It is also important to point out that capnometry/capnography are not foolproof. There have been a few isolated cases of failure, although most clinicians[18] agree that this technology is still the most reliable method of detecting unrecognized esophageal intubation in elective situations. Capnography alone is not totally reliable in emergency medical situations. A recent meta-analysis of over 2,000 emergency room intubations showed an aggregate sensitivity of 93% and specificity of 97% of capnography. These data indicate a 10% inaccuracy rate in emergency medical situations, which is unacceptable.[19] Therefore, one should not totally rely on capnography in emergency medical situations. We should also extend that philosophy to elective situations. Why is capnography so unreliable in emergency medicine? Capnography depends on the presence of carbon dioxide. If pulmonary blood flow is impaired, carbon dioxide will not be readily detected. The following box provides a list of false-negative and false-positive results leading to capnography misinterpretation (Boxes 7.1 and 7.2).

There are numerous other homemade devices for detecting inadvertent esophageal intubation that do not rely on the presence of CO_2 in exhaled gases. Negative-pressure devices are among the more interesting and are especially useful when end-tidal CO_2 monitoring is not available. Their principle is fairly simple, based

Box 7.1. False/Negative Results
(Tube in Trachea, Capnogram Suggests That Tube
Is in Esophagus)

1. Concurrent PEEP with ETT cuff leak
2. Severe airway obstruction
3. Low cardiac output
4. Severe hypotension
5. Pulmonary embolus
6. Advanced pulmonary disease

on the idea that the tracheobronchial tree is a semirigid structure and the esophagus is a collapsible one. Aspiration through a tube placed in the trachea is effective for removing respiratory gases, but aspiration through a tube in the esophagus is difficult because the negative pressure created by the aspirating syringe results in apposition of the muscular esophageal walls. Wee and Walker[20] have devised an esophageal detection device based on this principle. It consists of a 60 ml aspiration syringe connected to a catheter mount that, in turn, is connected to an endotracheal tube. The system must be airtight, lest false-negative results occur, but it is practical and cheap and all the necessary parts are readily available in every operating room (Fig. 7.16).

There is another esophageal detection device (EDD) available now called sonomatic confirmation of tracheal intubation (SCOTI). This is a handheld, battery-operated device used in emergency departments. It operates on the same principle as other EDDs. It does not require a ventilatory trial or exhaled carbon dioxide to provide a reading. Data is retrieved from the tip of the tube. There is an audible tone, a visual light-emitting diode (LED), and a numeric liquid crystal display (LCD). Feedback is instantaneous. A recent prospective, multicenter eval-

Box 7.2. False-Positive Results
(Tube Not in Trachea, Capnogram Suggests Tube
Is in Trachea)

1. Bag/valve/mask ventilation prior to intubation
2. Antacids in stomach
3. Recent ingestion of carbonated beverages
4. Tube in pharynx

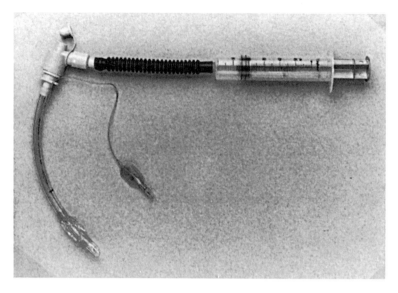

FIGURE 7.16. Negative-pressure esophageal detector device. (From Clyburn and Rosen,[24] with permission.)

uation of this device demonstrated a sensitivity of 93% and specificity of 98% in detecting correct endotracheal tube placement in the emergency setting.[21] However, this device is quite expensive.

In addition to using capnometry and other methods of continuously monitoring exhaled CO_2, you must confirm that the endotracheal tube is correctly positioned in the trachea. This is best achieved by auscultatory methods in an operating room setting and radiologically in an intensive care unit (ICU) setting. Immediately following intubation, first the tracheal placement of the tube is confirmed by capnometry and then the centimeter marking on the tube is noted at the level of the teeth. The distance from the teeth to midtrachea in the average adult is about 22 cm with the head in neutral position. If the centimeter marking is greater than 22 or less than 20, the tube should be adjusted before auscultation.

Auscultation is best performed by listening in the axillae while simultaneously ventilating the patient manually. In addition, you should observe chest wall movements (which are symmetrical when both lungs are being ventilated). Pulmonary compliance may appear diminished if the tube enters a mainstem bronchus, and peak inspiratory pressures will usually be well above the normal range of 15 to 25 cm because the complete tidal volume (normally shared by both lungs) is being forced into one lung (Fig. 7.17). These signs are not totally reliable, however, because they can also be observed in the presence of bronchospasm or pneumothorax. Nevertheless, auscultation remains the most practical method of confirming correct positioning of an endotracheal tube. Of course, fiberoptic bronchoscopy is a reliable method for confirming correct positioning of an endotracheal tube, especially when difficulties arise, and should be available in every operating suite.

FIGURE 7.17. Mainstem intubation.

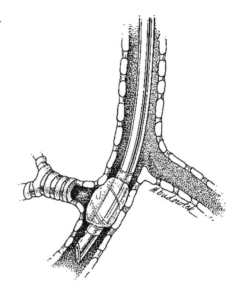

Pulse oximetry has become another indispensable monitoring device during airway intervention. Although it does not confirm correct or incorrect tube placement, it does act as a warning device and is particularly useful when teaching students airway management techniques. If during the course of endotracheal intubation the patient becomes hypoxic, you must strongly suspect incorrect tube placement or malfunction of a correctly placed tube; if there is any doubt about tube placement, remove the tube and ventilate by mask using 100% oxygen. Modern technology makes some of these decisions more difficult because the data obtained from capnography are very reliable. However, when faced with a crisis, you must revert to basic principles; and always remember the old adage "If in doubt, take it out." The longer you delay this process, the less time you will have to correct a problem; thus, be decisive and intervene early.

In most circumstances involving airway management there should be little hesitation about extubating a patient with suspected esophageal intubation. However, when an intubation has been especially difficult or the patient is extremely obese, there may be more reluctance than usual to extubate.

An alternative is to pass a tube changer, then extubate, and then perform mask ventilation with the tube changer in place. If the patient's condition improves with mask ventilation, you will have time to perform direct laryngoscopy again. The tube changer itself may be used to confirm whether the tube has been correctly placed. When a tube changer is advanced into the trachea, resistance is usually felt as its tip encounters the carina or mainstem bronchus at about 30 cm.[22] No such resistance is encountered at 30 cm when the changer is advanced into the esophagus. If indeed it was in the trachea initially, you may "railroad" another tube over it. Alternatively, you can apply mask ventilation with a "cutoff" tube in place.[23] If the patient's condition improves after mask ventila-

---

Box 7.3. Suspicion of Esophageal Intubation: Indications for Extubation

1. Poor or no chest movements
2. Cyanosis developing within 10 min of preoxygenation
3. Failure to oxygenate
4. Anomalous tube length
5. Tachycardia and hypertension
6. Increasing abdominal distension
7. Failure to palpate tube movement within the trachea
8. Absence of condensation in the expired gas
9. No CO_2 detected by capnograph

Source: Modified from Clyburn and Rosen,[24] with permission.

tion over an endotracheal tube, esophageal intubation is to be suspected. A number of other strategies may be used under these circumstances.[24] (Boxes 7.3 to 7.5).

Although the technique of endotracheal intubation becomes quite routine with practice, you should never undertake it lightly. The consequences of incorrect placement are devastating. The patient's cerebral function may be impaired for life, or his life ended. It would appear that the practice of auscultation of the chest following intubation is diminishing at least in the operating room setting. This is regrettable because there is no other reliable, practical way to detect endobronchial intubation. The most reliable method of confirming endotracheal tube placement in the trachea is to continuously monitor the concentration of CO_2 in exhaled gases. All other methods are either unreliable or impractical.

Box 7.4. Actions for Suspected Esophageal Intubation

1. Replace tracheal tube if laryngoscopy does not provide a good view of the larynx
2. Place a guide (bougie) through the tracheal tube if intubation was difficult and extubate; will permit reintubation if suspicion is unfounded
3. Extubate and do one of the following:
   a. Ventilate through mask
   b. Place a laryngeal mask airway
   c. Place an esophageal-tracheal Combitube
   d. Resort to failed-intubation drill

Source: Modified from Clyburn and Rosen,[24] with permission.

Box 7.5. Minimum Check After Placement of a Tracheal Tube

1. Auscultate over the trachea, lung apices, axillae, and epigastrium

    and *either*

2. Confirm that the CO_2 concentration is $> 4\%$

    or

3. Perform a negative-pressure test

Source: Modified from Clyburn and Rosen,[24] with permission.

Following is a list of the various methods used to verify tube placement in the trachea:

End-tidal CO_2 monitoring
Auscultation
Movement of the chest and epigastrium
Direct vision
Vital signs
Condensation in the tube
Videostethoscope
Negative pressure tests
Tube markings
Movement of the reservoir bag
Vocal silence (awake intubation)
Pulse oximetry
Fiberoptic bronchoscopy
Chest X ray
Tube changer
Cuff palpation
Transtracheal illumination
Sternal compression

Stabilization

Some novices are so overjoyed at successfully intubating a patient that they forget to secure the tube. Securing tubes may sound easier than it is. In an anesthetized patient it is easy, but on the ward it can be quite difficult. Often, when reoxygenated, a once comatose patient becomes revitalized and is distraught at finding a large plastic tube in his larynx. Patients have been known to bite the tube in half or to occlude it completely, preventing air from entering or leaving. Be prepared for this possibility. A combination of morphine and midazolam is

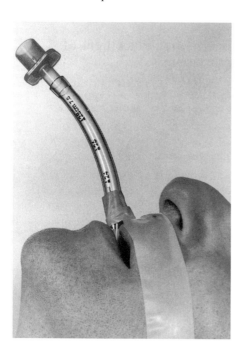

FIGURE 7.18. Securing the endotracheal tube.

usually quite effective in sedating such patients. If you are not planning to ventilate the patient, the dose of these drugs must be chosen very carefully. As a guide, morphine should be given in 2.5-mg increments and midazolam in 1-mg increments. As much as 15 mg of morphine and 10 mg of midazolam intravenously may be required for initial sedation in the average adult, but there is considerable variation. In securing the endotracheal tube, always use highly adhesive tape. The mandible is quite mobile; therefore, it is preferable to stabilize the tube to the maxilla (Fig. 7.18). If the tube is to be left in for some time, apply benzoin to the upper lip and recheck tube position after it has been stabilized.

Tape may not be adequate to secure the endotracheal tube under certain circumstances (e.g., oral, dental, or plastic surgery or burn debridements in the perioral region). There are a number of ways to secure it in these circumstances. You may wire it to a stable lower tooth or suture it to the tongue. If it is sutured, however, be sure to use sturdy suturing material and to introduce it horizontally through the median raphe of the tongue, lest it pull free.

Orotracheal Intubation by Direct Vision in an Adult (Miller Blade)

The Macintosh laryngoscope blade is widely used all over the world, especially in colonial countries. The straight blade, better known as the Miller blade, is quite popular in the United States. There is general agreement that the novice finds the Macintosh blade easier to use, which may explain its popularity. However, we are unable to see the larynx in up to 8% of cases when we use the Macintosh blade.[25] The curvature of the Macintosh blade impairs your vision when laryngoscopy is difficult. This deficiency led to the modification described in Figure 8.4B (improved vision Macintosh blade). The Macintosh laryngoscope blade tends to compress the tongue distally, causing posterior displacement of the epiglottis, thereby creating a soft tissue obstruction of the larynx.[26] There is a shallower learning curve with the Miller laryngoscope, but when you become familiar with its use, your ability to see the larynx improves. Your view is not obstructed by the curvature of the blade and because the tip of the blade is placed beneath the epiglottis, the tongue does not obstruct your view (Fig 7.19). There are some limitations to the Miller blade. It is rather narrow and if used incorrectly the tongue tends to overlap it. It is also sometimes difficult to pass the endotracheal tube when it is used. Henderson[27] has addressed some of these problems with a newly designed laryngoscope. The key to successful use of the straight laryngoscope blade is to introduce the blade at the right side of the mouth and keep it lateral to the tongue at all times (paraglossal approach).[28] Traditional teaching of laryngoscopy with the straight blade recommended introducing the blade in the midline, which invariably resulted in a difficult exposure because the tongue had a tendency to overlap. The newer designed Henderson straight blade hopefully will address some of the limitations of the Miller blade. New trainees should learn to perform laryngoscopy using both blades, bearing in mind that it is more difficult to master the straight blade.

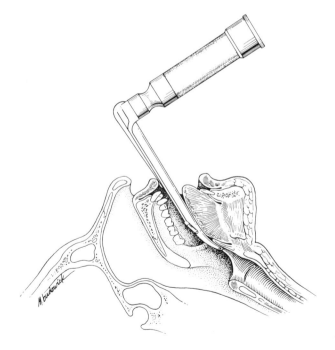

FIGURE 7.19. Direct laryngoscopy with a straight (Miller) blade.

Nasotracheal Intubation by Direct Vision in an Adult (Macintosh Blade)

Endotracheal tubes can also be introduced under direct vision through either nostril. This is slightly more difficult, however, and usually takes longer than orotracheal intubation. It is also more traumatic, and bleeding is quite common.

Preparation

In terms of equipment, the preparation for nasal intubation is basically the same as for orotracheal intubation. (See Chapters 4 and 5.) For emphasis, it should be restated that you should not perform nasotracheal intubation unless oxygen and suction are immediately available. Intubation trays should contain the same items. In addition, a Magill forceps is absolutely necessary for guiding the tube toward the glottis. Also, 0.25% phenylephrine, lidocaine, and a nebulizer should be available.

Before beginning nasal intubation, perform a cursory airway examination, paying specific attention to the nostrils. If the patient is conscious, check the patency of the nostrils and question him about any clotting abnormality. In some cases, the septum may be deviated or nasal polyps may be a problem. These factors will influence your choice. If time permits, spray both nostrils with a combination of 2% lidocaine and 0.25% phenylephrine or 4% cocaine. Sedation may or may not be required, depending upon the situation. Select an endotracheal tube whose internal diameter is a half-size less than would normally be used for an oral intubation. Lubricate the tube and selected nostril with K-Y Jelly.

Positioning

Position the head and neck as for orotracheal intubation, standing immediately behind the supine patient and extending his neck with your left hand.

Tube Insertion

Insert the tube, which should be connected to an oxygen source, into the nostril with the bevel pointing toward the septum (Fig. 7.20). Direct it vertically downward, at a right angle to the horizontal, until it reaches the oropharynx (Fig. 7.21). Some practitioners think that the nasal cavity is directed upward toward the brain. This misconception has led to the introduction of a nasogastric tube into the cranial cavity in a traumatized patient.[29]

Exposure

Open the mouth widely using the methods already described for orotracheal intubation.

Visualization

You can readily see the vocal cords in an average-sized patient using a Macintosh 3 laryngoscope blade.

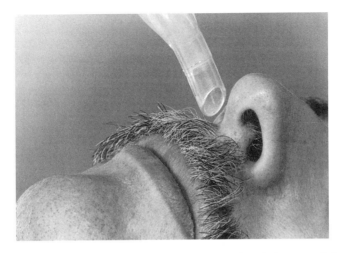

FIGURE 7.20. Nasotracheal intubation. Note that the bevel is pointing toward the septum.

Tube Placement

It is possible, in many instances, to direct the endotracheal tube toward and past the vocal cords manually by manipulating the tube from the top. More often than not, however, Magill forceps will be required to direct it toward the glottis.

Hold the forceps in your right hand and positioned as shown in Figure 7.22. Grip the tube towards its tip, above the point of attachment of the cuff (if possible), to avoid damaging the cuff. It can then be advanced by the assistant while you point it in the direction of the rima glottidis.

The tube should enter the trachea without difficulty. Occasionally, however, it will reach the vocal cords and not advance any further. In this situation, its distal end is probably impinging upon the anterior commissure, which lies nearly

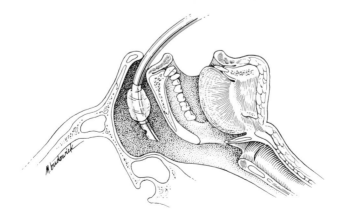

FIGURE 7.21. Introduction of the nasal endotracheal tube.

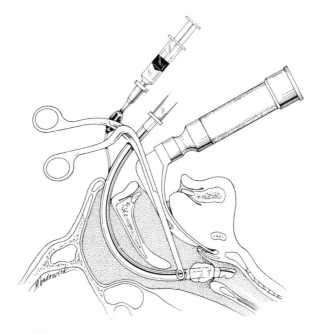

FIGURE 7.22. Nasotracheal intubation with the Magill (straight) forceps.

perpendicular to the axis of the trachea. The problem can be remedied by acutely flexing the cervical spine (Fig. 7.23). Another approach is to gently rotate the tube so that its concavity points toward the posterior trachea wall. If earlier attempts at nasotracheal intubation have been unsuccessful, do not withdraw the tube altogether but merely extract it far enough into the oropharynx to connect

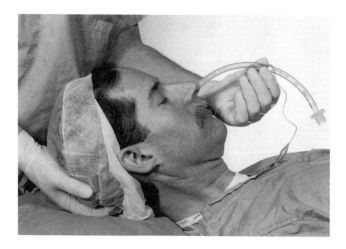

FIGURE 7.23. Flexion of the cervical spine facilitates nasotracheal intubation.

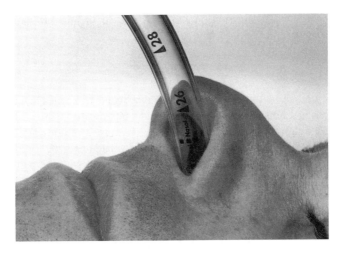

FIGURE 7.24. The average distance from the nose to the midtracheal region in an adult is about 25 cm.

it to an oxygen source. This will allow adequate oxygenation without undue trauma to the nasal mucosa. (In fact, the oxygen should be hooked up at all times during any intubation attempt.) The average distance from the nose to midtrachea is 25 cm in an individual with normal proportions weighing about 70 kg (154 lb) (Fig. 7.24).

Confirmation

The same rules apply for nasotracheal as for orotracheal intubation.

Stabilization

In addition to following previous advice about securing the tube, be particularly careful about securing one in an unconscious patient. The cartilaginous tip of the nose, because of its meager blood supply, is particularly vulnerable to pressure necrosis from an endotracheal tube. This problem can be allayed to some degree by using specifically designed tubes (nasal ring adhere Elwin [RAE]) and connectors that do not lean on the nasal rim during surgery.

Blind Nasotracheal Intubation

The technique of blind nasotracheal intubation, pioneered by Rowbotham and Magill[30,28] during World War I, has been replaced by improved direct and indirect methods, but in certain situations it remains invaluable. It is indicated when direct visualization of the airway is difficult or impossible because the mouth cannot be opened, or the instrumentation might damage teeth or other structures in the oropharynx. The preparation and equipment is identical to those used for the direct visualization approach.

Technique

The technique can be performed on an awake, sedated, or anesthetized patient. The only strict requirement is that the patient be capable of breathing spontaneously—although the use of succinylcholine has also been described.[31]

When performing the technique on an awake, sedated patient, spend a few moments explaining the procedure. It is usually performed with the patient supine, but when serious airway obstruction is present, it may be performed in the sitting position.

Spray both nostrils with 4% cocaine or a mixture of lidocaine and phenylephrine. The chosen nostril should be well lubricated. Place the tube, connected to an oxygen source, in the nostril and advance it into the oropharynx. More local anesthetic solution may be sprayed down the tube, whose tip should be pointing toward the glottis. Flex the cervical spine by placing a folded towel beneath the patient's head. Then extend the head and pull the mandible upward with your left hand. Occlude the mouth and free nostril at this time.

Next, to make the breath sounds more audible, disconnect the oxygen tubing. By lowering your left ear over the endotracheal tube, you will be able to hear and feel the breath sounds and can use them as an indicator of how close the tube tip is to the airway. Slowly advance the tube with the right hand. When it enters the airway, the patient usually coughs and a definite tubular sound replaces the harsher breath sound previously heard. A number of reports[32,33] refer to the use of a simple whistle, which can be attached to the tube connector during intubation attempts.

Blind nasal intubation is not always achieved on the first attempt and in some cases may require several attempts. If the tube does not enter the larynx, its tip is above the glottic opening, below it in the esophagus, or on either side of it in the piriform sinus. When the tube is excessively curved or when the patient's cervical spine is overextended, the tip of the tube tends to abut the anterior commissure. This can be remedied by withdrawing it slightly, flexing the neck, and advancing the tube slowly into the airway. The tube can also enter the esophagus if the patient's head is excessively flexed or the tube is too straight.

Occasionally, the tube will fail to go beneath the epiglottis and instead enter the vallecula. This problem can be remedied by withdrawing it slightly, pulling the mandible forward, and rotating the tube through 90°. An attempt should then be made to advance the tube into the glottis. One report[34] describes extrusion of the tongue as an aid to blind nasal intubation.

Finally, the tube may be deflected laterally toward either piriform sinus. Palpation of the neck will usually reveal to which side it is pointing. The tube should then be withdrawn slightly and rotated medially, its point directed toward the glottis.

Successful blind nasal intubation is usually heralded by a harsh "bovine" cough followed by vocal silence. However, other evidence of correct placement is also sought as described for orotracheal intubation.

In modern times the art of blind nasotracheal intubation is being rapidly replaced by fiberoptic laryngoscopy and bronchoscopy. Despite this new trend, however, physicians involved in airway management should be encouraged to learn the blind technique.

Summary

Nasotracheal intubation, whether by direct visualization or by the blind method, is usually more difficult to perform, more traumatic, and more time-consuming than orotracheal intubation. However, it has one important advantage—the presence of the tube in the nasopharynx allows oxygenation and sometimes ventilation during laryngoscopy while attempting intubation. (Complications of nasotracheal intubation are discussed in Chapter 9.)

Airway Maneuvers

Anesthesiologists and other experts in airway management employ some maneuvers to facilitate intubation or to protect patients against aspiration. Some of these maneuvers will now be described.

BURP

The BURP maneuver was first described by Knill in 1993[35] and is now a well-recognized aid to improve visualization of the airway during routine and difficult intubation. The maneuver has three distinct components:

1. Posterior pressure on the larynx against the cervical vertebrae (**B**ackward)
2. Superior pressure on the larynx as far as possible (**U**pward)
3. Lateral pressure on the larynx to the right (**R**ight)

By adding (**P**ressure) to the preceding terms, Knill came up with a memorable acronym, BURP.

The efficacy of this maneuver has been tested in 630 patients by Takahata et al and they concluded that it was a worthwhile maneuver and should be used routinely during attempts at laryngoscopy.[36]

OELM

Benumof et al[37] described a variation of the BURP maneuver referred to as Optimal External Laryngeal Manipulation, and it implies that one should experiment to find the optimal maneuver on the larynx to improve visualization.

Sellick's Maneuver (Cricoid Pressure)

Sellick's maneuver[38] is the name assigned to cricoid pressure applied during rapid sequence induction (RSI) of anesthesia to prevent passive regurgitation of gastric contents and aspiration. This maneuver has now become a standard of care in anesthesia in any situation in which patients are considered at risk for aspiration. It is not a universally accepted maneuver and its use has never been validated. The original experimental work was carried out on cadavers. There are many concerns about cricoid pressure. First of all, it is frequently applied incorrectly. It may distort one's view of the airway. It may damage the airway. It may increase the risk of regurgitation, and there are other issues as well. Brimacombe et al[39] recently published an extensive review of this topic.

Cricoid pressure is usually applied by an informed assistant during RSI of anesthesia. The single-handed method involves placing the thumb and middle finger on either side of the cricoid cartilage and the index finger above to prevent movement of the cricoid. A pressure of 20 N should be applied until loss of consciousness, at which time it is increased to 30 N.[40] The assistant is instructed to maintain pressure on the cricoid until instructed to release. Clearly, the operator must be assured that the endotracheal tube is in the trachea and is able to manually ventilate the patient, and that there is no leak.

Failed Intubation (Normal Anatomy)

Failed intubation in a patient with normal anatomy is most often caused by poor positioning of the head. Novices seem to have difficulty opening the mouth wide enough, and considerable time is lost trying to place the laryngoscope in the mouth. When they do succeed, they allow the tongue to overlap the laryngoscope blade, and this blocks their vision. Practitioners learning the technique often flex the wrist of their left hand in a pivoting motion, exerting excessive pressure on the patient's upper teeth. This does not help visualize the airway and it may damage the upper teeth. Instead, a firm but steady upward and forward motion should be used without flexing the wrist. Beginners are generally aware of the relative urgency of the situation and therefore rush. In contrast, some individuals are too timid in their approach and do not apply enough force.

The common causes of failed intubation in a patient with normal anatomy are as follows:

Incorrect positioning of the patient's head
Poor oral access
Tongue overlapping the laryngoscope blade
Pivoting laryngoscope against the upper teeth
Rushing
Being overly cautious
Inappropriate equipment

Summary

As with most endeavors, it becomes easier to manage orotracheal intubation when the technique is broken down into its component steps. To intubate a patient, flex the cervical spine, extend the atlantooccipital joint, open the mouth, insert a laryngoscope blade, displace the tongue, elevate the epiglottis, expose the vocal cords (preferably without chipping the patient's upper teeth), and guide the endotracheal tube through the rima glottidis—all within 30 seconds. Once the tube is inserted, confirm that it is in the proper place; ideally the tip should lie at the mid-tracheal level. Gurgling sounds in the epigastrium or asymmetry of breath sounds and chest wall excursion is a poor prognostic sign that necessitates repositioning of the tube. If there are any doubts about tube placement, they must be dealt with immediately. First, observe the end-tidal CO_2 monitor, then listen for breath sounds over the chest and epigastrium. If you are still not satisfied, immediately perform direct laryngoscopy. If doubt still remains, remove the tube and ventilate the patient by mask using 100% oxygen. When the tube is placed properly, inflate the cuff with sufficient pressure to seal off the trachea, but not so much that you burst the cuff or cause tracheal ischemia. (Unfortunately for the novice, the point at which these limits are reached may be best appreciated only in retrospect.) In addition, you must secure the endotracheal tube with adhesive tape, since tubes and patients have a natural tendency to become separated from each other.

The procedure for nasotracheal intubation via direct visualization is similar, except that you insert the tube into the nostril and then perform laryngoscopy to direct it through the rima glottidis. In blind nasotracheal intubation, which is used in patients who cannot undergo direct laryngoscopy, you must rely on the loudness of the breath sounds to guide the tube into the trachea.

There are numerous pitfalls in learning how to intubate, and most novices stumble into a few of them. It is of little consolation for the beginner to know that failure to intubate is usually the result of faulty technique rather than a faulty patient. (Nevertheless, as discussed in the next chapter, intubating patients with structural anomalies or certain diseases may prove difficult even for experienced anesthesiologists.) As your technique improves and you become more comfortable in performing intubations, both you and the patient will breathe more easily.

References

1. Berthoud M, Read DH, Norman J. Preoxygenation: how long? *Anaesthesia*. 1983;38: 96–102.
2. Baraka AS, Taha SK, Aouad MT, et al. Comparison of maximal breathing and tidal volume breathing techniques. *Anesthesiology*. 1999;91:612–616.
3. Nimmagadda U, Chiravuri SD, Salem MR, et al. Preoxygenation with tidal volume and deep breathing techniques: the impact of duration of breathing and fresh gas flow. *Anes Analg*. 2001;92:1337–1341.
4. Flaherty DO, Adams AP. Endotracheal intubation skills of medical students. *J R Soc Med*. 1992;85:603–604.
5. Safar P. *Cardiopulmonary Cerebral Resuscitation*. 1st ed. Philadelphia: WB Saunders; 1981.
6. Bannister PB, MacBeth RG. Direct laryngoscopy and tracheal intubation. *Lancet*. 1944;1:651–654.
7. Magill IW. Endotracheal anesthesia. *Am J Surg*. 1936;34:450–455.

8. Kirstein A. Autoskopie des larynx und der trachea. *Archive fur Laryngologie und Rhinologie.* 1895;3:156–164.

9. Jackson C. The technique of insertion of intratracheal insufflation tubes. *Surg Gynecol Obstet.* 1913;17:507–509.

10. Adnet F, Borron SW, Dumas JL, et al. Study of the "sniffing position" by MRI. *Anesthesiology.* 2001;94:83–86.

11. Chou HC. Rethinking the three axis alignment theory for direct laryngoscopy. *Acta Anaesthesiol Scand.* 2001;45:261–264.

12. Solazzi RW, Ward RJ. The spectrum of medical liability cases. *Int Anesth Clinics.* 1984;22:43–59.

13. ASA Committee on Professional Liability. Chicago, IL.

14. Barash PG, Cullen BF, Stoelting RK. *Clinical Anaesthesia.* 2nd ed. Philadelphia: JB Lippincott Co; 1992:739 [illustration].

15. Denman WT, Hayes M, Higgins D. The Fenem CO_2 detector device. *Anaesthesia.* 1990;45:465–467.

16. Linko K, Paloheimo M, Tammsto T. Capnography for detection of accidental esophageal intubation. *Acta Anaesthiol Scand.* 1983;27:199–202.

17. Sum Ping ST, Mehta MP, Symreng T. Reliability of capnography in identifying esophageal intubation with carbonated beverage or antacid in the stomach. *Anesth Analg.* 1991;73:333–337.

18. Deluty S, Turndorf H. The failure of capnography to properly assess endotracheal tube location. *Anesthesiology.* 1993;78:783–784.

19. Li J. Capnography alone is imperfect for endotracheal tube placement confirmation. *J Emerg Med.* 2001;20:223–229.

20. Wee MY, Walker AK. The esophageal detector device. *Anaesthesia.* 1988;43:27–29.

21. Li J. A prospective multicenter trial testing the SCOTI device for confirmation of endotracheal tube placement. *J Emerg Med.* 2001;20:231–239.

22. Kidd JF, Dyson A, Latto IP. Successful difficult intubation: use of gum elastic bougie. *Anaesthesia.* 1988;43:437–438.

23. Howells TH, Riethmuller RJ. Signs of endotracheal intubation. *Anaesthesia.* 1980;35:984–986.

24. Clyburn P, Rosen M. Accidental oesophageal intubation. *Br J Anaesth.* 1994;73:55–63.

25. Crosby ET, Cooper RM, Douglas MJ, et al. The unanticipated difficult airway with recommendations for management. *Can J Anaesth.* 1998;45:757–776.

26. Horton WA, Fahy L, Charters P. Factor analysis in difficult tracheal intubation: laryngoscopy-induced airway obstruction. *Br J Anaesth.* 1990;65:801–805.

27. Henderson JJ. Solutions to the problem of difficult tracheal tube passage associated with the paraglossal straight laryngoscopy technique. *Anaesthesia.* 1999;54:601–602.

28. Magill IW. Technique in endotracheal anaesthesia. *Ann Surg.* 1910;52:23–29.

29. Temple AP, Katz J. Management of acute head injury. *AORNJ.* 1987;46:1068.

30. Rowbotham ES, Magill IW. *Proc R Soc Med.* 1921;14:17.

31. Collins PD, Godkin RA. Awake blind nasal intubation: a dying art. *Anaes Int Care.* 1992;20:225–227.

32. Jantzen JP. Tracheal intubation—blind but not mute. *Anesth Analg.* 1985;64:646–653.

33. Dyson A, Saunders PR, Giesecke AH. Awake blind nasal intubation: use of a simple whistle. *Anaesthesia.* 1990;45:71.

34. Adams AL, Cane RD, Shapiro BA. Tongue extrusion as an aid to blind nasal intubation. *Crit Care Med.* 1982;5:335–336.

35. Knill RL. Difficult laryngoscopy made easy with a BURP. *Can J Anaesth.* 1993; 40:279–282.
36. Takahata O, Kubota M, Mamiya K, et al. The efficacy of the "BURP" maneuver during a difficult laryngoscopy. *Anesth Analg.* 1997;84:419–421.
37. Benumof JL, Cooper SD. Quantitative improvement in laryngoscopic view by optimal external laryngeal manipulation. *J Clin Anesth.* 1996;8:136–140.
38. Sellick BA. Cricoid pressure to control regurgitation of stomach contents during induction of anesthesia. *Lancet.* 1961;2:404.
39. Brimacombe JR, Berry A. Cricoid pressure. *Can J Anaesth.* 1997;44:414–425.
40. Vanner RG. Mechanisms of regurgitation and its prevention with cricoid pressure. *Int J Obst Anes.* 1993;2:207–215.

Suggested Readings

Applebaum EL, Bruce DL. *Tracheal Intubation.* Philadelphia: WB Saunders; 1976.

Gillespie N. *Endotracheal Anesthesia.* Madison, WI: University of Wisconsin Press; 1950.

Hagberg CA. Handbook of Difficult Airway Management. 1st ed. Philadelphia: Churchill Livingstone; 2000.

Latto IP, Rosen M. *Difficulties in Tracheal Intubation.* London: Bailliere-Tindall; 1985.

Roberts JT. *Fundamentals of Tracheal Intubation.* New York: Grune & Stratton; 1983.

8
The Difficult Airway

Our goals for this chapter are to provide you with basic information about the difficult airway. Most of the discussion will center around difficult intubation. However, we will also discuss difficult mask ventilation and difficult laryngoscopy. We will provide definitions for these terms. We will also present information about equipment available to deal with the difficult airway, but it will not be exhaustive. Finally, we will provide an update on the difficult airway algorithm and the application of this algorithm in various settings.

Intubation problems account for about a third of all deaths and serious injuries related to anesthesia.[1,2] In the Confidential Inquiry into Maternal Deaths in England and Wales, between 1973 and 1984,[3] 41% of all such mishaps attributable directly to anesthesia were linked to difficulties with tracheal intubation. Until quite recently, most anesthesiologists viewed difficult intubation as a minor setback and few considered it a serious issue. Consequently, the problem has been dealt with in a haphazard manner, without protocol or guidelines. In recent years the literature has come to contain more reports on the subject, and now most of us are aware that difficult intubation may be the harbinger of serious morbidity or even death. A difficult intubation needs to be managed like any other medical emergency. Most clinicians respond robotically to a cardiac arrest and quickly move through the ABCs of resuscitation without even thinking. We must adopt a similar attitude when dealing with difficult intubations.

In any busy operating room with patients undergoing routine elective surgery, there are usually one or two difficult intubations each week. However, over a 1-year period, the average anesthesiologist will be exposed to this emergency only a few times and a resident in training may encounter it even less frequently. Duncan et al[4] have estimated that a resident in training needs to be exposed to this emergency about 29 times before competency can be achieved. Few residency training programs are capable of providing this kind of experience. The problem is even greater in obstetrics, in which the need for general anesthesia has decreased dramatically during the past 25 years because the pattern of practice has changed predominantly to regional anesthesia (which is considered safer). Therefore, groups who work solely in obstetric anesthesia get very little exposure to difficult intubations and may not perform well when confronted with one. For this reason it is crucial that difficult airway drills be incorporated into routine practice guidelines and into residency training curricula.

In the past, we have relied heavily on our surgical colleagues to rescue us when we "lost the airway." Most of us believed that all surgeons could perform tracheostomy. The truth is most can, but the speed at which they do so varies greatly, and except for a few subspecialty groups who do it frequently, most surgeons cannot perform this operation quickly enough to prevent cerebral anoxia from occurring, simply because they are called upon so infrequently to do it.

There is one basic tenet in the practice of medicine that all physicians must adhere to: "We must not perform procedures on patients unless we are capable of dealing with the complications." Anesthesiologists, as a group, have not consistently adhered to this principle until recently, and even at this time there are some reluctant participants. Every anesthesiologist must be prepared to establish a surgical airway if conventional means fail. When airway problems occur and the oxygen supply is removed, every second counts. We cannot waste time waiting for the arrival of a surgeon to perform a tracheostomy. We must be prepared to deal with this problem ourselves. Residents in training therefore should be exposed to the necessary equipment and techniques required to establish a surgical airway and ideally be allowed to perform these procedures on animals during their training. Transtracheal jet ventilation (TTJV) and percutaneous cricothyrotomy are two procedures that all anesthesiologists should be able to perform. There are no reliable outcome data available yet to suggest that any one of these techniques is better than another; and, clearly, design of such a study would be extremely difficult. A number of cricothyrotomy kits are available on the market (and have been discussed in detail in Chapter 10).

One problem that we immediately encounter when discussing this topic is terminology. What do we mean by the *difficult airway*? To some, it means spending 10 or 15 minutes trying to intubate the trachea; to others it means difficult mask ventilation or failure to intubate. We will now attempt to provide you with definitions for these terms based on the literature.

Definition

The American Society of Anesthesiologists (ASA) task force[5] defined the difficult airway as a clinical situation in which a conventionally trained anesthesiologist experiences difficulty with mask ventilation, difficulty with tracheal intubation, or both. They define difficult mask ventilation as follows: "It is not possible for the unassisted anesthesiologist to maintain the oxygen saturation above 90% using 100% oxygen and positive pressure mask ventilation in a patient whose saturation was greater than 90% before the anesthetic intervention;

and/or it is not possible for the unassisted anesthesiologist to prevent or reverse signs of inadequate ventilation during positive pressure mask ventilation." Difficult laryngoscopy was defined as follows: "It is not possible to visualize any portion of the vocal cords with conventional laryngoscopy"; and they defined difficult endotracheal intubation as "proper insertion of the tracheal tube with conventional laryngoscopy requires more than 3 attempts or more than 10 minutes."[5] What do we mean by *conventional laryngoscopy*? Clearly, conventional laryngoscopy could apply to those who predominantly use a Macintosh or a Miller blade. There is some suggestion that the incidence of difficult laryngoscopy is less with the Miller blade.

The definition of *difficult intubation* has been challenged by at least one group on the basis that it should not be **time** nor **attempt** based because successful intubation can be achieved in less than 10 minutes or in less than 3 attempts in some cases, even when presented with a grade 4 laryngoscopic view.[6] Furthermore, the laryngoscopist, when presented with a grade 4 view, may immediately use an airway adjunct and successfully intubate the patient on the first attempt. They offer an alternative definition for difficult tracheal intubation as follows: "when an experienced laryngoscopist, using direct laryngoscopy, requires (1) more than one attempt with the same blade; (2) a change in blade or an adjunct to a direct laryngoscope (i.e., bougie); or (3) use of an alternative device or technique following failed intubation with direct laryngoscopy." Unfortunately, we will not obtain accurate data on this topic until we all agree on a universal definition.

Incidence of the Difficult Airway

We now have some good data on the incidence of difficult laryngoscopy, difficult intubation, failed intubation, and difficult mask ventilation (Table 8.1). Difficult laryngoscopy (defined as a Cormack and Lehane grade 3 or 4) occurs in 1.5% to 8.5% of cases. Difficult intubation occurs much less frequently than difficult laryngoscopy (Table 8.2).[7] Failure to intubate occurs in about 0.3% of cases and inability to mask occurs in about 0.01% of cases. These numbers vary depending upon the population studied. Obstetric patients have a higher incidence of difficult intubation than surgical patients,[8] and it is well known that the incidence of difficult intubation is less in children than in adults. Rose and Cohen have also shown that the incidence of difficult intubation is greater in males than females and in the 40 to 59 age group. In all of these discussions we are assuming that experienced individuals are performing these tasks (at least 2 years' experience).

Etiology

The causes of difficult intubation are discussed in some detail in Chapter 5. Instead of presenting a long list of diseases and syndromes that may cause problems, we will arbitrarily divide difficult intubation into three broad categories:

TABLE 8.1. The incidence of difficult airway—prospective reviews

Population (n)	Difficult/ failed ventilation	Grade 3/4 laryngeal view	Difficult intubation ($\geq$ 3 attempts)	Failed intubation	Reference
general surgical (18,500)	0.01%		2.5%	0.3%	5
obstetrical (1500)		1.8%	1.8%	0.13%	6
general surgical (3,325)		8.5%	1.9%		7
general surgical (6,477)		1.5%	1.7%		8
general surgical (3,312)			3.8%		9
general surgical (10,507)	0.07%	6.1%			10
general surgical + obstetrical (15,616)	0.025% (requiring tracheostomy)		1.15%	0.28%	11

Source: Crosby, Cooper, Douglas, et al,[6] with permission.

limited access to the oropharynx or nasopharynx; poor visualization of the larynx; and diminished cross-sectional area of the larynx or trachea.

Limited Access to the Oropharynx or Nasopharynx

Conventional methods of endotracheal intubation require the insertion of a laryngoscope blade into the oropharynx as a primary step. Any disease or condition that limits access to the oropharynx or nasopharynx may impair your ability to perform endotracheal intubation. (See Chapter 5.)

Inability to See the Larynx

Having gained access to the oropharynx, you must next move the soft tissues forward to allow the laryngeal opening to come into view. Failure to do so will make intubation difficult.

TABLE 8.2. Difficult intubation

Preoperative evaluation of airway	N	Easy (%)	Difficult (%)
Normal	8523	95.2	1.3
↓ Mouth opening	58	62.4	9.7
↓ Neck mobility	418	75.1	3.2
↓ Temporomandibular joint function	194	73.2	10.6
↓ Hypopharynx vision	332	81.8	5.2
2 abnormalities	254	62.1	6.8
$\geq$ 3 abnormalities	57	44.9	6.3

Source: Modified from Rose and Cohen,[7] with permission.

Diminished Cross-Sectional Area of the Larynx or Trachea

Finally, in some cases, although there may be no problems opening the mouth or seeing the larynx, for some reason you are unable to advance the endotracheal tube far enough into the trachea. Narrowing of the larynx and trachea may necessitate the insertion of a much smaller tube.

Equipment

Endotracheal intubation became a routine procedure in anesthesia when neuromuscular blocking drugs were introduced. Although the equipment used initially was quite rudimentary, tremendous advances have been made during the past 50 years, and now modern-day equipment is both sophisticated and versatile. Following is a brief description of some of these devices.

Endotracheal Tubes

There is a great variety of endotracheal tubes to choose from. The **Endotrol** has the appearance of a regular endotracheal tube but is equipped with a "built-in" stylet (see Fig. 3.35). Traction may be applied to the stylet by placing a finger in the loop and will cause the tube to become more curved by forcing its tip upward. The Endotrol is used to direct the tip of the endotracheal tube toward the glottis when the glottis is not readily visible or during an attempt at blind nasal intubation. It may also be used in a patient with cervical spine injuries.

Stylets

A stylet is an elongated metal or plastic rod with a smooth surface devoid of sharp edges (see Fig. 3.40). Ideally, it should be stiff yet flexible enough to let you alter the natural curve of an endotracheal tube. It must not be allowed to extend beyond the distal end of the endotracheal tube, and it must never be used to force entry into the trachea, lest complications occur (including submucosal dissection, lacerations, hemorrhage, hematomas, tracheal perforation, pneumothorax, and pneumomediastinum). The stylet may be lubricated to facilitate ease of entry and withdrawal from the endotracheal tube, and the tube may be preformed so that its distal end has the appearance of a hockey stick. This configuration allows one to direct the tube beneath the epiglottis toward the vocal apparatus (see Fig. 3.41).

Gum Elastic Bougies or "Tube Changers"

Gum elastic catheters or bougies (Fig. 8.1) have been used by clinicians in the UK for years to facilitate difficult intubations, especially when the posterior portion of the larynx is barely visible or the epiglottis cannot be elevated.[9] Many of these catheters are flexible and their distal end may be preformed to allow the tip to be

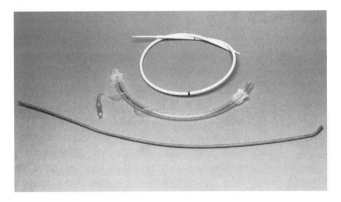

FIGURE 8.1. "Tube changers" or bougies.

directed beneath the epiglottis and into the airway. A small endotracheal tube is then advanced over the bougie into the glottis.[10] The bougie is then withdrawn and correct placement of the endotracheal tube is confirmed. We recommend using the laryngoscope to elevate the epiglottis as much as possible, lest the tube not pass easily over the bougie (which should be well lubricated before use). The Eschmann tracheal introducer is one of the most popular bougie devices. There is a characteristic "speed bump" sensation detected when the bougie is advanced into the trachea as it traverses the tracheal rings. Of course, this sensation will not be detected if the bougie enters the esophagus. Kidd et al[11] reported their experience with the bougie in a simulated setting. They studied 100 patients with a simulated grade 3 laryngoscopic view in 98 cases and genuine grade 3 view in 2 cases. They successfully entered the trachea in 78% of cases and entered the esophagus in 22%. The speed bump sensation was detected in 90% of the tracheal placements. They also noted a "holdup" at a certain point as the bougie was advanced into the trachea (usually noted between 24 and 40 cm), presumably due to encroachment on the smaller airways. This holdup was not detected if the bougie was in the esophagus. These are useful signs when using this "blind" technique. Kidd et al's study may not be a true reflection of reality, but it is the best information available on this topic.

A bougie can be used to change the endotracheal tube, especially when laryngoscopy is difficult. The hollow tube changers may be connected to an oxygen source or to a capnograph and will also facilitate jet ventilation (Fig. 8.2). Bougies or tube changers should be several centimeters longer than the endotracheal tube. They are not foolproof, however, and you may expect occasional failures especially when the airway anatomy is grossly distorted. A number of devices are commercially available.

Laryngoscopes

The basic components of laryngoscopes have been described in Chapter 3. In this section we will concentrate on blades, handles, and light sources that have been modified to facilitate intubation under difficult circumstances.

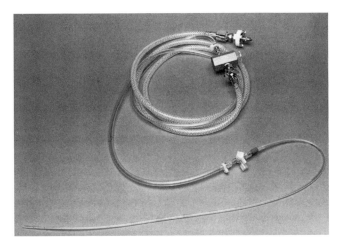

FIGURE 8.2. Hollow tube changer connected to jet ventilator.

Left-Handed Macintosh Blade

Left-handed Macintosh blades[12,13] are available not just for left-handed individuals but also for anatomical abnormalities on the right side of the face and mouth (Fig. 8.3).

Improved-Vision Macintosh Blade

This blade[14] (Fig. 8.4) is very similar to the regular Macintosh except that its midportion (which is normally curved) is concave, allowing improved vision.

Polio Blade

The polio blade is also a modification of the Macintosh, made by altering the angle between the blade and the handle (Fig. 8.5).[15] It was originally designed

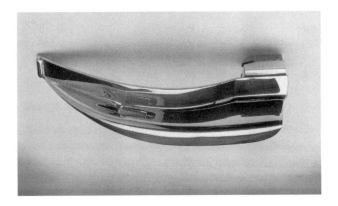

FIGURE 8.3. Left-handed Macintosh blade.

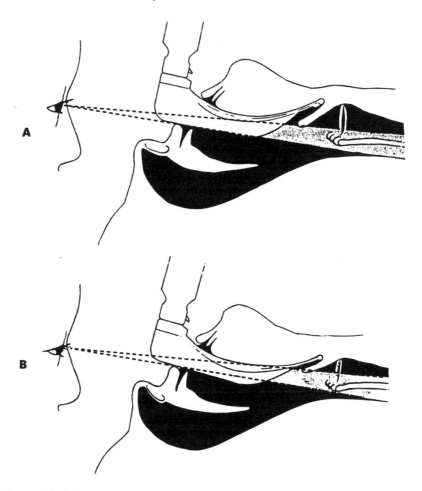

FIGURE 8.4. **A.** Regular Macintosh. **B.** Improved-vision Macintosh blade. (From Racz,[14] with permission.)

for use in patients confined to the Drinker respirator (iron lung). It may now be used when the anteroposterior diameter of the chest is such that insertion of a laryngoscope into the mouth is impossible. Its main disadvantage is that all mechanical advantages of the conventional blade are lost.[16] Alternatively, a regular Macintosh blade with a "stunted" handle may be used.

Oxiport Macintosh

This Macintosh blade has been modified to include an oxygen port (Fig. 8.6), allowing the oxygenation of patients during intubation attempts.

Tull Macintosh

In the Tull modification, suction is applied to the airway (Fig. 8.7).

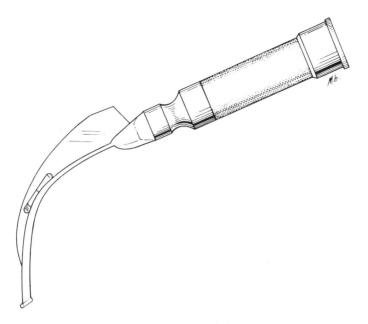

FIGURE 8.5. Polio blade.

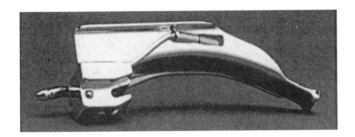

FIGURE 8.6. The Oxiport Macintosh.

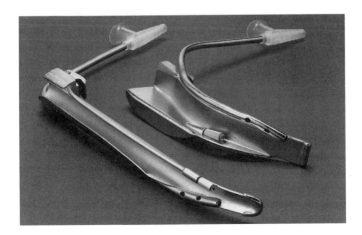

FIGURE 8.7. The Tull Macintosh. A suction port is attached to the blade.

Huffman Modification

A prism can be attached to a Macintosh laryngoscope blade (Huffman modification)[17-19] to refract the light, allowing you to literally see "around corners" (Fig. 8.8). Although being able to see the airway does not always ensure successful intubation, it will at least give you some idea of the general direction in which to point the endotracheal tube.

Siker Blade

The Siker blade is a reflecting surface that may help you see the anterior larynx. The laryngoscope is awkward to use, however, and you need to remember that the image of the larynx is inverted.

Howland Adapter

The Howland adapter is another example of how the laryngoscope handle may be modified to aid exposure of the larynx. This modification decreases the angle that the blade makes with the horizontal axis of the patient, giving you a definite mechanical advantage. However, because of the design of the handle, it may be difficult to insert the blade into the mouth, especially in patients with an increased anteroposterior chest diameter. Ideally, the Howland adapter should have a shorter handle (Fig. 8.9).

Racz-Allen Blade

The Racz-Allen blade is straight with a curved tip (Fig. 8.10). The straight portion is hinged and held in place by a spring that allows lateral movement of the straight portion.

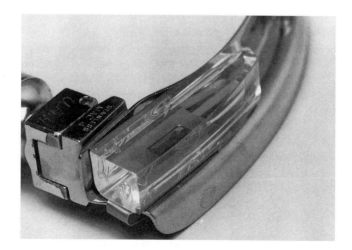

FIGURE 8.8. The Huffman modification. A prism is attached to the blade.

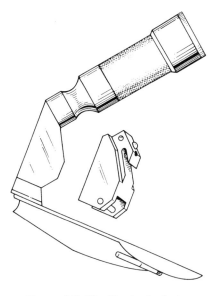

FIGURE 8.9. The Howland adapter.

Choi Blade

The double-angled Choi blade [20,21] was designed to enhance your ability to lift the epiglottis. It is angled in two places and has no flange, which allows more room to pass a tube into the trachea (Fig. 8.11).

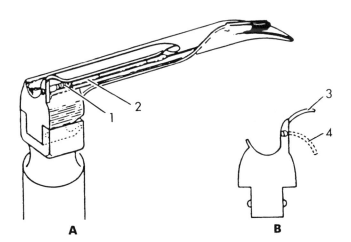

FIGURE 8.10. The Racz-Allen blade. **A.** Side view. **B.** Back view. *1*, Spring; *2*, threaded screw; *3*, normal position; *4*, full displacement of portion that flexes. (From Racz,[14] with permission.)

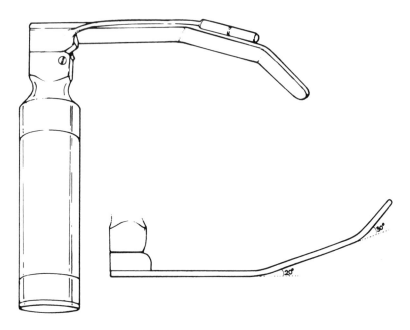

FIGURE 8.11. The double-angled Choi blade. (From Choi,[20] with permission.)

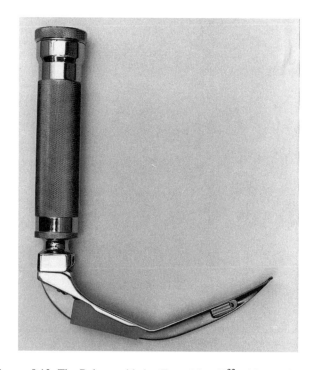

FIGURE 8.12. The Belscope blade. (From Mayall,[22] with permission.)

Belscope Blade

This laryngoscope blade[22,23] is a modified straight blade that has been bent to form a wide V-shaped angle. It is designed to reduce dental trauma. To improve vision, a prism may be attached (Fig. 8.12).

McCoy Levering Laryngoscope[24]

This is another modification of the standard Macintosh blade that enables you to have a better view of the vocal apparatus. Its tip is hinged, and the angle of the hinged portion can be altered by a lever attached to the handle (Fig. 8.13). The main advantage of this modification is improved visualization without altering the axis of the handle. The efficacy of the McCoy blade has been evaluated in a small clinical trial involving about 50 patients. The difficult airway was simulated by neck immobilization in the neutral position. Laryngoscopic views improved by one grade in 70% of patients with a grade 2 view and 83% of patients with a grade 3 view, compared with the view obtained with the standard Macintosh blade. However, no improvement occurred with a grade 4 view.[25] These results have been corroborated by other investigators.[26,27]

Bullard Laryngoscope

The Bullard laryngoscope[28,29] was designed for difficult intubations. Consisting of a rigid curved blade with a fiberoptic bundle posteriorly, it may be used in both adults and children. It is battery operated or may be connected to a light

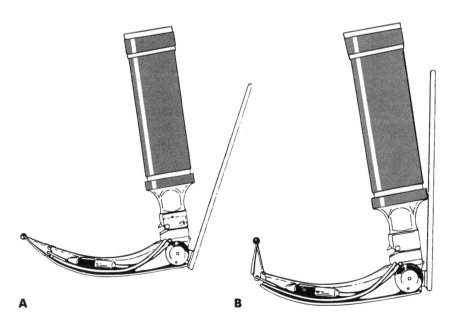

A   **B**

FIGURE 8.13. The levering laryngoscope. **A.** Normal position. **B.** Tip elevated. (From McCoy,[24] with permission.)

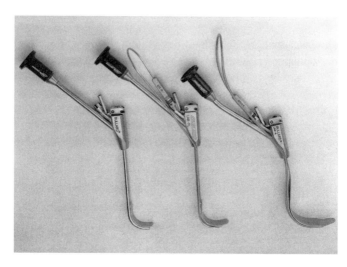

FIGURE 8.14. The Bullard laryngoscope. (From Borland[28] and Bjoraker,[29] with permission.)

source. It comes with an eyepiece attached to the main body of the scope at a 45° angle, and a teaching head is also available. The Bullard device is not immediately user-friendly, however, and practice on normal airways is recommended first (Fig. 8.14).

Some studies have shown that the learning curve for the Bullard laryngoscope is similar to that required to learn fiberoptic assisted intubation.[29,30] The Bullard laryngoscope functions well with the head and neck in the neutral position and when there is limited mouth opening. It has two ports, one for oxygen, suction, or injection and the other to house a malleable, intubating stylet. A number of studies have reported high success rates when the Bullard is used in difficult airway situations by experienced personnel.[31]

A number of straight laryngoscope blades have been modified to facilitate difficult intubation. For more details about laryngoscope blades and airway equipment, refer to Dorsch and Dorsch[32] and McIntyre.[33]

Fiberoptic-Assisted Intubation

Fiberoptically assisted intubation is one of the most important advances in airway management since the introduction of the laryngoscope. It allows endotracheal intubation to be performed even in the most difficult circumstances. Details about this equipment and use appear in Chapter 4.

Rigid Bronchoscope

Each difficult intubation tray should have a rigid bronchoscope to enable you to ventilate the patient with tracheal wall abnormalities or one with intraluminal pathology using transtracheal jet ventilation.

Laryngeal Mask Airway

Complete details about the LMA can be seen in Chapter 13.

Combitube

The Combitube, or ETC (esophagotracheal Combitube), is a variation of the esophageal obturator airway that may be useful in the presence of a difficult intubation or the "can't intubate, can't ventilate" situation.[34,35] It is a double-lumen tube with a closed distal end that is inserted blindly orally, and it has versatility in that it can be used regardless of which orifice is used. If it enters the esophagus (Fig. 8.15A), which is the most likely destination following a blind insertion, the esophageal cuff is inflated to prevent regurgitation around the tube. The proximal cuff occupies the pharynx above the airway and prevents leakage externally through the mouth and nose. Perforations in the esophageal lumen allow ventilation of the airway. If the ETC enters the trachea (Fig. 8.15B), ventilation may take place via the tracheal lumen.

This device is a major advance over the esophageal obturator airway, which proved to be quite dangerous if accidentally inserted into the airway. The major disadvantage of the ETC is that it does not allow suctioning of the trachea if it enters the esophagus.

The efficacy of the Combitube has been tested in field management of the airway by Rumball et al.[36] They compared successful insertion of the Combitube, the pharyngotracheal lumen airway (PTLA), the LMA, and an oral airway by EMTs in 470 cardiac arrest victims. The Combitube was inserted successfully and ventilation achieved in 86% of patients, compared with 82% with the PTLA and 73% with the LMA. The Combitube may be more advantageous in the field and the emergency room, where those performing airway management are more familiar with it and where patients are more likely to regurgitate. The LMA may be more advantageous in an operating room setting, where anesthesiologists are more familiar with its use and where passive regurgitation is less likely to occur. There is a greater risk of damage to the airway, the pharynx, or the esophagus when the Combitube is used by inexperienced personnel.[37]

Illuminating Stylets or Light Wands

Transillumination of the soft tissues of the neck[38,39] to blindly intubate the trachea was first suggested by the Japanese. Since that time, a number of devices have been tested and many improvements made. These devices are now available for both orotracheal and nasotracheal intubation.

The following guidelines for use are recommended:

1. The shaft of the stylet should be lubricated, as should the wall of the endotracheal tube. The stylet/tube combination should be preformed into a "hockey stick" configuration.
2. The patient's head should be placed in the sniff position (with the neck slightly extended). The jaw should be lifted upward, toward the ceiling (Fig. 8.16).

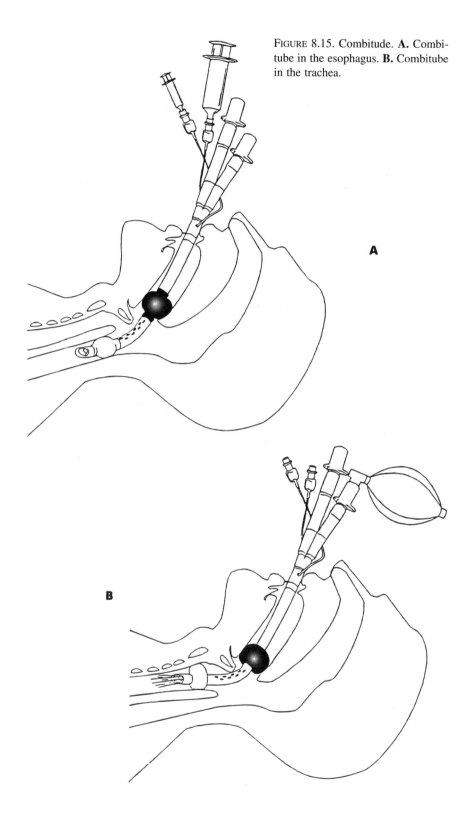

FIGURE 8.15. Combitude. **A.** Combitube in the esophagus. **B.** Combitube in the trachea.

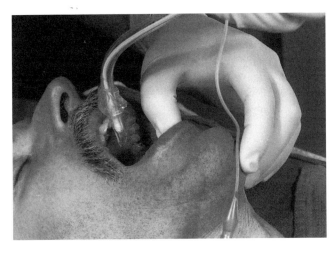

FIGURE 8.16. Positioning the patient for insertion of the light wand.

3. The light source is usually bright enough to preclude reducing ambient lighting conditions.
4. The light wand may be inserted in the awake state or under general anesthesia.
5. Experience with the light wand should be acquired in patients with a normal airway. The light wand may be a useful approach, especially with the unanticipated difficult intubation in an anesthetized patient.
6. The light wand may also be inserted nasally.

Trachlight and the Light Wand are two such devices commonly used in North America. Hung et al[40] have tested the Trachlight in 265 patients. Two hundred and six of these patients had a history of difficult intubation or were evaluated to have a difficult airway, and 59 had an unanticipated difficult intubation. Intubation was successful in 204 of the group with anticipated difficulty using the Trachlight. The mean time to intubation in that group was 25.7 ± 20.1 s. Intubation was successful in all of the patients with unanticipated difficulty. The mean time to intubation in that group was 19.7 sec ± 13.5 s. One of the main advantages of Illuminating stylets is that their insertion does not require laryngoscopic instrumentation. Therefore, they are very useful when access to the mouth is limited. They are also useful when there is some risk to dental structures. The disadvantage of Illuminating stylets is that they are inserted blindly and may damage diseased structures.

Invasive Equipment

Occasionally a retrograde catheter-assisted or transtracheal jet ventilation, or a cricothyrotomy or tracheostomy, will be required to deal with the difficult intubation. For this situation the equipment is very specific and is discussed in Chapter 10.

Difficult Airway Kit

Each operating or emergency suite should have a dedicated difficult airway kit. Operating and emergency suites all over the world have their own airway management culture and traditions; therefore, it would be impossible to come up with a generic kit that satisfies all groups. The following items are considered essential and then individual preferences can be added:

Basic Essentials of an Airway Kit

1. A variety of straight and curved laryngoscope blades
2. A gum elastic catheter or bougie and an airway exchange catheter, such as that manufactured by Cook Critical Care (Bloomington, IN)
3. A fiberoptic bronchoscope
4. An illuminating stylet or Bullard laryngoscope
5. An LMA or Combitube
6. A transtracheal airway kit

Routine endotracheal intubation for anesthesia has been in vogue for close to 50 years and the need for practice guidelines has been raised numerous times. In 1992 the ASA commissioned a task force to establish practice guidelines for managing the difficult airway, and their recommendations were published in 1993. These guidelines are required reading for any serious student of airway problems, and although they do not give comprehensive details about each possible airway problem, they are extremely useful.

ASA Difficult Airway Algorithm

Tunstall et al[41] was among the first to suggest an algorithm for the difficult airway in obstetric anesthesia. Benumof[42] advanced this issue further in 1991 and created so much interest in the topic that the ASA developed official guidelines, which were published in 1993.[43] These guidelines were modified further in 1996[44] and it is likely that we will see ongoing changes to the algorithm as new technologies are introduced (Fig. 8.17). The Canadians[6] published a very good set of guidelines on the difficult airway in 1998 that did not differ remarkably from those published by the ASA (Fig. 8.18). We have emphasized the importance of careful preoperative evaluation of the airway in order to reduce the number of unanticipated difficult intubations; however, despite these warnings, compliance among anesthesiologists is poor. Rose et al[7] noted inadequate preoperative evaluation of the airway in 50% of cases in a large series of 18,500 cases. Furthermore, even when difficult airways are identified, there seems to be a great reluctance to perform awake intubations. Duncan et al[4] have estimated that residents in training need to be exposed to 29 separate difficult airway scenarios in order to become proficient. Few training programs

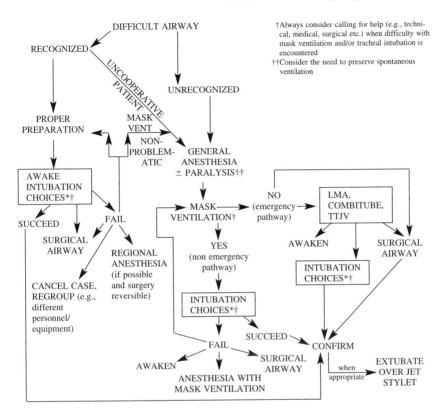

†Always consider calling for help (e.g., technical, medical, surgical etc.) when difficulty with mask ventilation and/or tracheal intubation is encountered

††Consider the need to preserve spontaneous ventilation

FIGURE 8.17. The ASA Difficult Airway Algorithm. Nonsurgical tracheal intubation choices consist of laryngoscopy with a rigid laryngoscope blade (many types), blind orotracheal or nasotracheal technique, fiberoptic/stylet technique, retrograde technique, illuminating stylet, rigid bronchoscope, percutaneous dilational tracheal entry. (From ASA Task Force on Management of the Difficult Airway, 1993; and *Anesthesiology*. 1996;84: 686–694.)[43,44]

can offer that kind of experience to trainees on a random basis. Few training programs offer formal difficult airway training in anesthesiology. Koppel et al[45] noted that only 27% of 143 programs in the United States offered formal training in the difficult airway, and when training was offered it mostly consisted of didactic lectures. It seems ironic that we have neglected to tackle this problem more vigorously in view of the number of airway-related anesthetic deaths that have been reported in the Closed Claims Study. More than 200 anesthesia-related airway deaths have been reported in the United States since 1975, and the results are equally poor if not worse in other countries. Therefore, we must continue to campaign within our departments to avoid unnecessary chances when dealing with the airway, and we must promote formal airway training within our programs.[46]

234

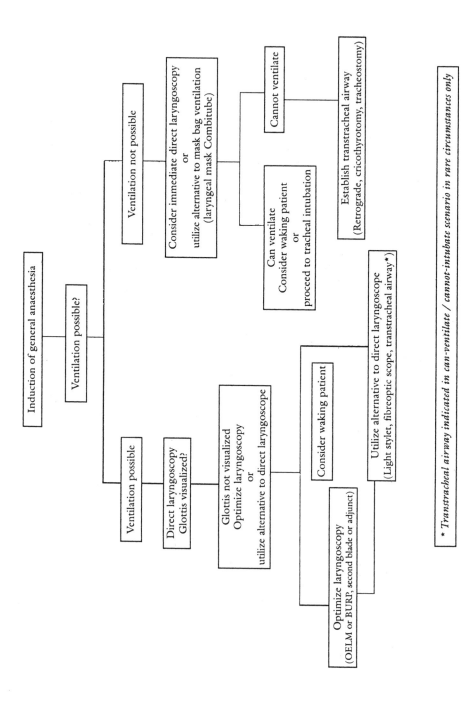

FIGURE 8.18. Algorithm for the proposed management of the unexpected difficult airway. (From Crosby et al. The Unanticipated Difficult Airway with Recommendations for Management. *Can J Anaesth.* 1998;45(8):757–776, with permission.)

Anesthesia Implications of the Difficult Airway

We have already discussed in detail the importance of preoperative evaluation in detecting the difficult airway. Even though there is no absolutely reliable way to detect all difficult airway cases, we can detect the vast majority of them by making a few simple observations. We can then safely secure the airway in most of these cases by performing awake or asleep intubation under controlled circumstances.

Structured Approach to the Difficult Airway

Failed Awake Elective Intubation

Occasionally you will be unable to perform awake intubation, due to a lack of preparation, an uncooperative patient, equipment failure, or anatomic limitations. In elective situations your options are postponement and further evaluation. It is very important to place a time limit on your efforts to secure the airway in all circumstances, not just for humane reasons but also for safety reasons. As a general rule you should abandon your efforts after a maximum of 30 minutes or at any time that you are unable to adequately oxygenate or ventilate the patient. You should also abort your efforts to secure the airway if the patient is endangered in any way from your intervention.

You may consider inducing general anesthesia if patient cooperation is an issue. Before doing so, however, you must have reasonable assurance that mask ventilation will be easy. Difficult airways are invariably managed under general anesthesia in children. The LMA is a useful crutch in some situations because your hands are free to solve the problem and the patient can breathe an inhalation agent spontaneously. There are several options open to you at this time, and individuals usually select the airway adjunct that they are most familiar with. Following are some of these options:

1. Direct laryngoscopy using a straight or curved blade
2. Bougie with direct laryngoscopy
3. The Bullard laryngoscope
4. Illuminating stylets
5. Fiberoptic-assisted intubation
6. Intubating laryngeal mask
7. Retrograde catheter techniques

Regional anesthesia may also be an option in the event of failed awake intubation; however, these techniques should never be used to sidestep a difficult airway. If there is even a remote possibility that airway intervention may be required, the airway should be secured first. It would be unwise to embark on major abdominal, thoracic, or vascular surgery, under regional anesthesia, if there was a problem with the airway. Regional anesthesia can be safely performed in patients with difficult airways if, in the event of intraoperative failure of regional anesthesia, the procedure can be easily terminated or completed with local anesthesia supplementation. We do not agree with the ASA Difficult Airway Algorithm on this issue. They suggest that it is reasonable to proceed with surgery under regional anesthesia in the presence of a difficult airway even when surgery cannot be terminated quickly, provided there is good access to the airway and the patient accepts regional anesthesia. A surgical airway may be the first option in some cases with anticipated difficult intubation. An example of this would be a patient presenting with a laryngeal tumor scheduled for a radical neck dissection.

Elective, *Unanticipated* Difficult Airway

This is one of the most common airway emergencies encountered in the operating room. The usual scenario is as follows: On induction of general anesthesia and the administration of a muscle relaxant, you are unable to see the vocal apparatus. Your priority at this point is maintenance of adequate oxygenation. Assuming that you can ventilate and oxygenate the patient, your next priority is to maintain anesthesia and relaxation. At this point you should ask for the difficult airway cart and ask for an assistant if you do not already have one. You should try to figure out why you are unable to see the vocal apparatus. You should ask yourself if you are using the appropriate size and type of laryngoscope blade. Then you should try to determine what the problem is. It is important to do something different with every new attempt. There is a tendency to keep doing the same thing over and over. Before you make your second attempt you should do the following:

1. Check suction
2. Try a smaller styletted tube
3. Check the head position
4. Ask the assistant to be ready to apply pressure on the larynx
5. Repeat laryngoscopy
6. Attempt to place a bougie or ventilating stylet

With each failed attempt, the risk of trauma increases and the presence of blood in the mouth interferes with your ability to recognize structures. Furthermore, laryngeal edema with repeated attempts can lead to difficult mask ventilation. Most difficult intubations are successful on the second attempt, because initial failures are often due to inadequate preparation or head position. Some airway experts suggest that we should use airway adjuncts after the first failure, and it is difficult to argue against that approach, but from a practical point of view, it usually takes some time before the difficult airway cart becomes available and by then most impatient clinicians will have made a second attempt. It would be reasonable to attempt to pass a bougie at this stage. Should failure occur on the second attempt, you should ask for help. Occasionally you will receive an offer of help to intubate from an individual who has little training or expertise in airway management. It is wise to decline the offer (Fig. 8.19). Once again, go back to the basics. Make sure that you can still oxygenate and ventilate the patient, and prepare to move to the next step. At this stage, you should consider abandoning conventional laryngoscopy and consider using one of the following devices:

1. Illuminating stylet
2. Bullard laryngoscope
3. Intubating laryngeal mask
4. Fiberoptic-assisted intubation
5. Retrograde catheter device

Most of these techniques have all been discussed in other chapters. The majority of anesthesia departments will stock some if not all of the equipment needed. Each department tends to have its own culture, and there are also international differences. Bougie techniques, for example, are traditionally more popular in the UK as a first-line approach. Fiberoptic techniques are more popular in North America. You also might consider using some of these techniques as a **first line** of approach when confronted with a difficult airway.

If the airway cannot be secured after three or four good attempts by an experienced person in a purely elective situation, it is advisable to postpone the case. Few would argue with this philosophy. The longer you persist, the greater the likelihood of morbidity. Allow spontaneous ventilation and consciousness to return, and be sure to visit the patient subsequently to explain the circumstances. Some anesthesiologists will have difficulty accepting failure. Never allow your ego to stand in the way of good medical practice. Always do what is best for the patient.

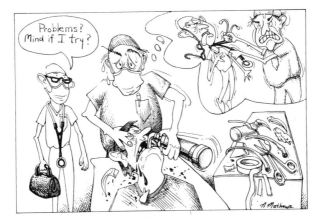

FIGURE 8.19. Beware of the inexperienced, ambitious clinician who offers to help.

Following is the summarizing algorithm for what has been presented:

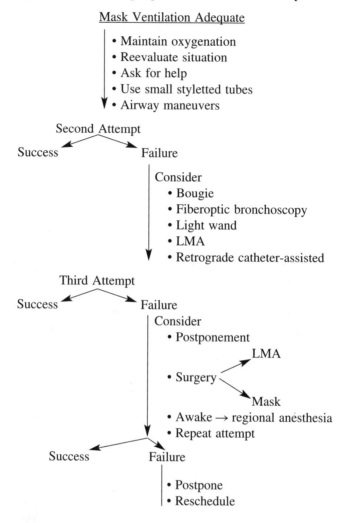

Mask Ventilation Adequate
- Maintain oxygenation
- Reevaluate situation
- Ask for help
- Use small styletted tubes
- Airway maneuvers

Second Attempt

Success   Failure

Consider
- Bougie
- Fiberoptic bronchoscopy
- Light wand
- LMA
- Retrograde catheter-assisted

Third Attempt

Success   Failure

Consider
- Postponement

          LMA
- Surgery
          Mask
- Awake → regional anesthesia
- Repeat attempt

Success   Failure

- Postpone
- Reschedule

Unanticipated Difficult Intubation in *Emergency Surgery*

An unanticipated difficult intubation will occasionally be encountered in a patient scheduled for emergency surgery. The same rules apply. But, in addition, this patient presents the risk of aspiration of gastric contents. The option to postpone no longer exists.

A more aggressive approach must be taken from the outset. You must prevent regurgitation while the patient is unconscious (continuous cricoid pressure), and you must allow the patient to regain consciousness. Then, an awake fiberoptically assisted intubation must be considered. If the option for regional anesthesia exists, it should be given every consideration. In life-threatening emergencies (e.g., difficult intubation in the face of massive hemorrhage), a surgical approach may be required from the outset.

Following is an algorithm:

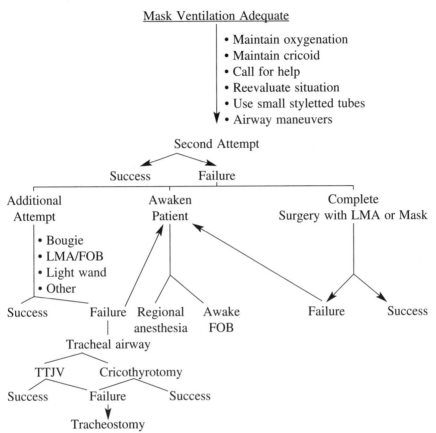

Mask Ventilation Adequate
- Maintain oxygenation
- Maintain cricoid
- Call for help
- Reevaluate situation
- Use small styletted tubes
- Airway maneuvers

Second Attempt

Success   Failure

Additional Attempt   Awaken Patient   Complete Surgery with LMA or Mask
- Bougie
- LMA/FOB
- Light wand
- Other

Success   Failure   Regional anesthesia   Awake FOB   Failure   Success

Tracheal airway

TTJV   Cricothyrotomy

Success   Failure   Success

Tracheostomy

Elective or Emergency, Anticipated

If difficult intubation is anticipated in an elective or emergency situation, awake techniques are usually recommended—except in pediatric practice, where general anesthesia is often induced while the ability to breathe spontaneously is not interfered with. If in doubt as to your ability to intubate a patient, avoid using neuromuscular blocking drugs. However, if for some reason you must use them, be certain to select only short-acting agents (10 to 20 mg succinylcholine IV/70 kg) and keep the dose small so that adequate ventilation can recur within a minute.

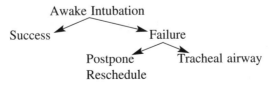

Awake Intubation

Success   Failure

Postpone Reschedule   Tracheal airway

Airway Problems in Obstetric Patients

The confidential enquiries into maternal deaths in England and Wales[47,48] have found airway emergencies a common feature, and on one occasion anesthetic deaths were ranked as the third most frequent cause of mortality. It has been estimated[49] also that 10 to 13 obstetrical deaths occur in the UK every year as a result of complications of anesthesia, and airway problems feature prominently in most of these disasters. Fortunately, the incidence of maternal death related to anesthesia has declined significantly within the last 10 years; however, the majority are still airway related. There was only one anesthesia-related maternal death in the most recent triennial report available from the UK (1994–1996). Hawkins et al[50] compiled the American experience of anesthesia-related maternal mortality from 1979 to 1990. The results were somewhat similar to those in the UK. Anesthesia complications were the sixth most common cause of maternal death in the United States. From 1979 to 1981 there were 4.3 maternal deaths per million live births, and from 1988 to 1990 there were 1.7 maternal deaths per million live births. Most of the deaths were linked with cesarean section (82%). The decline in maternal mortality rate in the United States was credited to the increased use of regional anesthesia for operative obstetrics and to a reduction in the number of deaths related to regional anesthesia. Unfortunately, the number of deaths related to general anesthesia remained the same.

Several studies have shown that the incidence of failed intubation is higher in obstetrics than in the general surgical population. Pilkington et al[51] reported an increased Mallampatti score with advancing pregnancy, probably related to fluid retention. Lyons and Hawthorne[52] reported a 0.33% incidence of failed intubation in 1984 and a 0.4% incidence in 1994. Samsoon et al[8] suggested that the incidence of failed obstetrical intubation was approximately 10 times that in surgical patients. More recent prospective data from surgery patients, however, suggest that the incidence may be similar (0.3%).[6] Nevertheless, most clinicians agree that difficult intubation in an obstetrical patient carries with it far greater risk of morbidity and mortality in both mother and fetus because of their diminished oxygen reserves and the other physiological changes associated with pregnancy.

Besides the usual anatomical airway abnormalities seen in nonpregnant women, obstetrical patients have some added risk factors. The caliber of the airway may be smaller and anatomical structures may be difficult to identify because of edema, especially if the woman is preeclamptic. Furthermore, weight gain is a common feature of late pregnancy, adding further to diminished respiratory reserves and poor visualization of the airway.

Advances in regional anesthesia within the past 20 years have been such that general anesthesia is infrequently used for operative obstetrics in the developed world. Consequently, individuals who subspecialize in obstetrical anesthesia are exposed to difficult airways even less frequently than most anesthesiologists. This clearly has training implications for both residents and staff, who must find other ways to maintain their skills.

The ASA and other groups have published guidelines for the management of difficult airways, but these are quite generic and do not address specific problems. Tunstall and Sheikh[41] have suggested guidelines in obstetrics that are well worth reading. However, a number of important advances have taken place since and are worthy of discussion.

Suggested guidelines for difficult intubation in obstetrical patients are as follows: Responsibility for the administration of general anesthesia should be delegated to an individual with specialty qualifications in anesthesia. Although a resident may actually administer the anesthetic, an attending anesthesiologist should be present. A difficult airway kit must be immediately available and should be checked daily. All patients presenting for operative obstetrics should be carefully evaluated by an anesthesiologist and undergo thorough scrutiny of the airway. Whenever possible, regional anesthesia should be selected. The main reasons for general anesthesia are: patient preference, sepsis, coagulopathy, fetal distress, fixed cardiac output states, and maternal hemorrhage. Patients who demand general anesthesia should clearly understand the implications. Fetal distress per se is **not** necessarily an indication for general anesthesia. In fact, an anesthesiologist skilled in modern regional anesthesia techniques can administer a spinal anesthetic as quickly as a general. Nor are the risks of hemorrhage and fixed cardiac output states considered absolute contraindications to regional anesthesia, especially in patients with a known difficult airway. In elective situations with a known difficult airway, some clinicians feel more comfortable securing the airway first, whereas others will elect to use regional anesthesia. You should select the technique that you feel most comfortable with.

If while administering a general anesthetic to an obstetrical patient you find you cannot intubate, how do you proceed? The algorithm for failed intubation in emergency surgery should be applied. However, some aspects of management must be emphasized. Obstetrical patients desaturate rapidly. Oxygenation is the top priority, and you should not hesitate to apply positive pressure ventilation while maintaining cricoid pressure. But remember: Cricoid pressure, applied inappropriately, may interfere with your ability to see the larynx, and thus its temporary release may be of benefit. It is also possible to apply cricoid pressure and backward/upward right pressure (BURP) simultaneously. Edema of the airway is quite common in late pregnancy, so you should always select a **small** endotracheal tube for the first attempt (7.0 mm ID). A styletted 6.0-mm ID cuffed tube also should be used following a failed first attempt.

Your first attempt at intubation is always your best chance, so do not squander it by being unprepared. Each time you attempt intubation following a failed attempt, you expose the patient to increased risk. The introduction of the laryngeal mask airway[53,54] has changed our whole attitude toward this problem. Therefore, you should not hesitate to insert the LMA following a failed second attempt at intubation. The ProSeal LMA offers some additional advantages over the conventional LMA; however, its efficacy has not yet been fully tested. The LMA functions optimally when patients are adequately anesthetized. Consideration should also be given to completing the surgical procedure with the LMA in place.

The LMA can serve as a conduit through which fiberoptically assisted intubation is performed. Alternatively, a bougie may be passed through the LMA into the airway and an endotracheal tube may be advanced over that. Finally, a small endotracheal tube (6.0 mm ID) may be passed blindly into the airway through an LMA. Consideration should be given to letting the patient recover from the effects of general anesthesia and muscle relaxants, and then, depending upon the circumstances, you can perform awake intubation or regional anesthesia. If at any point oxygenation of the patient becomes a problem, a more aggressive stance must be taken—two-handed mask ventilation with an assistant holding the airway in both hands. Oral and nasal airways should be inserted and mask ventilation attempted with the aid of an assistant. The Combitube, if available, should be inserted; if it is not successful, alternative approaches to the airway should be attempted. These include transtracheal jet ventilation and cricothyrotomy. The anesthesiologist must be prepared to perform these procedures and not rely on surgical colleagues who might not be familiar with either the circumstances or the equipment. If TTJV or needle cricothyrotomy is successful, tracheostomy will be required to protect the airway from aspiration. If TTJV or cricothyrotomy is not successful, cardiopulmonary bypass may be necessary and must be considered if and when facilities are available.

Following is an algorithm for failed obstetrical intubation:

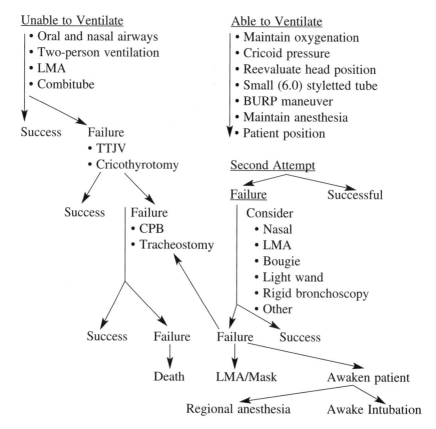

In summary, airway problems in the parturient are among the most challenging. When problems ensue, there is even less time than usual to act, and the lives of both mother and her infant are at stake. The consequences of failure to secure the airway are loss of life in many cases, and in some, permanent brain damage in mother and child.

Difficult Intubation in the Emergency Room Setting

The same basic rules apply to difficult intubations regardless of geography. However, it is important to point out that anesthesiologists are also called upon to deal with challenging airway problems outside the operating room. Emergency room physicians occasionally require our assistance. Emergency room intubations are usually more challenging because invariably there is a greater sense of urgency and the anesthesiologist is usually not familiar with the personnel, equipment, or surroundings. Patients usually have injuries that need urgent attention and may be uncooperative because of hypoxemia, mind-altering substances, or head injuries. There is rarely sufficient time to do a thorough evaluation of the airway, and quite often uncertainty exists about treatment because of a lack of information. Finally, the situation is often dynamic and can change within minutes. In the next few pages examples of challenging airway problems in the emergency room will be discussed.

Head Injury

A patient presenting with head injuries may require the expertise of the anesthesiologist. In a life-threatening situation, emergency intubation is usually required because of inadequate oxygenation/ventilation. More frequently, however, intubation is required to reduce the risk of aspiration of gastric contents in a patient who is semicomatose. Occasionally, hyperventilation will be required to reduce intracranial pressure. Sometimes, general anesthesia is necessary because the patient is so uncooperative that appropriate diagnostic work cannot be performed. General anesthesia is preferable in a patient with serious head injury (unless difficult intubation is anticipated) because the intracranial pressure increases dramatically during attempts at awake intubation. Thiopental and lidocaine are frequently used as induction drugs, and both decrease intracranial pressure. Cervical spine injuries occur in 1.5% to 3% of all major trauma victims and in up to 3% of all head injuries in adults.[55-59] Therefore, this matter should be considered when general anesthesia is being administered to these patients.

Cervical Spine Injury

Approximately 6,000 people die from cervical spine injury (CSI) and 5,000 new quadriplegics are reported in the United States each year.[60] Most victims are males ranging in age from 15 to 35 years. Cervical spine injury is most frequently associated with accidents involving motor vehicles, diving, contact sports, riding horses, falls, and blunt head and neck trauma. Most CSIs are not immediately fatal. Injuries occur primarily at one of three levels of the cervical spine: C2, C6, or C7. If you encounter an accident anywhere, how do you decide who needs cervical spine precautions? Alert victims, devoid of neck pain and tenderness, numbness, or weakness in the arms or legs, should not require cervical spine evaluation or special precautions. Any victim who reports even the slightest symptom of neck discomfort or anyone who is not fully alert should have cervical spine precautions (Table 8.3).[61]

Airway management in the presence of CSI is often a challenging prospect. In emergency situations, the anesthesiologist may be forced to intervene without information about the cervical spine. It has been demonstrated over and over again that intubation even in the presence of CSI is safe—provided proper precautions are taken, which include in-line stabilization and appropriate caution during laryngoscopy. The debates continue as to the optimal way to handle a patient with CSI (e.g., awake vs. general anesthesia, nasotracheal vs. orotracheal intubation). Intuitively, it would appear that awake fiberoptically assisted oral or nasal intubation is the ideal method because head or neck movement is not required. However, there are no data comparing these techniques with other methods.[62,63] The most important consideration is that the anesthesiologist secure the airway using the most familiar techniques. There is no room for dogma in dealing with these cases. Direct laryngoscopy is perfectly safe provided reasonable precautions are taken. Awake intubation may be dangerous in an uncooperative patient or one who is semicomatose. There is a suggestion that neck muscles act as a splint in the awake state and this is lost when general anesthesia is used with muscle relaxants.

The trauma victim's neck must be immobilized as soon as possible after injury, and the most reliable method of doing this is to secure the victim on a hard board. If possible, place sandbags at each side of the neck and a rigid collar around the neck. These will reduce movement significantly though not completely. All airway maneuvers, including cricoid pressure, widen the disc space to some degree. Patients with unstable C_1C_2 fractures seem most vulnerable to neurological damage from intubation. Despite the potential for serious neuro-

TABLE 8.3. Risk of cervical-spine injury

Known injury	High-risk group ($> 10\%$)	Moderate-risk group (1%–2%)	No-risk group
Positive C-spine roentgenogram or CT scan Neurologic deficit	Front-end MVA > 35 mph without seatbelt Head-first fall Equivocal C-spine roentgenograms	MVA Head injury Non-head-first fall Contact sport injury High-risk group with C-spine roentgenograms negative for injuries	Alert patient without neck pain or tenderness Negative C-spine roentgenograms (3 views) Negative C-spine CT scan

CT, computed tomography; MVA, motor vehicle accident.
Source: From Hastings,[61] with permission.

logical deficit during airway manipulation, however, the actual incidence is extremely rare. Few reports[64] have appeared dealing with serious injury after intubation and they are rarely published. The patient is at greatest risk of neurological injury when CSI is not recognized. Reid et al[65] found that new neurological deficits were 7.5 times more common if an injury went unrecognized. It is important to remember that up to 8% of C-spine fractures are not recognized radiologically, even when **three** views are taken. Radiological clearance may give you a false sense of security. In one study involving 128 patients with suspected CSI, both the senior radiologist and emergency medicine physician missed the diagnosis of CSI in 25% of cases.[66] It has been suggested that the anesthesiologist should be able to read the ABCs of cervical spine films as well. This involves alignment of the vertebrae, the condition of the bones and cartilage, and the width of the soft tissue and intervertebral spaces (Fig. 8.20). Therefore, when obtaining a history, even if there is only the remotest hint of neck injury, handle the patient with extreme care if airway manipulation is required.

Whenever possible, obtain radiological clearance before allowing airway manipulation to take place. The three standard views (cross-table lateral, anterior-posterior [AP], and through-the-mouth) should be obtained,[67] and all seven vertebrae must be visible (Fig. 8.21). The "swimmer's view" may be necessary. Fractures at $C_1.C_2$ may not be reliably diagnosed on plain films but require a CT scan. Widening of the cervical soft tissue space may be the only evidence of an injury at $C_1.C_2$ and should alert the anesthesiologist to the possibility of difficult intubation caused by airway encroachment (Fig. 8.22A and B).[68,69]

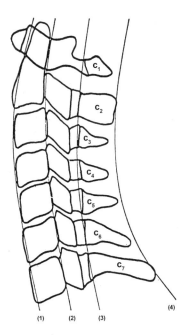

FIGURE 8.20. Diagram of the lateral view of the cervical spine demonstrating normal alignment. Lines drawn through the anterior margins of the vertebral border: (*1*), the posterior margins; (*2*), the junction between the lamina and spinous processes; (*3*), and the tips of the spinous processes; (*4*) should be smooth curves. Lines (*2*) and (*3*) are the approximate boundaries of the spinal canal. (From Williams C, Bernstein T, Jelenko C. Essentiality of the lateral cervical spine radiograph. *Ann Emerg Med.* 1981;10:198–204, with permission.)

A difficult intubation in the presence of CSI is probably the ultimate airway challenge facing anesthesiologists. Cricothyrotomy and tracheostomy are obvious options. Retrograde catheter-assisted techniques may also help. Transtracheal jet ventilation is valuable in desperate situations, but it does not protect the airway against aspiration. The laryngeal mask may also be a useful temporizing measure in some cases.

In summary, CSIs present some unique challenges. No one technique of airway management appears to be any better than another. In view of the multiple

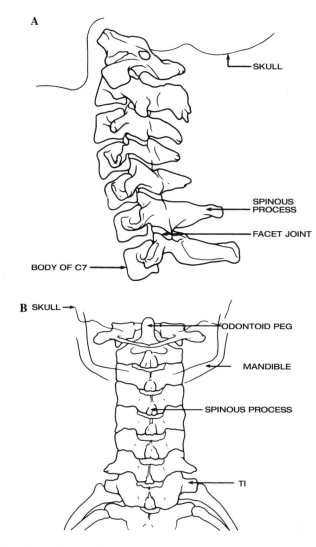

FIGURE 8.21. Cervical spine line drawings. **A.** Lateral X ray. **B.** Anterior-posterior.

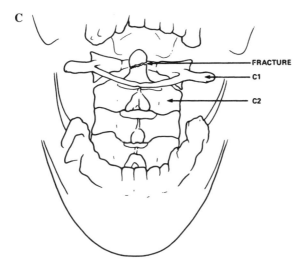

FIGURE 8.21. *Continued.* **C.** Through-the-mouth showing C1, C2. (From Doolan LA and O'Brien JF. Safe Intubation in Cervical Spine Injury. *Anaesth Intens Care*, 1985;13: 319–324, with permission.)

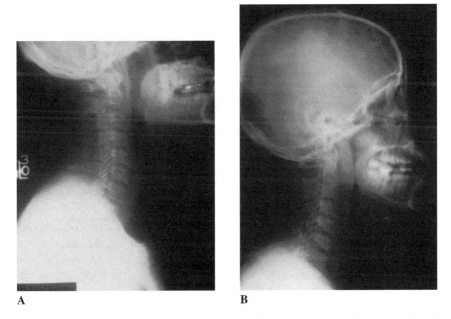

FIGURE 8.22. Cervical spine soft tissue films. **A.** Normal with cervical prevertebral soft tissue. **B.** Abnormal swelling of cervical prevertebral soft tissue.

disciplines involved, it would make sense to establish clinical guidelines for optimal management of these cases.

Airway Burns

The anesthesiologist may be called upon to assess the airway of a burn victim. Patients presenting with airway burns may have carbon monoxide poisoning, which can be difficult to diagnose clinically because the usual clinical signs (pallor, clamminess) are masked by carbonaceous material staining the skin. Carboxyhemoglobin (CO) levels should be determined and treatment is required if quantities around 15% are detected. Levels near 50% are usually fatal. Oxygen therapy (100%) via an endotracheal tube or nonrebreathing bag rapidly reduces the half-life of CO from about 4 hours in room air to 40 minutes.

A patient with burns around the head and neck is at risk of developing upper airway obstruction. Coughing episodes and hoarseness in the presence of singed facial and nasal hair are often symptomatic of airway burns. One of the most reliable ways to assess the airway is to perform fiberoptic bronchoscopy following topical anesthesia and sedation. Intubation should be performed if there is any suspicion of airway burn. The anatomy of the airway becomes grossly distorted following fluid resuscitation, making intubation extremely difficult at times. Eschar formation may limit chest expansion and compromise ventilation.

The presence of burn scars in a patient with chronic burns may restrict mouth opening, access to the nasal passages, and limit flexion and extension of the neck, making endotracheal intubation very difficult. Airway burns are among the most challenging airway problems in medicine.

Facial Trauma

In a facial trauma victim the airway reflexes may be impaired by associated head injuries or inebriation, and aspiration of vomitus, blood, teeth, or bony fragments is a real possibility. Edema and swelling in the vicinity of the airway may lead to airway obstruction even in the presence of intact airway reflexes. Nasotracheal intubation may be difficult in a patient with Lefort II or III fractures because bony fragments may encroach on the nasal airway. Cerebrospinal fluid leakage following a basal skull fracture is contraindication to nasotracheal intubation because of the risk of meningitis. Trauma to the mandible, especially in the region of the condyle, limits a person's ability to open the mouth because of disruption of temporomandibular joint function. Mouth opening may also be limited by trismus associated with mandibular fractures. Access to the oropharynx may be impeded by a knife impaled in the vicinity of the airway. Endotracheal intubation may also be difficult in these cases because the anatomy is distorted or concealed by blood and secretions. It is advisable to discuss the preferred route of intubation, if and when it is required, with the surgeon. In maxillary and mandibular fractures the surgeon frequently wires the mandible and maxillae together; thus oral intubation would be contraindicated. Occasionally the degree of destruction and swelling is so great that the surgeon will elect to perform a tracheostomy.

Cardiac Arrest

Cardiac arrest is the most common indication for emergency intubation outside the operating room. Oxygenation and ventilation are priorities and are achieved best by endotracheal intubation. Bag/valve/mask ventilation cannot be reliably carried out during chest compression, and regurgitation of gastric contents is very common during cardiac arrest.

Bag/Valve/Mask Ventilation

The importance of bag/valve/mask ventilation has been overshadowed over the years by the inherently more attractive technique of intubation. The average anesthesiologist in full-time clinical practice may intubate as many as 500 patients per year. Bag/valve/mask ventilation is a component of the intubation process and is frequently used before intubation. It is, in fact, one of the first contingencies called upon when difficulties arise. Thus, your ability to perform it must be assessed before attempting endotracheal intubation. Effective bag/valve/mask ventilation in many cases requires much more practice than intubation and a number of factors can interfere with your ability to do it efficiently:

Morbid obesity
Bearded patient
Laryngospasm
Anatomical distortion of the mouth or nose
Airway obstruction from any cause
Poor access to the mouth or nose
Edentulous state
Inappropriate equipment
Asthma
Pneumothorax
Pleural effusion
Bronchospasm

"Cannot Intubate, Cannot Ventilate"

Fortunately, "cannot intubate, cannot ventilate" situations are rare. Ironically, this places anesthesiologists at a bit of a disadvantage in that few have had much experience treating this serious problem.

In the past we have relied heavily on our surgical colleagues to establish a surgical airway. Most of us are now of the opinion that time does not permit this luxury and we must be prepared to manage the problem aggressively ourselves (see algorithm). If bag/valve/mask ventilation fails, four-handed ventilation should be attempted (two hands holding the mask, two squeezing the bag). The difficult airway kit should be immediately available. Also consider inserting the LMA or a Combitube. If these methods fail, TTJV or cricothyrotomy must be performed immediately. (These techniques are described in detail in Chapter 10.) There are no objective data on the safety and efficacy of these techniques in emergency airway management. We recently conducted a survey of the use of transtracheal jet ventilation in emergency situations, receiving data on 16 patients, and found a success rate of 25%, with 75% failure and a death rate of 25%. Subcutaneous air was a serious and frequent complication.

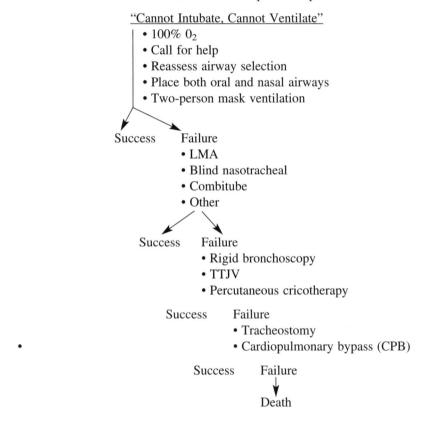

"Cannot Intubate, Cannot Ventilate"
- 100% O_2
- Call for help
- Reassess airway selection
- Place both oral and nasal airways
- Two-person mask ventilation

Success   Failure
- LMA
- Blind nasotracheal
- Combitube
- Other

Success   Failure
- Rigid bronchoscopy
- TTJV
- Percutaneous cricotherapy

Success   Failure
- Tracheostomy
- Cardiopulmonary bypass (CPB)

Success   Failure

Death

Summary

There are no clear-cut guidelines that you can apply to all difficult intubations. Each case is different. Obviously, a failed intubation in a patient with rapidly progressive airway obstruction is a much more urgent problem than a failed attempt in elective surgery. The only requirement common to all cases is that oxygenation must be maintained at all times. The experience of the individual dealing with the problem is also important. Experienced practitioners tend to be more aggressive from the outset. Do not underestimate the value of vigorous manipulation of the airway by an experienced colleague. We have not emphasized this aspect sufficiently in algorithms. Unfortunately, we frequently do not have good assistance when we encounter difficult airways.

In recent years bougies have become much more popular and are often used as a first line of defense when difficulties arise. We endorse this approach, especially since one of the drawbacks of fiberoptic techniques is the fact that you invariably need time to prepare.

Remember also the old adage that "a difficult oral is often an easy nasal intubation." However, if you do attempt nasal intubation during a failed oral intubation, you must take appropriate precautions to prevent nasal bleeding. Most anesthesiologists are reluctant to follow this course because of the risk of hemorrhage. A brisk nasal hemorrhage not only makes it impossible to see the airway but may also precipitate a "cannot intubate, cannot ventilate" scenario.

The most important advance in airway management in recent years was the introduction of the laryngeal mask airway and its many modifications. The LMA has a particular value in the difficult airway situation for a number of reasons. In some cases the problem may be solved by placing an LMA. One can only speculate on the number of difficult intubations that have been preemptively avoided as a result of the introduction of the LMA. The LMA is a noninvasive approach to the difficult airway and allows you time to regroup and reevaluate a difficult situation. The LMA may also act as a conduit for subsequent endotracheal intubation. The ProSeal variation of the LMA comes close to a replacement for endotracheal intubation.

Your must always be prepared to deal with **complete airway obstruction.** Many centers have special "difficult intubation" trays complete with all the necessary equipment. Certainly do not attempt intubation unless the ability to deliver oxygen and apply suction is immediately at hand.

We have seen a tremendous increase in the number of technical devices that have become available to facilitate difficult intubation and mask ventilation in the past two decades. Each department of anesthesia across the globe seems to develop its own culture when it comes to using these devices. It would be difficult to attain competence in the use of all of these devices; however, one should strive to master at least two or three of them.

Ultimately, knowledge and competence in handling difficult intubations will be acquired only by managing patients. In fact, you will learn most when placing the endotracheal tube seems like an unattainable goal and the best course of action is not clear. As an astute observer once said, "Good judgment comes from experience, and experience comes from bad judgment."

The next chapter will discuss some complications of intubation, which also come from bad judgment and bad technique (or plain bad luck).

References

1. Benumof JL, Scheller MS. The importance of transtracheal jet ventilation in the management of the difficult airway. *Anesthesiology.* 1990;72:828–833.

2. Bellhouse CP, Dore C. Criteria for estimating likelihood of difficulty of endotracheal intubation with Macintosh laryngoscope. *Anaesth Intensive Care.* 1988;16:329–337.
3. *Report on Confidential Enquires into Maternal Deaths in England and Wales, 1976–78.* DHSS London: Her Majesty's Stationery Office; 1982.
4. Duncan PG, Cohen MM, Yip R. Clinical experiences associated with anaesthesia training. *Ann R Coll Physicians Surg Can.* 1993;26:363–367.
5. Caplan RA, Benumof JL, Berry FA, et al. Practice guidelines for the management of the difficult airway. A report by the American Society of Anesthesiologists Task Force on the Management of the Difficult Airway. *Anesthesiology.* 1993;78:597–602.
6. Crosby ET, Cooper R, Douglas MJ, et al. The unanticipated difficult airway with recommendations for management. *Can J Anaesth.* 1998;45:757–776.
7. Rose DK, Cohen MM. The airway: problems and predictions in 18,500 patients. *Can J Anaesth.* 1994;41;5:372–383.
8. Samsoon GLT, Young JRB. Difficult tracheal intubation: a retrospective study. *Anaesthesia.* 1984;39:1105–1111.
9. Macintosh RR. An aid to oral intubation. *Brit Med J.* 1949;1:28.
10. Nolan JP, Wilson ME. An evaluation of the gum elastic bougie. *Anaesthesia.* 1992;47:878–881.
11. Kidd JF, Dyson A, Latto IP. Successful difficult intubation: use of the gum elastic bougie. *Anaesthesia.* 1988;43:437–438.
12. McComish PB. Left sided laryngoscopes. *Anaesthesia.* 1965;20:372.
13. Lagade MRG, Poppers PJ. Use of the left-entry laryngoscope blade in patients with right-sided orofacial lesions. *Anesthesiology.* 1983;58:300.
14. Racz GB. Improved vision modification of the Macintosh laryngoscope. *Anaesthesia.* 1984;39:1249–1250.
15. Legade MRG, Poppers PJ. Revival of the polio laryngoscope blade. *Anesthesiology.* 1982;57:545.
16. Bourke DL, Lawrence J. Another way to insert a Macintosh blade. *Anesthesiology.* 1983;59:80.
17. Huffman J. The application of prisms to curved laryngoscopes: a preliminary study. *J Am Assoc Nurse Anesth.* 1968;35:138–139.
18. Huffman J, Elam JO. Prisms and fiber optics for laryngoscopy. *Anesth Analg.* 1971;50:64–67.
19. Huffman J. The development of optical prism instruments to view and study the human larynx. *J Am Assoc Nurse Anesth.* 1970;38:197–202.
20. Choi JJ. A new double-angle blade for direct laryngoscopy. *Anesthesiology.* 1990; 72:576.
21. Benumof JL. Management of the difficult adult airway. *Anesthesiology.* 1990;72:576.
22. Mayall RM. The Belscope for management of the difficult airway. *Anesthesiology.* 1992;76:1059–1060.
23. Bellhouse CP. An angulated laryngoscope for routine and difficult tracheal intubation. *Anesthesiology.* 1988;69:126–129.
24. McCoy EP, Mirakhur RK. The levering laryngoscope. *Anaesthesia.* 1993;48:516–519.
25. Uchida T, Hikawa Y, Saito Y, et al. The McCoy levering laryngoscope in patients with limited neck extension. *Can J Anaesth.* 1997;44:674–676.
26. Laurent SC, de Melo AE, Alexander-Williams JM. The use of the McCoy laryngoscope in patients with simulated cervical spine injuries. *Anaesthesia.* 1996;51:74–75.
27. Gabbott DA. Laryngoscopy using the McCoy laryngoscope after application of a cervical collar. *Anaesthesia.* 1996;51:812–814.

28. Borland LM, Casselbrant M. The Bullard laryngoscope: a new indirect oral laryngoscope (pediatric version). *Anesth Analg.* 1990;70:105–108.

29. Bjoraker DG. The Bullard intubation laryngoscopes. *Anesthesiol Rev.* 1990;17:64–70.

30. Dyson A, Harris J, Bhatia K. Rapidity and accuracy of tracheal intubation in a mannequin: comparison of the fiberoptic with the Bullard laryngoscope. *Br J Anaesth.* 1990;65:268–270.

31. Mendel P, Bristow A. Anaesthesia for procedures on the larynx and pharynx: the use of the Bullard laryngoscope in conjunction with high frequency jet ventilation. *Anaesthesia.* 1993;48:263–265.

32. Dorsch JA, Dorsch SE. *Understanding Anaesthesia Equipment.* 3rd ed. Baltimore: Williams & Wilkins; 1994.

33. McIntyre, JWR. Laryngoscope design and the difficult adult tracheal intubation. *Can J Anaesth.* 1989;36:94–98.

34. Brain AIJ. The development of the laryngeal mask—a brief history of the invention, early clinical studies and experimental work from which the laryngeal mask evolved. *Eur J Anaesthesiol.* 1991;4:5–17.

35. Frass M, Frenzer R, Rauscha F, et al. Evaluation of esophageal tracheal Combitube in cardiopulmonary resuscitation. *Crit Care Med.* 1987;15:609–611.

36. Rumball CJ, MacDonald D. The PTL, Combitube, laryngeal mask, and oral airway: a randomized prehospital comparative study of ventilatory device effectiveness and cost-effectiveness in 470 cases of cardiorespiratory arrest. *Prehosp Emerg Care.* 1997; 1:1–10.

37. Klein H, Williamson M, Sue-Ling HM, et al. Esophageal rupture associated with the Combitube™. *Anesth Analg.* 1997;85:937–939.

38. Ellis DG, et al. Guided orotracheal intubation in the operating room using a lighted stylet: a comparison with direct laryngoscopic technique. *Anaesthesia.* 1986;64:823–826.

39. Mehta S. Transtracheal illumination for optimal tracheal tube placement. *Anaesthesia.* 1989;44:970–972.

40. Hung OR, Pytka S, Morris I, et al. Lightwand intubation, II. Clinical trial of a new lightwand for tracheal intubation in patients with difficult airways. *Can J Anaesth.* 1995;42:826–830.

41. Tunstall ME, Sheikh A. Failed intubation protocol: oxygenation without aspiration. *Clin Anesthesiol.* 1986;4:171–187.

42. Benumof JL. Management of the difficult airway. *Anesthesiology.* 1991;75:107–110.

43. Practice Guidelines for Management of the Difficult Airway: a report by the ASA Task Force on Management of the Difficult Airway. *Anesthesiology.* 1993;78:597–602.

44. *Anesthesiology.* 1996;84:686–699.

45. Koppel JN, Reed AP. Formal instruction in difficult airway management: a survey of anesthesiology residency programs. *Anesthesiology.* 1995;83:1343–1346.

46. Caplan RA, Posner KL, Ward RJ, et al. Adverse respiratory events in anesthesia: a closed claims analysis. *Anesthesiology.* 1990;72:828–833.

47. *Report on Confidential Enquiries into Maternal Deaths in England and Wales, 1982–84.* London: Her Majesty's Stationery Office; 1989.

48. *Report on Confidential Enquiries into Maternal Deaths in England and Wales, 1988–90.* London: Her Majesty's Stationery Office; 1994.

49. The Association of Anaesthetists of Great Britain and Ireland and the Obstetric Anaesthetists Association. *Anesthetic Services for Obstetrics: A Plan for the Future.* London: 1987.

50. Hawkins JL, Koonin LM, Palmer SK, et al. Anesthesia-related deaths during obstetric delivery in the US, 1979–1990. *Anesthesiology.* 1996;86:277–284.
51. Pilkington, Scarli F, Dakin MJ, et al. Increase in Mallampatti score during pregnancy. *Br J Anaesth.* 1995;74:638–642.
52. Hawthorne L, Wilson R, Lyons G, et al. Failed intubation revisited: 17-year experience in a teaching maternity unit. *Br J Anaesth.* 1996;76:680–684.
53. McClure S, et al. Laryngeal mask airway for cesarean section. *Anaesthesia.* 1990;45:227–228.
54. Chadwick IS, Vohra A. Anaesthesia for emergency cesarean section using the Brain laryngeal airway. *Anaesthesia.* 1989;44:261–262.
55. Bachulis B, et al. Clinical indications for cervical spine radiographs in the traumatized patient. *Am J Surg.* 1987;153:473–477.
56. Bryson B, et al. Cervical spine injury: incidence and diagnosis. *J Trauma.* 1986;26:669.
57. Cadoux C, et al. High-yield roentgenographic criteria for cervical spine injuries. *Ann Emerg Med.* 1987;16:738–742.
58. Bayless P, Ray CG. Incidence of cervical spine injuries in association with blunt head trauma. *Am J Emerg Med.* 1989;7:139–142.
59. Kreipke D, et al. Reliability of indications for cervical spine films in trauma patients. *J Trauma.* 1989;29:1438–1439.
60. Ivy ME, Cohen SM. Addressing the myths of cervical spine injury management. *Am J Emerg Med.* 1997;15:591–594.
61. Hastings RH, Marks JD. Airway management for trauma patients with potential cervical spine injuries. *Anesth Analg.* 1991;73:471–482.
62. Meschino A, et al. The safety of awake tracheal intubation in cervical spine injury. *Can J Anaesth.* 1992;39:114–117.
63. Crosby ET. Tracheal intubation in the cervical spine-injured patient [editorial]. *Can J Anaesth.* 1992;39:105–109.
64. Hastings RH, Kelley SD. Neurologic deterioration associated with airway management in a cervical spine injured patient. *Anesthesiology.* 1993;78:580–583.
65. Reid DC, et al. Etiology and clinical course of missed spine fractures. *J Trauma.* 1987;27:980–986.
66. Blahd WH Jr, Iserson KV, Bjelland JC, et al. Efficacy of the posttraumatic cross table lateral view of the cervical spine. *J Emerg Med.* 1985;2:243–249.
67. Doolan LA, O'Brien JF. Safe intubation in cervical spine injury. *Anaesth Intensive Care.* 1985;13:319–324.
68. Biby L, Santora AH. Prevertebral hematoma secondary to whiplash injury necessitating emergency intubation. *Anesth Analg.* 1990;70:112–114.
69. Gopalakrishnan KC, et al. Prevertebral soft tissue shadow widening: an important sign of cervical spinal injury. *Injury.* 1986;17:125–128.

Bibliography

Benummof JL. *Airway Management: Principles and Practice.* St. Louis: Mosby; 1996.
Hagberg CA. *Handbook of Difficult Airway Management.* Philadelphia. Churchill Livingstone; 2000.
Latto IP, Rosen M. *Difficulties in Tracheal Intubation.* 1st ed. London: Bailliere-Tindall; 1985.

9
Complications of Endotracheal Intubation

Teeth
Laryngeal injuries
Pharyngeal injuries
Esophageal trauma
Tracheal/bronchial injuries
Lung
Hypoxemia
Acute hypoxic encephalopathy
Failure of oxygen at the source
Failure of oxygen at the delivery site
Improper procedure
Inability to intubate or ventilate
Vomiting and aspiration
COMPLICATIONS ARISING IMMEDIATELY AFTER INTUBATION
Hypoxemia
Accidental esophageal intubation
Ingestion of laryngoscope lightbulb
Accidental endobronchial intubation
Bronchospasm
Difficulty with ventilation
Laryngeal intubation
Accidental extubation
Rupture of the trachea or bronchus
Tension pneumothorax
Hypertension, tachycardia, and arrhythmias
Elevated intracranial pressure
COMPLICATIONS ARISING UPON REMOVAL OF ENDOTRACHEAL TUBE
Hypoxemia
Laryngospasm
Airway obstruction
Vomiting and aspiration
Sore throat
Temporomandibular joint dysfunction
Vocal cord injury
Postintubation croup
Difficult extubation
Arytenoid dislocation
Cord avulsion
Neural injury
Recurrent laryngeal nerve injury
Lingual, hypoglossal, and mental nerve damage
Mental nerve
COMPLICATIONS ARISING FROM LONG-TERM INTUBATION
Ulceration of the mouth, pharynx, larynx, and trachea
Granuloma formation

The routine use of endotracheal tubes in anesthesia occurred following the introduction of the neuromuscular blocking drugs by Griffith and Johnstone in 1942.[1] Few will dispute the importance of endotracheal anesthesia; however, the technique is associated with a myriad of complications, ranging from minor injuries to lips and teeth to permanent brain damage and death. The process of endotracheal intubation involves bag/valve/mask ventilation, insertion of airways, the use of various aids, laryngoscopy, and endotracheal intubation. Complications can occur at any stage of the process, but the majority of serious complications occur in association with the insertion or failure to insert an endotracheal tube. Therefore, most emphasis will be placed on complications arising from endotracheal intubation. We would like to start out by providing information on airway management complications from studies in various countries worldwide.

Airway Management Complications Summarized from Anesthesiology Morbidity Studies

Over the years anesthesiologists have sought to catalog the types of airway-related injuries as well as to establish causes. Understanding the problems and causes and implementing changes of technique, pharmacology, and equipment have led to improved patient safety. Guidelines and protocols are published to disseminate information and to standardize and improve care.

Anesthesiologists have led the way in establishing safer airway management practices. Worldwide, professional organizations, researchers, and teachers dedicate a very large portion of their time, expense, and effort toward improving airway management practices. Organizations such as the Society of Airway Management (Chicago) were founded, in part, to establish a forum dedicated to this aspect of medicine, which is important to all practitioners, not just anesthesiologists.

In the past, morbidity studies have been rather limited in scope, anecdotal, and even biased. Poor outcome implied blame. A litigious social environment did not encourage the practitioner to broadcast shortcomings. Because poor anesthesia-related outcome is so rare, large, prospective, controlled, randomized studies would be very expensive to conduct. None has been undertaken to date.

But recently, several ongoing studies have been reporting morbidity statistics that are gathered utilizing different methods. Some of the studies are large and have been retrieving and analyzing data for many years. Other studies are unique because of methodology or more focused scope. While many aspects of anesthesia morbidity are dealt with in these studies, only complications related to airway management will be described in this section. Hopefully, the lessons learned by anesthesiologists will be useful to other practitioners of airway management.

American Society of Anesthesiologists (ASA) Closed Claims Study

The American Society of Anesthesiologists (ASA) Closed Claims Study was initiated in 1985 by the ASA Committee on Professional Liability.[2] The study analyzes closed insurance claims. A **claim** is a financial demand made to an insurance company by a person alleging injury sustained from medical care. Once the claim is resolved, the claim is **closed.** Through the years, the ASA has gained the cooperation of 35 medical liability insurance companies and has gathered over 5,400 claims into its database.[3] Dental claims are not included in the study. A closed claim file typically includes the hospital and anesthesia records, narratives from involved personnel, "expert and peer reviews, deposition summaries, outcome reports, and the cost of settlement or jury awards."[4] The file is examined on site at the insurance company office by volunteer practicing anesthesiologists using standardized forms with specific instructions. The claims are further reviewed by project investigators and other anesthesiologists to establish reliability of the review process.[4(p553)] The study characterizes claims according to two basic features: **damaging events** and **adverse outcomes.** There are more adverse outcomes than damaging events "because some patients display injuries for which a specific damaging event cannot be identified in the records."[2(p1)]

The project managers and authors reporting data from the study admit that there are limitations to the study's design that must be considered when reviewing the published findings. Most notably, these limitations include the following:

Limitations of the Closed Claims Study[4(pp552–553)]

1. The study does not provide a denominator for calculating the risk of injury
2. The study is voluntary
3. The insurance carriers cover approximately 14,500 of the 23,000 practicing anesthesiologists in the country
4. The study is retrospective
5. Some injured patients do not submit claims

6. Data may be conflicting or incomplete

Despite these limitations, the study can be used to define specific types of morbidity and to establish hypotheses concerning the mechanism and prevention of anesthetic injuries.

Following are various findings from the Closed Claims Study relating to **airway management complications.**

Respiratory System

Since the study began, damaging events related to respiration have been the single leading source of injury. These accounted for 27%[2(p1)] of the total claims reported in 2000 and 38% of the claims for death and brain damage[4(p555)] reported in 1999. The three most common mechanisms of injury, accounting for 75% of all respiratory claims involved, are as follows:[2(p4)]

1. Inadequate ventilation (38% of cases)
2. Esophageal intubation (18% of cases)
3. Difficult intubation (17% of cases)

Respiratory-related claims were associated with severe outcomes (85% death or brain damage) and costly payments (median $200,000).[2(p4)]

An interesting conclusion of the study published in 2000 states that "most adverse respiratory outcomes were considered preventable with pulse oximetry, capnometry, or a combination of these two monitors."[2(p4)] This assertion presents a hypothesis that demands future research.

Management of the Difficult Intubation in Closed Malpractice Claims

A report published in 2000 analysed 4,459 claims and deals specifically with the management of difficult intubation.[5] Table 9.1 lists the most common **damaging events** reported in the study.

Brain damage or death was the outcome of 57% of the claims involving difficult intubation, compared to 43% of the claims concerning other **damaging events.**

Demographically, the claims involving difficult intubation tended to represent older, sicker, and more obese patients.

Disconcertingly, the study revealed that in nearly half of the claims involving

TABLE 9.1. Most common damaging events, ASA Closed Claims Study, number of claims: 4,459, year reported: 2000

Difficult intubation—6.4%
Esophageal intubation—4.5%
Inadequate ventilation/oxygenation—7%
Wrong drug or dose—4%
Other claims—78.5%

difficult intubation, **difficulty was not anticipated.** In fact, a preoperative airway history was not taken and a preoperative airway physical examination was not conducted in 25% and 22% of the claims respectively. **When airway difficulty was anticipated, 28% of the claims contained no information concerning airway management strategy.**

This report also introduced a new "difficult airway" subset generated from data gathered on a collection form based on the ASA Difficult Airway Algorithm. Ninety-eight claims fell into this category. (These claims were collected before the LMA was commonly used in difficult airway scenarios.)

Analysis of these 98 claims revealed that the "cannot intubate and cannot ventilate" situation occurred in nearly half of the reports. Hopefully, the Closed Claims Project will expand this subset's database and report more findings in the future.

Aspiration in Closed Malpractice Claims[6]

A report published in 2000 reviewing 4,459 claims states, "Of the total database, aspiration was either the primary or secondary **damaging event** (mechanism of injury) in 158 claims (3.5%). Aspiration was noted as the primary cause of the adverse event in about $1/2$ of the 158 patients."[6(p5)] Table 9.2 summarizes associated factors in the aspiration claims.

The incidence of death and brain damage in aspiration-related claims is 60%, compared to 43% of the remainder of the claims in the database. This high percentage of severe morbidity of aspiration-related claims may reflect the fact that most aspiration complications are readily treatable and that only in those cases in which extremely poor outcome ensues is legal action instigated.

Gas Delivery Equipment and Closed Malpractice Claims[7]

Gas delivery equipment in the operating room, the recovery room, and the ICU were associated with 72 of 3,791 closed claims analyzed and reported in 1997. Table 9.3 lists the site of occurrence of the equipment problem.

Misuse of the equipment rather than failure was implicated in 75% (n = 54) of the claims.

TABLE 9.2. Associated factors in 158 (of 4,459) aspiration-related claims, ASA Closed Claims Study, year reported: 2000

Phase of anesthesia	n = 158	%
Induction	67	42
Maintenance	28	18
Emergence/PACU	17	11
Obstetrical-related	33	21
Difficult intubation	20	13
Cricoid pressure	17	11
History of reflux	4	3

Source: From Cheney,[6] with permission.

TABLE 9.3. Equipment problems

Equipment group	Operating room	Recovery room	ICU
Breathing circuit (n = 28)	26	1	1
Vaporizer (n = 15)	15	0	0
Ventilator (n = 12)	8	2	2
Supply tanks or lines (n = 8)	8	0	0
Anesthesia machine (n = 5)	5	0	0
Supplemental oxygen tubing (n = 4)	0	3	1
Total (n = 72)	62 (86%)	6 (8%)	4 (6%)

Site of occurrence of equipment problem, ASA Closed Claims Study, 3,791 claims analyzed: 1997.
Source: From Caplan,[7] with permission.

The three most common damaging events identified were: breathing circuit misconnects (19%), breathing circuit disconnects (15%), and supply tank problems, most notably oxygen switches (10%).

The reviewers judged that 78% of the claims could have been prevented if better monitoring had been used. Overall, 38% of the claims were deemed preventable if capnography, pulse oximetry, or both monitors had been used.

Ambulatory and Office-Based Anesthesia and Closed Claims[3,8]

Claims involving ambulatory surgery and office-based anesthesia practices are increasing as the database incorporates more recently gathered information. As of 2001, 14 office-based claims and 666 ambulatory surgery anesthesia claims in which damaging events could be identified have been recorded. Damaging events involved the respiratory system in 22% of the ambulatory claims and 50% of the office-based claims. Damaging events associated with ambulatory claims included difficult intubation, inadequate oxygenation or ventilation, and airway obstruction. In the office, damaging events included airway obstruction, bronchospasm, inadequate oxygenation-ventilation, and esophageal intubation. While the numbers are small, it was judged that in the office, 50% of the claims involved substandard care while 46% of the claims were judged preventable if better monitoring was utilized.

Airway Injury during Anesthesia

A review of 4,460 closed claims found 266 (6%) that were associated with airway injury. The sites of the injuries are tabulated in Table 9.4.[9]

Laryngeal injuries included vocal cord paralysis (34%), granuloma (17%), arytenoid dislocation (8%), and hematoma (3%). Most laryngeal injuries were associated with short-term intubation.

Pharyngeal injuries included perforation (37%), lacerations and contusions (31%), localized infection (12%), sore throat without physical evidence of injury (12%), and miscellaneous (8%). Pharyngeal perforations were also caused by other equipment such as the nasogastric tube, suction catheter, and jet ventilator.

The most common esophageal injury was perforation (90%). Esophageal per-

TABLE 9.4. Anatomic site of airway injury

Site	Number of cases (% total)
Larynx	87 (33%)
Pharynx	51 (19%)
Esophagus	48 (18%)
Trachea	39 (15%)
Temporomandibular joint	27 (10%)
Nose	13 (5%)

ASA Closed Claims Study, (266 of 4,460 claims: 1999)
Source: From Domino,[9] with permission.

forations were also caused by a nasogastric tube, esophageal dilator, esophageal stethoscope, and surgical manipulation of a laryngoscope.

Tracheal injuries included injury from the creation of a tracheotomy (64%), perforation (33%), and infection (3%).

With respect to the perforation claims, early signs (pneumothorax and subcutaneous emphysema) were present 51% of the time. Late signs (retropharyngeal abscess and mediastinitis) were present 63% of the time.

The payment for esophageal injuries (median: $138,975) was higher than for any other class of injury.

"Injuries to the esophagus and trachea were more frequently associated with difficult intubation. Injuries to the temporomandibular joint and the larynx were more frequently associated with nondifficult intubation."[9(p1703)]

In conclusion, the ASA Closed Claims Study has been a very useful instrument to help anesthesiologists understand the types and mechanisms of airway-related morbidity. The information generated from the study will help researchers design prospective studies that could establish cause and effect relationships between specific injuries and the mechanisms leading to the injuries. Information reported by the study has guided anesthesiologists to propose protocols and guidelines designed to promote safer patient care.

Australian Incident Monitoring Study (AIMS)

The AIMS began in 1988. The study is administered by the Australian Patient Safety Foundation. The purpose of AIMS is to collect data documenting incidents that could or did cause patient injury in the practice of anesthesia in Australia. The anesthesiologist involved in the incident voluntarily submits a confidential form concerning the incident to the AIMS staff, who then process the data. While the methodology of the study shares some of the limitations of the ASA Closed Claims Study, the AIMS design may offer more clinically relevant and accurate data for a few noteworthy reasons. First, the clinician involved with the incident personally and promptly submits the data. The data is supplied firsthand. Second, investigators do not have to wait for an alleged victim to instigate data collection either through a malpractice suit or an insurance claim. Third, the

TABLE 9.5. Circuitry incidents, AIMS

Type of incident	1993 (2,000 incidents)	2000 (6,000 incidents)
Leak	129	474
Disconnect	148	437
Rebreathing	0	130
Misconnection	36	115
Disruption of gases	0	77
Overpressure	0	71
Other	6	404
Total	**319***	**1,708**

*In two cases, more than one circuitry component was involved.
Source: Russell, et al,[11] 1993; Petty,[12] 2000.

form submitted in the proper fashion is complete. It is designed to minimize incomplete data collection. Fourth, reviewers are not biased by narratives from self-proclaimed medical experts, nor confused by trying to interpret court proceedings, nor influenced by financial awards.

In 1993, the first 2,000 incidents of the AIMS were reported in a landmark symposium in the journal *Anaesthesia and Intensive Care.*[10] Following is a summary of the information reported in the symposium that is related to airway management complications. Information concerning equipment and monitors has been included, since the proper use and maintenance of both types of devices help to insure safe airway management. Updates to the 1993 data are made where available.

Many incidents involved problems with the airway circuitry. These are listed in Table 9.5.

Table 9.6 documents which circuitry component was involved in the incident reported.

TABLE 9.6. Circuitry involved in the incident, AIMS

Component	1993 (2,000 incidents)	2000 (6,000 incidents)
Endotracheal tube	4	550
Tubing or connection	5	392
Vaporizer	4	231
Ventilator	32	218
Absorber	4	159
Patient circuit valve (unidirectional valve)	46	144
Common gas outlet	0	112
Gas supply	6	74
Flowmeter	0	73
Humidifier	0	50
Scavenging system	0	43
Patient relief valve	0	24
Oxygen bypass	0	15
Laryngoscope	2	0
Other	6	225
Total	**109**	**2,310**

Source: Petty,[12] 2000; Webb,[13] et al, 1993.

TABLE 9.7. Airway incidents, AIMS

Type of incident	1993 (2,000 incidents)	2000 (6,000 incidents)
Obstruction	35	686
Nonventilation	12	408
Endobronchial intubation	79	203
Difficult intubation	85	—
Failed intubation	17	174
Extubation	0	130
Esophageal intubation	35	104
Trauma	0	70
Misplaced tube (not in trachea or esophagus)	7	0
Inappropriate tube choice	5	0
Other	0	606
Total	**275**	**2,381**

Table 9.7 summarizes information from multiple studies related to difficult intubation, esophageal intubation, and endotracheal tube problems.[12,14–16]

The classification nomenclature was slightly different for the two years reported. In 1993, a subset of "difficult intubation" was described. In 2000, only a "failed intubation" category of incidents was presented. By implication, difficult intubations are included in this group.

The paper entitled "Difficult Intubation"[16] will be discussed in more detail. The authors analyzed 2,000 incidents and reported 85 (4%) cases of difficult intubation. One cardiac arrest was reported in this subset of cases, while there were no deaths. Of the 85 cases reported, in 27 (32%) difficult intubation was not predicted. In 22 (26%) preoperative evaluation of the airway predicted difficulty. In 17 (20%) of the cases intubation failed. Switch to regional anesthesia was made in 6 of the failures, surgery was cancelled in 5 cases, and in 6 cases an emergency airway procedure was instituted. Various aids to intubation were utilized to help secure the difficult airway (Table 9.8).

Many factors contributed to the intubation's classification as difficult. These are listed in Table 9.9.

Finally, the complications that were associated with the 85 cases of difficult intubation are listed in Table 9.10.

The authors of the study suggested that a more thorough preoperative assess-

TABLE 9.8. Aids to intubation, AIMS, 1993 (2,000 incidents)

Aid used	Number of cases
Gum elastic bougie	24
Introducer	15
Fiberoptic endoscope	11
Magill forceps	3
Rigid bronchoscope	1
Blind nasal intubation (all failed)	7

Source: Williamson et al,[16] with permission.

TABLE 9.9. Factors contributing to difficult intubation, AIMS, 1993 (2,000 incidents)

Contributing factor	Number of reports
Obesity	14
Limited neck mobility	12
Limited mouth opening	11
Inadequate assistance	9
Teeth limiting access	5
Equipment deficiencies	5
Inexperienced intubator	4
Beard	2
Incorrect cricoid pressure	2
Wrong drug administered	2
Laryngeal tumor	1
Facial carcinoma	1
Masseter spasm	1
Ruptured trachea	1

Source: Williamson et al,[10] with permission.

ment of the airway and more readily available emergency airway equipment would be appropriate steps to help avoid and to manage difficult airways. Finally, the authors presented an algorithm that could be used to deal with difficult airway situations (Fig. 9.1).

Monitors and the AIMS (1993: 2,000 incidents)[17–19]

Of the 2,000 incidents under consideration, in 1,256 (63%) the authors signified that the role of the device used to monitor the patient undergoing general anesthesia was applicable to the study. They determined that the monitor detected the incident in

TABLE 9.10. Complications reported in association with difficult intubation, AIMS,1993 (2,000 incidents)

Complication	Number of reports
Esophageal intubation	18
Arterial desaturation	15
Central cyanosis	7
Esophageal reflux	7
Bronchospasm	5
Laryngospasm	4
Intubation right mainstem bronchus	2
Loosened tooth	2
Epistaxis	1
Ruptured tube cuff	1
ECG ischemic signs	1
Esophageal tear	1
Lacerated tongue	1
Cardiac arrest	1
Annoyed theater staff	1

Source: Williamson et al,[10] with permission.

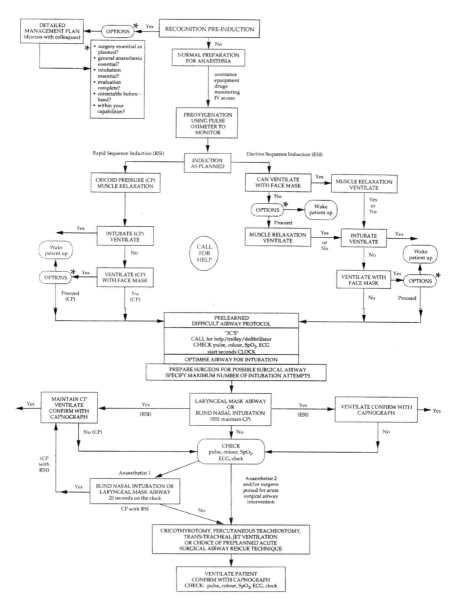

FIGURE 9.1. A suggested sequence for management of a difficult airway. It is assumed that ventilation is with 100% oxygen at all times. Special additional considerations may apply for obstetric and neonatal patients. Emphasis has been placed upon avoidance of entering a "no-win" situation, and upon the necessity for seeking early and skilled assistance. (From Williamson et al,[10] with permission.)

52% of the cases. The oximeter detected the incident in 27% of the cases, the capnography in 24% of the cases; this was followed by the ECG (19%), the blood pressure monitor (12%), low pressure (circuit) alarm (8%), and the oxygen analyzer (4%). The authors predicted that the oximeter used alone would have detected 82% of the incidents, 65% before organ damage occurred. Subsequent studies vindicate the guideline that both an oximeter and a capnograph be used on all patients undergoing any type of anesthetic. Oximeters should also be used to monitor sedated patients preoperatively as well as patients admitted to the recovery room after surgery.

AIMS and Obstetric Anesthesia[20]

An analysis of the first 5,000 AIMS incidents was published in 1999 which explored obstetric patients undergoing anesthesia and analgesia. There were 203 reports of 226 incidents related to anesthesia. Seven groups of incidents were reported. Twenty-six reports were related to equipment problems (12.8%), 18 related to difficult or failed intubation (8.9%), and 16 related to problems with the endotracheal tube (7.8%). Equipment failure included problems with the anesthesia machine, circuit disconnects, central gas (oxygen) system failure, and one case of laryngoscope blade breakage. Difficult intubation was reported in 18 cases; intubation failed completely in 12 of these cases. Nine of the 12 cases occurred in the emergency setting. Other airway-related incidents dealt with single cases of aspiration, bronchospasm and hypoventilation, and desaturation of oxyhemoglobin to 89%.

In conclusion, the AIMS is an ongoing, large-scale study that continues to gather and report studies related to patient safety.

Deaths Attributed to Anesthesia in New South Wales: 1984–1990[21]

A study published in 1996 concerning anesthesia-related deaths from the years 1984 to 1990 reported data collected under more stringent methodological conditions than those imposed by the ASA Closed Claims Study or the AIMS. Under government mandate, all deaths that occurred under, as a result of, or within 24 hours of an anesthetic had to be reported to the coroner. The coroner then notified the specialty committee investigating each death. The secretary of the committee would write the anesthetist to request that a questionnaire concerning details of the case be completed. The response rate for the years involved in the study was 93%. The New South Wales Special Committee Investigating Deaths Under Anaesthesia analyzed and reported the data. During this period, it was estimated that 3.5 million anesthetics had been performed in New South Wales. Confidentiality regarding the committee's activities has been legally guaranteed.

When considering the results of the study, the reader should recall that the data represent, at least in part, rather old findings. Many of the drugs, the equipment (such as the LMA), and the techniques (such as fiberoptically guided intubation) were not available or widely used in the early years of the study. Popular airway management protocols had not been published. However, since entry into the study was mandatory and a reasonable denominator had been established, the risk of mortality associated with anesthesia could be estimated. Unfortunately, the types and causes of less severe morbidity was not analyzed in the study.

The committee identified 1,503 deaths occurring in the years 1984 to 1990. The overall mortality rate per 10,000 anesthetics was calculated to be 4.4 (6.6 for males, 2.8 for females). Sixty percent of the deaths were considered inevitable, while 4% were considered accidental. The committee classified 172 deaths as "wholly or partly attributable to anaesthesia."[21(p66)] The airway-related conclusions of the study are reported here.

The first manifestation of crisis was respiratory in 22% of the deaths. Interestingly, the respiratory problem was first detected either in the recovery room or at another postoperative location in three quarters of the cases. Problems with the airway were the first indicators of crisis in 10 of the 172 cases. Most frequently, these airway problems occurred during surgical anesthesia, but 4 of these 10 cases occurred in the recovery room or in another postoperative location. The types and causes of the respiratory and airway problems were not specified in the study.

An important conclusion of the study was that postoperative care of the patient should include more vigilant airway and ventilation monitoring.[21(p73)]

This study is unique for its methodological design. Hopefully, in the future, the study will be updated and the types and causes of injury will be more specifically reported. Perhaps less morbid outcomes could also be defined and analyzed.

The Pediatric Perioperative Cardiac Arrest Registry (POCA)[22]

In an attempt to determine factors and outcomes associated with cardiac arrest in anesthetized children, the POCA Registry was established in 1994. Institutions that provide anesthesia to children (patients 18 years or younger) voluntarily provide data to the Registry. Cardiac arrest is "defined as the need for chest compressions or as death."[22(p6)]

In the year 2000, data from the Registry's first four years of collection were published. There were 289 cases of cardiac arrest reported. Results pertinent to airway management are summarized in Table 9.11.

The POCA Registry represents a new vehicle to collect, analyze, and report data related to one outcome of anesthesia practice. Its limitations are similar to those of the ASA Closed Claims Study. However, as more cases are reported, more insights into the airway-related causes of pediatric cardiac arrest and anesthesia will be gleaned.

TABLE 9.11. Respiratory system problems leading to cardiac arrest and POCA. 30 respiratory-related cases of 289 total cases (20%)

Mechanism	Number
Laryngospasm	9
Airway obstruction	8
Difficult intubation	4
Inadequate oxygenation	3
Inadequate extubation	2
Presumed respiratory	2
Inadequate ventilation	1
Bronchospasm	1

Source: From Mooray,[22] with permission.

TABLE 9.12. Factors associated with dental injury and anesthesia, Mayo Clinic

- General anesthesia
- Tracheal intubation
- Preexisting poor dentition
- Difficult intubation
- Previous difficult intubation
- Limited cervical range of motion
- Preexisting craniofacial abnormalities

Source: From Warner,[23] with permission.

Perianesthetic Dental Injuries[23]

Dental injuries were not included in the ASA Closed Claims Study. Dental injuries, though, remain at the top of the list of anesthesia and airway management–related morbidity. A recent study, reviewing the anesthetic records of 598,904 consecutive patients at one institution, established risk statistics for dental injury in the patient population under consideration. Findings pertinent to airway management are reported here.

The study identified 132 cases of dental injury. The overall risk of dental injury was approximately 1:4,500 of patients receiving anesthesia service. One half of the injuries occurred during laryngoscopy and tracheal intubation. For patients undergoing general anesthesia, the dental injury rate was 1:2,805 vs. 1:7,390 for intubated vs. nonintubated patients. Interestingly, three patients who received either local anesthesia or local with monitored anesthesia care received dental injury. The upper incisors were the most commonly injured teeth. Most frequent injuries were crown fractures and partial dislocations. More than one tooth was involved in 13% of the cases. The median cost of repair (in 1997 dollars) was $782 (range, $88–$8,200). Finally, the study identified factors that made the probability of dental injury more likely (Table 9.12).

NCEPOD (National Confidential Enquiry into Perioperative Deaths)

In the United Kingdom, an ongoing study has been updated and published since 1990. It is known as the NCEPOD. "The National Confidential Enquiry into Perioperative Deaths is a registered charity whose aim is to review clinical practice and identify potentially remediable factors in the practice of anaesthesia, surgery and other invasive medical procedures."[24] NCEPOD is an independent body with executives, a steering group, clinical coordinators, and local reporters in each of the participating hospitals. The steering group is composed of representatives from medical associations, colleges, and faculties in England, Wales, and Northern Ireland. Scotland conducts its own enquiry. All hospitals in the National Health Service and Defence Secondary Care Agency and public hospitals in Guernsey, Jersey, and the Isle of Man are included in the Enquiry, as well as many hospitals in the independent healthcare sector.[40(Appendix)] Confidentiality is guaranteed.

The authors of the report specifically state that NCEPOD is "not a research study based on differences against a control population and does not produce any kind of comparison between clinicians or hospitals."[24] The Enquiry does not look at the causation of death.[24]

For the 2000 report, all deaths that occurred within 30 days of a surgical procedure between April 1, 1998, and March 31, 1999, were included in the present Enquiry. Ten percent (10%) of the cases were randomly selected for analysis. A questionnaire was sent to each surgeon or anesthesiologist with whom a case was identified. The physician had until December 31, 1999, to return the questionnaire. Since April 1999, the government has made it mandatory for physicians in the National Health Service (NHS) to return the questionnaires. Enquiry staff members try to assure full compliance. In the present study, anesthetists returned 85% of the questionnaires, while surgeons returned 83%.[24(General Data)]

Because of the Enquiry's design, no specific airway-related information was reported with respect to causation of morbidity. The study listed "critical events" during anesthesia or recovery and compared these to events reported in the 1990 report. The events related to airway management are summarized in Table 9.13.

Other data documented that the recent trend was toward increased utilization of oxygenation and ventilation monitoring both in the operating room and especially in the recovery room.

TABLE 9.13. Critical events during anesthesia or the immediate recovery period, (airway related), NCEPOD 2000,[25] number of cases: 431

Critical event	1998/1999 (%)	1990 (%)
Airway obstruction	2	2
Bronchospasm	1	4
Hypoxemia (< 90% sat)	17	6
Misplaced tracheal tube	<1	1
Pneumothorax	1	1
Pulmonary aspiration	2	1
Respiratory arrest (unintended)	2	4
Ventilatory inadequacy	9	*

*Not reported.

NCEPOD 1996/1997 Report

Two airway-related recommendations published in a previous NCEPOD report are the following:

1. "A fibreoptic intubating laryngoscope should be readily available for use in all surgical hospitals. Several anaesthetists working in a department should be trained for, and competent at, awake fibreoptic intubations."
2. "The technique of tracheostomy should be taught to trainee surgeons. The indications for performing this procedure under local or general anaesthesia should also be taught."[26]

The NCEPOD is a very large study in which participation is mandatory. Perhaps the steering group should change the aim of the study and begin to ask questions that are included in the ASA Closed Claims Study and the AIMS. Then, specific mechanisms of injury as well as clinical practice patterns that lead to morbidity could begin to be defined in a population with a known denominator. This would be a very important step toward understanding anesthetic (and airway-related) morbidity and mortality.

SAMS (Scottish Audit of Surgical Mortality)

In Scotland, a mortality report similar in scope and design to NCEPOD is published annually. While "adverse factors"[27] are discussed and there is an "anaesthetics overview"[27(pp31–32)] section in the latest report reviewed (1999), no specific mechanisms of injury are documented. This is not a criticism of the report, as its aims were not to define causative factors related to surgical mortality. However, as with the NCEPOD, should the future goals of the study be changed to include more detailed questions concerning the mechanisms of injury, another significant step toward understanding airway-related morbidity and mortality would have been taken.

Danish Morbidity Study: 1994–1998[28]

The Danish National Board of Patients' Complaints (NBPC) was founded in 1988. The board receives complaints from patients or relatives against personnel employed by the Danish Health Care System. The board collects and reviews information concerning the complaint through a regional medical officer, expert reviews, comments from the involved parties, and a review of the medical records. The board reaches a final decision concerning the complaint after review by a committee consisting of a chairman, a judge, two laymen, and two professional members. The board may issue a reprimand, may turn the case over to the police or medical-legal council, or it may decide that the person or persons named in the complaint were not guilty of any violation of the standards of care.

From 1994 to 1998, the NBPC received 8,869 complaints. Three percent (n = 284) involved anesthesia or intensive care personnel. Complaints involving dental damage not associated with difficult intubation were excluded from analysis in a study that summarized the Danish morbidity findings.

TABLE 9.14. Danish National Board of Patients'
Complaints: 1994–1998, Total complaints: 8,869,
Respiratory complaints: 60

Category	Number
Misuse of anesthetic equipment	5
Neonatal resuscitation	8
Pulmonary aspiration	7
Uncomplicated intubation	8
Difficult intubation	15
Miscellaneous causes	17
TOTAL	**60**

Of the 284 complaints, 60 involved the respiratory system. They are summarized in Table 9.14.

Outcomes

Of the 60 respiratory complaints reported by the NBPC, "Thirty patients died, thirteen suffered permanent damage, and nine patients had temporary minor damage." In 32% of the complaints, treatment was ruled to have been substandard.

Difficult Endotracheal Intubation

Ten of fifteen difficult intubations were not anticipated. Nine patients died. Two cases were associated with caesarean section. Poor communication and inadequate assessment of existing medical records in the preoperative period contributed to poor outcome.

Complaints Related to Uncomplicated Endotracheal Intubation

Many different complaints involving the airway were lodged. These included hoarseness, temporomandibular joint pain, tracheal stenosis, and neurological symptoms involving the cervical spinal cord. No criticism was made about the anesthetic treatment in this subgroup of complaints.

Conclusions

The Danish study shares many design features with the American Closed Claims Study. However, the Danish study has confirmed, once again, that adverse respiratory events occur in the anesthesia–intensive care setting. The mechanisms of the different types of injuries are documented in this study. Finally, the study should lead to the establishment of educational strategies and programs that are designed to improve patient care.

Summary

The information presented in this section of the book clearly establishes the fact that airway management complications associated with the practice of anesthesia are myriad. Many complications are serious. Many problems involve the most basic airway maneuvers, such as ventilation, intubation, and observation of the patient. Many difficult airways are not predicted. Moreover, studies report that even when difficulty is predicted, strategies to deal with the anticipated difficulty are not documented. Problems with equipment and monitors are more likely to result from misuse rather than failure.

As a result of the lessons learned, anesthesiologists have established protocols, guidelines, and training strategies that are designed to improve patient safety. Hopefully, practitioners in other fields of medicine who are involved with airway management will learn from their anesthesia colleagues.

Complications Arising During Intubation

Trauma

Eyes

Occasionally during intubation attempts, a watch strap or ring may graze the cornea, leading to a corneal abrasion. Intraocular pressure rises significantly during endotracheal intubation, especially in patients who are improperly anesthetized. Succinylcholine, a depolarizing neuromuscular blocking agent, is also associated with increases in intraocular pressure.[29] However, bucking and coughing during attempts at intubation are the most common causes of significant increases in intraocular pressure. Sudden surges in intraocular pressure may be associated with extrusion of the lens or vitreous in patients presenting for anesthesia with open-eye injuries.

Upper Lip

Careless laryngoscopy often results in damage to the upper lip in the form of hematomas, lacerations, and teeth marks. During laryngoscopy, the upper lip tends to become trapped between the laryngoscope blade and the teeth. This problem is best avoided by manually clearing the upper lip from the laryngoscope blade. Such trauma is usually self-limiting, but its disfigurement can be annoying to the patient. Artificial airways are frequently placed in the oropharynx prior to extubation. Semiconscious patients emerging from anesthesia sometimes vigorously bite down on these airways, and if the airway has not been properly positioned, self-inflicted, unsightly bite marks to the lips occur.

Mucous Membranes of the Oropharynx

During laryngoscopy, the blade may inadvertently tear the mucous membranes in the region of the tonsillar bed. This is a common complication, most often seen on the right side, and is usually associated with inexperience. It is self-limiting and may be partly responsible for the sore throat often observed in the post-intubation period. Trauma to mucous membranes in the region of the larynx, however, is more serious, and may result in subcutaneous air or, worse, tension pneumothorax and pneumomediastinum. Subcutaneous air is an ominous sign and should alert the clinician to the possibility of tension pneumothorax and mediastinal air. A chest X-ray view must be obtained as soon as possible, and systemic antibiotics administered immediately. Positive-pressure ventilation is extremely hazardous in these patients. In elective situations, intubation and positive-pressure ventilation should be deferred if possible.

Koh and Coleman[30] recently reported a 5-mm ulceration in the oropharynx most likely caused by an overheated laryngoscope lightbulb. The laryngoscope was in the "cocked" position for several minutes before laryngoscopy. This anecdotal report reminds us of the importance of an equipment check before attempted intubation.

Teeth

Dental damage is the single most common complication resulting in litigation against anesthesiologists. A review of data from St. Paul Fire and Marine Insurance Company[31] indicated that it accounted for 15.3% of all litigious actions against anesthesiologists during 1985. There were 42 suits, with an average claim of $3,400.00. Some 29% of all successful malpractice claims against anesthesiologists are the result of dental damage occurring during the course of administering an anesthetic. It is interesting and surprising to note that oral airways accounted for 55% of all injuries to teeth. Anesthesiologists are not very knowledgeable about dental issues in general, despite the risks involved. Preoperative evaluation of patients must include a discussion about dental risk, and a record of that discussion should be entered on the chart.

It is difficult to obtain accurate information about all aspects of dental damage associated with anesthesia. Most of the data we have access to are retrospective and involve small numbers of patients.

The most recent information available on the topic of perianesthetic dental injury comes from the Mayo Clinic (see page 268).[23]

Even though this was a retrospective study, it was well designed, had good controls and high surveillance rates at 24 hours and 7 days, and was carried out in a single, large institution.

The introduction of the LMA predictably should reduce the incidence of dental damage associated with anesthesia. It is best to avoid laryngoscopy in patients who present with multiple crowns. Intubation can be readily achieved in these cases using blind techniques, for example, the lighted stylet.

Restorative dentistry has become quite sophisticated in recent years,[32] and a number of innovative techniques have been introduced to replace missing teeth. Some patients present with removable bridgework. These appliances are held in place by retainers and can be easily removed by the anesthesiologist or the patient. Butterfly bridges are now being used with increasing frequency. They lack the durability of a fixed bridge and are readily broken, and their "wings" are bonded to adjacent teeth and easily broken. Titanium implants are now frequently used by dentists. If dental trauma is anticipated, these appliances may be removed by the dentist before the procedure and replaced post-operatively.

Despite the frequency of claims against anesthesiologists for dental damage, insufficient attention has been paid to this problem. Evaluation of the airway should always include a thorough assessment of dental risk. If a patient is particularly vulnerable, alternative methods of anesthesia must be considered. Protective dental guards are available and may be inserted prior to laryngoscopy. Oral airways, which account for a large percentage of injuries, should be avoided whenever possible in those at risk. When dental damage occurs, the incident must be recorded in the patient's chart and the patient informed as soon as possible.

Laryngeal Injuries

Some laryngeal injuries occur at the time of intubation but are usually not evident until extubation or even later. In the Closed Claims Study,[9] 34% of laryngeal injuries involved paralysis of the vocal cords; granuloma occurred in 17% of cases and arytenoid dislocation in 8% (see Table 9.4). The vast majority of traumatic injuries (80%) were associated with routine tracheal intubation that was short term. These issues will be discussed in more detail later in the chapter.

Pharyngeal Injuries

The best source of information on these injuries comes from the Closed Claims Study.[9] The most common pharyngeal injuries in that study were:

Pharyngeal perforation (37%)
Lacerations and contusions (31%)
Localized infection (12%)
Sore throat (no obvious injury) (12%)
Miscellaneous injury (8%)

More than 50% of all pharyngeal injuries and 68% of pharyngeal perforations were associated with difficult intubation. Pharyngeal perforations were attributed to nasogastric tubes, jet ventilation, and suction catheters in equal number, and the cause was not determined in 50% of cases. Death occurred in 81% of pharyngeal perforations (5/6) and was caused by mediastinitis.

Esophageal Trauma

Esophageal perforation was the most common esophageal injury in the Closed Claims Study[9] (90%) and was clearly linked with difficult intubation in the majority of cases (62%). Esophageal perforation was strongly linked with female gender and age over 60 years. Instruments causing esophageal perforation included nasogastric tubes, esophageal dilators, esophageal stethoscope, and laryngoscope. Nineteen percent of patients presenting with esophageal injury died as a result of the complication.

The problem with both pharyngeal and esophageal perforation is that it is difficult to diagnose. Early signs of perforation include pneumothorax or subcutaneous emphysema. These signs were present in only about 50% of the cases. In many cases there was no history of difficult intubation. A chest X ray must be performed in all cases of difficult intubation and perhaps should be repeated 24 hours later. Typical symptoms of pharyngoesophageal perforation include severe sore throat, deep cervical or chest pain, and fever; and patients presenting with these symptoms following difficult intubation or nasogastric tube placement are prime candidates for mediastinitis, especially if aged 60 or over and female.

Tracheal/Bronchial Injuries

The majority of tracheal injuries reported in the Closed Claims Study[9] were in association with injuries that occurred following tracheostomy for difficult intubation. These injuries included tracheal perforation and infection.

Marly-Ané et al[33] recently described 6 cases of membranous tracheal rupture following endotracheal intubation. Overinflation of the endotracheal tube cuff was deemed to be the cause of this problem. The diagnosis was suspected on the basis of the following signs: subcutaneous emphysema, respiratory distress, pneumomediastinum, and pneumothorax.

A number of reports, mostly letters to the editor, discuss the concern about increased endotracheal tube cuff pressures when nitrous oxide is used. In some of these reports, it is suggested that we monitor intra-cuff pressures in intubated patients.

Tu et al[34] showed that cuff pressure changes due to N_2O could be minimized by using the same mixture of gases in the cuff that is used to anesthetize the patient.

Karasawa et al[35] showed that when N_2O is used in the cuff of the endotracheal tube, serious cuff leaks occurred when N_2O was withdrawn.

Lung

Pneumothorax may occur as a result of overzealous manual or mechanical ventilation in normal lungs, or normal manual or mechanical ventilation in diseased lungs. Endobronchial intubation is a risk factor for barotrauma in normal and diseased lungs.

Hypoxemia

Hypoxemia is an abnormally low tension of oxygen in arterial blood. In normal individuals breathing room air, the tension of oxygen in arterial blood is between 90 and 100 mm Hg. When the quantity of oxygen delivered to the tissues falls below metabolic demand, hypoxia occurs despite adequate perfusion.

Acute Hypoxic Encephalopathy

Acute hypoxic encephalopathy is a global insult to the brain from lack of oxygen that results in an arrest of aerobic metabolic activity, which is necessary to sustain the function of the Krebs cycle and the hydrogen ion transport system. The degree of permanent damage is variable and unpredictable, but generally, oxygen deprivation for more than 3 minutes is likely to result in some permanent brain damage. Every effort should be made to prevent hypoxic episodes because damaged brain cells cannot regenerate. If a significant hypoxic insult occurs, every effort should be made to minimize the damage. The patient's circulation and oxygenation must be restored as soon as possible. Hyperventilation and steroids are recommended to reduce cerebral edema. Anticonvulsants should be used if seizure activity occurs. Barbiturates reduce the cerebral metabolic rate and have been recommended by some authorities. In Haldane's words, "Oxygen lack not only stops the machine, but wrecks the machinery."

Failure of Oxygen at the Source

Very rarely, there may be failure of the oxygen supply at the central source. These central banks are usually situated in a remote part of the hospital in the open air. Severe weather conditions may cause excessive buildup of ice on the piping, which may interfere with oxygen delivery. Historically but, fortunately, rarely, serious plumbing errors have occurred whereby oxygen lines have been interchanged with nitrous oxide lines—with serious consequences. Defects such as these can be readily detected by using oxygen analyzers. If oxygen has failed at the source, the safety officer, the chiefs of anesthesiology and respiratory therapy, and the executive director of the hospital should all be contacted immediately.

Failure of Oxygen at the Delivery Site

The inability to deliver oxygen when needed is an emergency. The inability to deliver oxygen to patients who are apneic is a dire emergency. The most common cause of this problem is a breach in the delivery system close to the patient (e.g., a ventilator disconnect or an actual leak). Decreased oxygen concentration can also occur if the oxygen flowmeters are faulty. Furthermore, because of inexperience or inattention, the clinician may select a hypoxic mixture. Modern anesthesia machines are designed so that it is next to impossible to deliver a hypoxic mixture.

In case of oxygen failure, remember the basics: If an endotracheal tube is not in place already, begin mouth-to-mouth ventilation immediately. If an Ambu bag is available, use it. If an endotracheal tube is in place, deliver a tidal volume directly into it. In an operating room, each anesthesia machine should be equipped with two E-cylinders of oxygen that will allow a 10-liter flow of oxygen for 2 hours.

Improper Procedure

Because of failure to ventilate and oxygenate patients before and during attempts at intubation, hypoxemia may occur in the course of an intubation. Prevention of hypoxemia should always be your **main** priority when attempting endotracheal intubation.

Inability to Intubate or Ventilate

There are occasions when, for one reason or another, you will be unable to intubate or ventilate a patient. These patients are at great risk of hypoxemia and the aspiration of acid gastric contents. Risk factors for difficult mask ventilation (DMV) include: obesity, age, macroglossia, beard, edentulous state, short thyromental distance, history of snoring, and increased Mallampati grade III or IV.[36]

Vomiting and Aspiration

Aspiration of gastric contents into the tracheobronchial tree is one of the most feared complications in anesthesia, and a number of preventative strategies are routinely used to prevent this complication.

Blitt et al[37] suggested that for every 1,000 patients undergoing elective surgery, six would aspirate, and that the presence of a cuffed endotracheal tube was no guarantee against aspiration. Engelhardt et al[38] published a very comprehensive review of this important topic recently, and in that learned treatise they challenged a number of the accepted medical doctrines that we have been practicing for years. While the true incidence of aspiration pneumonitis is difficult to determine, it is clear from recent reports that the incidence of this malady is low and mortality following pulmonary aspiration in surgery is extremely rare (Table 9.15). These data should not encourage us to be complacent. We should still continue to take precautions to prevent aspiration. There are no data demonstrating that there is improved outcome following the use of antacids, H_2 receptor blocking agents or proton pump inhibitors. However, serious side effects, though rare, associated with their use. So we must question the routine use of these agents in at-risk groups. The critical volume and pH of gastric aspirant triggering a serious pneumonitis was established by Roberts and Shirley[39] almost 30 years ago (pH 2.5 and volume 0.4 mL/kg). Those values have recently been challenged. Schwartz et al[40] have shown that serious pneumonitis can occur in animals when the pH is as high as 7. They also suggested that the critical volume required to trigger a serious pneumonitis is 1 mL/kg. There are three pathophysiologic processes associated with aspiration of gastric contents:

1. Particle related complication—Patients might develop acute airway obstruction, severe hypoxemia, or be at risk for death. Particles must be rapidly cleared from the airway to prevent acute asphyxiation.

TABLE 9.15. Incidence of aspiration

Publication	Period of assessment	Method of assessment	Patient group	Number of anesthetics	Number of aspirations	Incidence of aspiration per 10,000	Factors thought to contribute to the risk of aspiration
Olsson, 1986 (1)	1967–1970 1975–1985	Retrospective study from database at Karolinska Hospital, Sweden	Children and adults	185,358	87	4.7	Emergency; abdominal surgery; history of delayed gastric emptying; pregnancy; obesity; pain; stress; raised intracranial pressure
Warner, 1993 (3)	1985–1991	Retrospective study from database at Mayo Clinic, Rochester, New York	Adults	215,488	67	3.1	Emergency; lack of coordination of swallowing; depressed conscious level; previous esophageal surgery; recent meal; laryngoscopy; tracheal extubation
Brimacombe, 1995 (7)	1988–1993	Meta-analysis of 101 publications on the Laryngeal Mask Airway	Children and adults	12,901	3	2.3	Emergency; Trendelenberg position; bronchospasm and light anesthesia
Mellin-Olsen, 1996 (2)	1989–1993	Prospective study from database at Trondheim University Hospital, Norway	Children and adults	85,594	25	2.9	Emergency; general anesthesia
Borland, 1998 (5)	1988–1993	Retrospective study from database at Children's Hospital of Pittsburgh, Pennsylvania	Children	50,880	52	10.2	Increased severity of illness; intravenous induction; ages 6 to 11; emergency
Ezri, 2000 (6)	1979–1993	Retrospective study from a hospital database	Adult females Peripartum period, except Cesarean Sections	1870	1	5.3	—
Warner, 1999 (4)	1985–1997	Prospective study from database at Mayo Clinic, Rochester, New York	Children	63,180	24	3.8	Emergency; depressed conscious level; gastroinestinal problems such as gastroesophageal reflux, ileus, bowel obstruction, hemoperitoneum, recent meal; sepsis; shock
Lockey, 1999 (8)	1999	Prospective study of the London Helicopter Emergency Medical Service	Adults Severe trauma from road traffic accidents and falls from heights	53	18	3,396.2	Emergency

Source: From Engelhardt T, et al,[38] 1999.)

279

2. Acid-related complications—These occur in two phases: (a) immediate tissue injury, and (b) a later inflammatory response. Most cases of aspiration are a combination of particle- and acid-related injuries that, when combined, have a synergistic effect on pulmonary capillary leaks.
3. Bacterial-related complications—Gastric and pharyngeal contents usually contain bacteria; however, prophylactic antibiotics are not routinely recommended as a preventative measure following aspiration of gastric contents.

Preventative Measures

The use of antacid therapy, endotracheal intubation, rapid sequence induction, and Sellick maneuver are now standards of care in anesthesia, even though we do not have data to support these measures. However, common sense tells us that some of these preventative measures do not need definitive proof. However, the risk/benefit ratio of routine antacid therapy must be challenged.

For treatment of pulmonary aspiration, the following measures are recommended:

1. Administer 100% oxygen by mask. Place the patient in 30° Trendelenburg
2. Thoroughly suction all gastric material from the oropharynx and trachea
3. Intubate patient and suction down the endotracheal tube
4. Apply positive pressure ventilation (PPV) with PEEP
5. Administer 100% initially
6. Obtain an arterial blood gas (ABG)

Steroids or antibiotics are not routinely recommended as prophylactic measures.

When intubating patients on a ward, never ignore the fact that they are at great risk for aspiration. In fact, in a number of these cases, aspiration of gastric contents is frequently the reason for intubation. Unlike patients presenting for routine surgery, few of these patients are prepared. Many will have ingested food recently. Furthermore, their reflexes may be impaired to some degree through illness and infirmity. Always be prepared to deal with this emergency. Oxygen and suction must be at hand. In patients who are particularly at risk, do not hesitate to conscript a bystander to apply cricoid pressure (Sellick maneuver).[41] However, be sure that you give clear instructions as to how this is done. Cricoid pressure is performed most effectively by placing the thumb and index finger of either hand on the cricoid cartilage, in the midline, and pressing firmly downward. Patients should be in the supine position. Also, the person applying cricoid pressure must not release it until instructed to do so, i.e., until correct tube placement has been confirmed and the cuff inflated. It seems ironic that the very procedure that is implemented to prevent aspiration and regurgitation (intubation) is often associated with this serious complication. On rare occasions, a tooth, tiny lightbulb, or other foreign body will enter the pharynx during attempted intubation. Be sure that the teeth or such foreign bodies lost in this manner are not aspirated or swallowed by the patient.

Recent data from the Closed Claims Study[6] remind us of the serious nature of aspiration pneumonitis and should encourage us to take every precaution to protect the airway in those who cannot protect themselves.

Complications Arising Immediately After Intubation

Hypoxemia

Accidental Esophageal Intubation

Despite advances in monitoring technology during the past 20 or 30 years, intubation of the esophagus is still a major cause of cerebral damage or death in anesthesia. Adverse respiratory events accounted for 27% of all cases in one Closed Claims Study[2(p1)] and these were invariably associated with either brain damage or death. About one fifth were due to esophageal intubation (conservative estimate). In 750 cases reported to the Medical Defence Union in the United Kingdom between 1970 and 1982,[42] in which patients sustained either cerebral damage or death, 100 were due to complications associated with tracheal intubation. In a recent study by Keenan and Boylan involving 163,240 patients, over a 15-year period[43] there were 27 cardiac arrests thought to be due solely to anesthesia, and four of these (15%) were due to esophageal intubation. One of the most disturbing observations about esophageal intubation is that it frequently occurs in relatively young, healthy patients. Data from the Closed Claims Study[44] indicated that the mean age of those who died or who were injured was 39 years and the median ASA status was 2.

Endotracheal intubation is readily performed in the majority of patients and esophageal intubation seldom occurs. It can be considered a forgivable mistake provided it is detected in time, before cerebral damage occurs. But do not become complacent about this seemingly simple procedure, and definitely do not rely solely on the usual clinical means to verify correct placement of an endotracheal tube. When a tube is correctly placed in the trachea, you cannot guarantee it will remain there. The consequences of failure to detect esophageal intubation are so grave that every effort must be made both to verify correct placement initially and to monitor placement continuously while the tube is in the trachea. The most reliable method of continuously monitoring tracheal intubation and tracheal tube placement is by using **capnometry.** Capnometry has become the standard for use during endotracheal intubation in most parts of the developed world, and though it is not foolproof, it is the most reliable technology available today.

Details about the principles of capnometry/capnography are beyond the scope of this text, so only the basics will be mentioned. The key to capnometry is the presence or absence of carbon dioxide. Carbon dioxide concentrations in exhaled air are usually around 5%, and in inhaled air they are about 0.04%. There are many ways to detect carbon dioxide. You should be able to not only detect the presence or absence of the gas but also quantitate it numerically (see a wave form via capnography). The use of capnometry does not relieve you of the responsibility of performing the usual clinical chores associated with endotracheal intubation, however. Although capnometry clearly verifies the presence of an endotracheal tube in the trachea in all but exceptional circumstances, it does not verify correct tube placement. Thus, you still need to rely heavily on clinical means to verify both that the tube is in the tracheobronchial tree and that it is correctly placed in the trachea, above the carina. This is best done by listening over the axillae and the epigastrium. And yet, even the presence of breath sounds at auscultation is not foolproof evidence that the tube has been correctly placed. For example, breath sounds over the epigastrium may be absent in a patient who has had a major gastric resection, despite the fact that the tube is in the esophagus. The consequences of an incorrectly placed endotracheal tube usually become evident within 1 to 2 minutes.

However, there are numerous anecdotal reports about delayed diagnoses of esophageal intubation. We are aware of a situation in which 40 minutes elapsed after the initial intervention before esophageal intubation was diagnosed. A number of factors may delay the diagnosis:

A preoxygenated patient with good respiratory function may recover from paralysis and breathe spontaneously for several minutes before hypoxia becomes evident. Some authors have even suggested that for this very reason, routine preoxygenation should be avoided. The logic of avoiding preoxygenation to make an earlier diagnosis of esophageal intubation, however, is difficult to accept.

An accidental extubation may occur with movement of the patient, especially movement of the head or neck.

An endotracheal tube may slide up and down in the trachea (by as much as 5 cm according to radiologic studies.)[45]

A patient may be accidentally extubated during attempts to place a nasogastric tube.

If the vital signs of a recently intubated patient suddenly deteriorate, esophageal intubation must first be ruled out. There may be great reluctance to remove an endotracheal tube in some cases, especially when the initial intubation was difficult or when the patient has a full stomach or is morbidly obese. Nevertheless, the best advice to give under these circumstances is "if in doubt, take it out," and the sooner this decision is made the better.

The consequences of esophageal intubation include asphyxia (especially if the patient is paralyzed), regurgitation of gastric contents (enormously increased and a frequent cause of death), and acute gastric and intestinal distension (which becomes very obvious after several minutes of delivering about 5 L of gas per minute into the stomach).

Esophageal intubation is a preventable complication. Ideally, capnometry/capnography should be performed on every patient who is intubated, because there is no guarantee that an endotracheal tube, correctly placed initially, will remain in that position after intubation.

Occasionally, an accidental esophageal intubation will become a "gastric" one, as demonstrated in Figure 9.2. In this particular case, the endotracheal tube disappeared following an intubation attempt in a neonate and was later retrieved

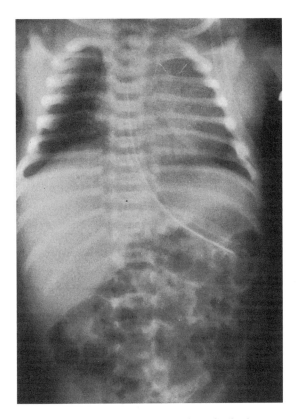

FIGURE 9.2. "Disappearing" endotracheal tube.

during esophagoscopy. This potentially serious complication can be prevented by being certain that the 15-mm adapter is always connected to the tube before intubation is attempted.

Accidental deglutition of endotracheal tubes is well documented in the neonatal and pediatric literature but rarely seen in adults. Block et al[46] reported such a case in a 28-year-old patient with head trauma. Attempts at intubation in the field by paramedics were unsuccessful. He was later intubated in the hospital. He made a full recovery and was discharged soon thereafter. Two years later, an incidental chest X ray revealed an endotracheal tube in the stomach, which was surgically removed.

Ingestion of Laryngoscope Lightbulb

Ince et al[47] reported an accidental ingestion of a lightbulb during laryngoscopy. The infant vomited a few hours later and the lightbulb was retrieved from the vomitus. This complication would have been far more serious if the lightbulb was aspirated. Part of the equipment check before intubation should include scrutiny of all the detachable parts of the laryngoscope.

Accidental Endobronchial Intubation

In the early stages of learning the technique of endotracheal anesthesia, most students have a natural tendency to advance the tube too far. Because of the anatomical layout of the trachea and mainstem bronchi, there is a greater tendency to advance the tube into the right mainstem bronchus. The right upper lobe bronchus arises, in many cases, about 2.5 cm from the carina. Thus, right mainstem intubations are quite often associated with collapse of both the left lung and the right upper lobe (see Fig. 7.18).

This complication is easily detected provided you follow the basic instructions of auscultation after placing an endotracheal tube. Notice also whether compliance of the lungs is significantly diminished. With a keen eye, you can detect asymmetrical movement of the chest wall. In addition, endobronchial intubation is often associated with "bucking" and straining by the patient and a few will become cyanotic. With the tube in the right mainstem bronchus, you are attempting to deliver the complete tidal volume into one lung, causing a significant increase in peak inspiratory pressure; this should alert you to the diagnosis. Also look at the centimeter marking on the tube. In an adult patient, it should be about 25 cm at the level of the nose during nasotracheal intubation, and about 21 cm at the level of the teeth during orotracheal intubation. You may also notice that it takes higher concentrations of inhalational agents to keep the patient anesthetized. Finally, pulse oximetry and end-tidal CO_2 monitoring can be used to detect misplacement of the tube in a more timely fashion.

Bronchospasm

Asthmatic patients are very sensitive to any type of airway manipulation and, unless properly handled, will develop bronchospasm that is sometimes so severe as to cause life-threatening hypoxemia. Bronchospasm may be described as an increased tone in the bronchial smooth muscles, leading to narrowing of the bronchi and bronchioles. The diagnosis is made when high-pitched rhonchi are detected at auscultation of the chest. The etiology is not clearly known but may be related to an excessive discharge from the nerves that supply the smooth muscles of the bronchi. It may also be chemically mediated. These patients are a particular challenge to the anesthesiologist. If there is even a hint of bronchospasm, elective surgery must be postponed because invariably it will become more intense during anesthesia, possibly due to an increased production of bronchial secretions and increased bronchomotor tone. Preoperative preparation is optimally facilitated by priming patients with aerosolized bronchodilators, anticholinergics, and, in severe cases, steroids. Endotracheal intubation should be performed only after the patient is deeply anesthetized. Bronchospasm may be the first manifestation of pneumonitis following aspiration of acidic material from the stomach.

Difficulty with Ventilation

Successfully placing an endotracheal tube in the glottis does not guarantee successful ventilation. If, after connecting the oxygen source, you are unable to effectively ventilate a patient, you must evaluate the situation systematically. First deliver 100% oxygen and auscultate the chest. The most common problems are endobronchial tube placement, bronchospasm, and undiagnosed pathology (e.g., pleural effusions or pneumothorax). Difficulty with ventilation may occur following esophageal intubation, especially in the last stages, and the aspiration of gastric contents may go unnoticed, though it usually presents with signs of bronchospasm. In the delivery room, you may encounter a neonate with diaphragmatic hernia. Pulmonary compliance is so poor that ventilation is almost impossible.

When confronted with difficulty in ventilating a patient, ask yourself four questions:

Is the problem related to disease process in the patient?
Is it related to tube placement?
Is it due to obstruction of the tube?
Is it caused by the oxygen delivery system?

Time permitting, each of these questions should be answered satisfactorily. Obstruction of the endotracheal tube may occur secondary to any of the following:

Kinking
Biting
Cuff herniation
Foreign body in the lumen
A small-diameter tube
Blood and secretions blocking the lumen
Manufacturing defects

Laryngeal Intubation

This is not strictly a complication, but it could become one. Typically, you are called to the ward to replace an endotracheal tube because of excessive air leak around the cuff. Before doing so, however, you should investigate further. It is always a good idea to note the centimeter marking on the tube at the level of the teeth, which will give you a reasonable clue as to the depth of the tube. In situations such as this, the tip of the tube is indeed below the vocal cords, but the cuffed portion may be partly outside and partly inside the larynx. Thus, large volumes of air are required to seal the leak. The nurse may inform you that as much as 30 cc have already been injected, but it is always a good idea to perform simple laryngoscopy. If your diagnosis is correct, you will notice a large globular, transparent (balloonlike) object in the oropharynx. A timely laryngoscopy at this stage may save you the trouble, and the patient the inconvenience, of an unnecessary repeat intubation. If the problem is not corrected, the patient is at risk for regurgitation and aspiration of gastric contents into the pulmonary tree as well as complete extubation.

Accidental Extubation

Failure to secure the endotracheal tube properly may result in an untimely extubation, which could be serious in an anesthetized patient undergoing surgery, especially if he or she is obese and in an odd position such as the prone jackknife!

Rupture of the Trachea or Bronchus

Rupture of the trachea or bronchus in association with endotracheal or endo-bronchial intubation is a rare and devastating complication. Most of the problems seem to arise in association with endobronchial tubes.[48–50] Sukuragi et al[51] reported a case of rupture of a mainstem bronchus during insertion of a double lumen (DL) tube. Rupture occurred in the membranous portion of the DL tube, which was advanced too far into the left mainstem. The patient was a very small, elderly female. Even though very little force was used, the tracheal portion of the DL tube was too large for the bronchus and ruptured it at its weakest point. In many instances, the etiology is poorly understood. Predisposing factors include:

Trauma
Age
Preexisting disease
Nitrous oxide diffusion
Tissue fragility

The diagnosis may be suspected when patients present with:

Subcutaneous emphysema
Decreased pulmonary compliance
Tension pneumothorax
Hemorrhage
Unexplained air leak
Surgical exposure

To avoid such complications, the following guidelines should be used in placing endotracheal or endobronchial tubes:

Never use force
Be careful with stylets
Do not overinflate the cuff
When using nitrous oxide, be sure to intermittently deflate the cuff
Deflate the cuff also during esophagoscopy
Use fiberoptic bronchoscopy to verify tracheal placement of the tube

Tension Pneumothorax

Tension pneumothorax is a life-threatening complication that may occur in association with endotracheal intubation. The diagnosis is made clinically, and you should not waste valuable time getting radiologic confirmation. (Despite the correct diagnosis and needle aspiration, a significant pneuomothorax was still present in this infant (Fig. 9.3). The cardinal signs are:

1. Marked cyanosis
2. Deteriorating vital signs
3. Diminished breath sounds
4. A marked decrease in pulmonary compliance

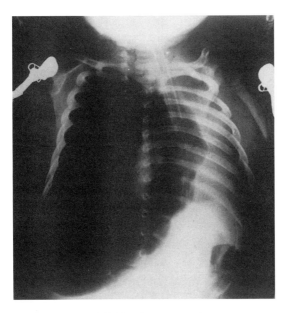

FIGURE 9.3. Tension pneumothorax.

Immediate treatment consists of inserting a large-bore needle into the affected side of the chest beneath the second rib. Patients improve dramatically within a matter of seconds.

Hypertension, Tachycardia, and Arrhythmias

Laryngoscopy and intubation are powerful stimuli to patients even in the anesthetized state. The most significant stimulus occurs when the endotracheal tube enters the trachea. A marked surge in blood pressure and heart rate may occur in the hypertensive patient unless he or she is deeply anesthetized or unless a vasodilator is used. Arrhythmias may also occur during and following intubation. Occasionally, the rate/pressure product (heart rate $\times$ systolic blood pressure) increases so much that ischemic changes are noted on the electrocardiogram. Persistent changes of this nature must be treated aggressively. Fortunately, ischemic changes are usually transient. Hypertension and tachycardia in the setting of intubation are likely due to systemically mediated vasomotor center stimulation. Hemodynamic responses to intubation in children are quite different from those in adults, especially those in the younger age groups. They frequently experience bradycardia during intubation, which is probably vagally mediated.

Elevated Intracranial Pressure

Endotracheal intubation often provokes a significant increase in intracranial pressure, which could be dangerous in an individual who has an intracranial aneurysm, cerebral edema, intracranial bleeding, or raised intracranial pressure. Every effort therefore must be made to control intracranial pressure in susceptible patients. Changes in intracranial pressure can be minimized with hyperventilation and blood pressure control and by the prevention of coughing and straining. Anesthetic drugs (e.g., thiopental and lidocaine) reduce intracranial pressure and may be useful in this situation.

Complications Arising upon Removal of Endotracheal Tube

Hypoxemia

Laryngospasm

Laryngospasm is a functional form of airway obstruction that, to date, has defied definition. It is poorly understood and often mislabeled. A physiologic mechanism has not yet been elucidated. The term *laryngospasm* has been loosely connected with any "crowing" sound emanating from the larynx. Fink,[51] who has shed more light on this interesting condition than most others, suggests that crowing emanating from the airway is due to apposition of the "true" vocal cords (which are readily separated by positive-pressure ventilation). The phenomenon is otherwise known as "shutter spasm" and is often a harbinger of true laryngospasm. Fink suggests that true laryngospasm is a form of airway obstruction caused by contraction of the extrinsic muscles of the larynx, which encroach on the airway in a ball valve–like fashion (Fig. 9.4). He maintains that the extrinsic muscles of the larynx come together much like an accordion, and in contrast to shutter spasm or stridor, the application of positive pressure may make the obstruction worse by forcing air into the piriform fossae (Fig. 9.5).

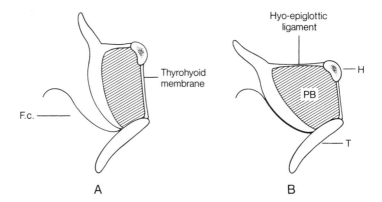

FIGURE 9.4. Sagittal section showing the action of a laryngeal ball valve. **A.** Open; **B.** Closed. During laryngeal closure the preepiglottic body (*PB*) is squeezed between the hyoid bone (*H*) and the thyroid cartilage (*T*). The paraglottis buckles and is forced against the upper surface of the false cords (*FC*). (Adapted from Fink,[52] with permission.)

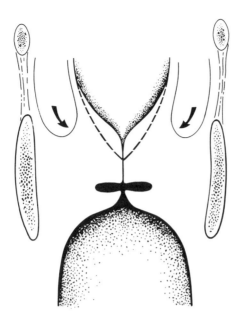

FIGURE 9.5. Effect of bag pressure on the closed larynx. Attempted inflation of the lungs distends the piriform fossae (*arrows*) and reinforces the closure. (From Fink,[52] 1956, with permission.)

Incidence

Laryngospasm has a predilection for younger individuals.[53] The incidence in all age groups has been estimated to be 8.7 per 1,000 persons studied and 17.4 per 1,000 between the ages of 0 and 9 years. The highest incidence seemed to be in infants between 1 and 3 months of age. While most anesthesiologists view it as a self-limiting condition devoid of serious morbidity, the literature reveals that 5/1,000 patients who develop laryngospasm have a cardiac arrest.

The following factors influence its development:

Inadequate anesthesia
Premature extubation
Semicomatose state
Aspiration
Presence of a nasogastric tube

The highest incidence has been reported in children with upper respiratory tract infections (95.8/1,000).

Clinical Features

The onset of laryngospasm is usually quite sudden. It may occur in any age group, but children are especially vulnerable. Premature extubation is the usual offending stimulus. Typically, there is very little warning and the patient rapidly desaturates. Effective positive-pressure ventilation is rarely possible until either a neuromuscular blocking drug is administered or profound hypoxia ensues. Premature application of a tourniquet or a rectal examination in a lightly anesthetized patient may be sufficient to induce it. Light anesthesia with either a barbiturate or an inhalation agent may sensitize laryngeal reflexes to develop spasm.

Laryngospasm typically occurs with unusual rapidity following stimulation of the airway in a lightly anesthetized patient. In contrast to stridor, which is manifested by a crowing sound of varying pitch, laryngospasm is a relatively silent phenomenon characterized by strenuous respiratory efforts similar to those observed in a choking victim. There is no obvious movement of air and O_2 saturation falls rapidly. Positive-pressure ventilation is generally ineffective under these circumstances. Laryngospasm usually breaks when profound hypoxia occurs. Most anesthesiologists intervene, however, before profound hypoxemia ensues. Although PPV is probably ineffective under these circumstances, few authors would argue with its use, because when the spasm eventually does abate O_2 may be immediately delivered. Small doses of neuromuscular blocking drugs IV (succincylcholine 10 mg/70 kg) are usually rapidly effective in breaking the spasm. An anticholinergic is recommended when succinylcholine is administered under these circumstances. (An intramuscular [IM] injection may be necessary in the absence of IV access.) Fink has suggested that laryngospasm may be relieved by performing the triple airway maneuver (which serves to disengage the supraglottic body from its locked position on the glottis).

Larson[54] recently published a letter to the editor in *Anesthesiology* in which he described the best treatment of laryngospasm. His description of the maneuver is as follows: "The technique involves placing the middle finger of each hand in what I call the laryngospasm notch. This notch is behind the lobule of the pinna of each ear. It is bounded anteriorly by the ascending ramus of the mandible adjacent to the condyle, posteriorly by the mastoid process of the temporal bone, and cephalad by the base of the skull (Fig. 9.6). The therapist presses very firmly inward toward the base of the skull with both fingers, while at the same time lifting the mandible at a right angle to the plane of the body (i.e., forward displacement of the mandible or 'jaw thrust'). Properly performed, it will convert laryngospasm within one or two breaths to laryngeal stridor and in another few breaths to unobstructed respirations."

The author convincingly reported the high degree of success he had experienced when he applied this maneuver in cases of laryngospasm but was unable to explain the mechanism and gave credit to a former mentor for this important "pearl."

Laryngospasm may be life-threatening in patients with limited cardiorespiratory reserve and should be avoided in all patients, not just those who are particularly vulnerable. It is impossible to quantitate the long-term effects of brief episodes of hypoxemia, but common sense suggests you strive to maintain good oxygenation in any patient who has entrusted you with this responsibility. Therefore, every effort should be made to prevent laryngospasm. Negative pressure

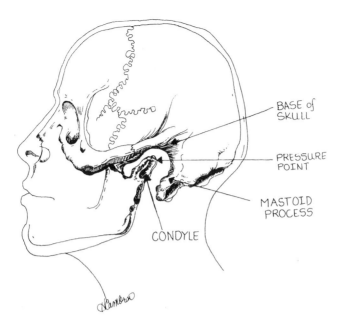

FIGURE 9.6. Schematic illustration of laryngospasm notch bounded anteriorly by the condyle of the mandible, posteriorly by the mastoid process, and superiorly by the base of the skull. Digital pressure is applied firmly inwardly and anteriorly on each side of the head at the apex of the notch (see pressure point arrow), which is slightly cephalad to the plane of the earlobes (not shown). (From Larson,[53] with permission.)

pulmonary edema may develop in spontaneously breathing patients following laryngospasm. Therefore, every effort must be made to prevent laryngospasm. Extubation should be carefully timed especially in children and all external stimuli should be avoided in a child who is emerging from anesthesia. Ideally, the child should be able to open his eyes and make purposeful movements before extubation. And, if deep extubation is required, be sure that the child is indeed deep. Lidocaine 2 mg/kg IV within 2 to 3 minutes of extubation may reduce the tendency toward laryngospasm. If a child is bucking on the endotracheal tube or has a conjugate gaze, it is advisable to allow him to wake up before extubation. It is also important to allow regular respirations to occur before extubation.

In summary, laryngospasm is a relatively common clinical situation in pediatric anesthesia. Serious morbidity rarely occurs but healthy patients may become profoundly hypoxic for brief periods. The problem can be prevented by obeying some simple rules when the patient is emerging from anesthesia.

Airway Obstruction

Airway obstruction may occur immediately upon removal of the endotracheal tube if done prematurely. For example, a patient may not have recovered fully from anesthesia, narcotic and sedative drugs, or neuromuscular blocking agents.

Inadequate tone in the muscles of the jaw and tongue allows the tongue to approach the posterior pharyngeal wall, causing obstruction of the airway. Patients who develop airway obstruction following extubation should be given high O_2 concentrations; bag/valve/mask ventilation may be required, and occasionally patients may require reintubation.

Vomiting and Aspiration

If a patient's reflexes are impaired upon removal of the endotracheal tube, vomiting and regurgitation can result in aspiration.

Sore Throat

Sore throat is probably the most common complaint that patients have following intubation, especially in association with anesthesia. The incidence varies somewhere between 5% and 100%, depending on the author.[55] There have been some interesting observations in the literature. First, the incidence is doubled in patients who are intubated during anesthesia versus those who are not. Second, it is greater in patients who have a nasogastric tube in place. Third, it is greater in female than in male patients. And fourth,[56] its incidence and severity are proportional to the internal diameter of the endotracheal tube.

Abrasions and lacerations of the oropharynx and nasopharynx can occur, especially lacerations of the palatopharyngeal and the palatoglossal folds, when intubation is attempted by inexperienced personnel.

Steward[57] reviewed the problem in children undergoing outpatient anesthesia and reported a 59% incidence. He also found that the incidence was proportional to the duration of surgery: 24% when an oral airway was in place, and 8.5% when neither an oral airway nor an endotracheal tube was used. A more recent study by Monroe et al[58] of adults showed that the presence of a hard, plastic oropharyngeal airway did not appear to influence the incidence of sore throat, although the incidence of sore throat was increased relative to the incidence of pharyngeal trauma from any cause.

Vigorous suctioning of the oropharynx may contribute significantly to the incidence of postoperative sore throat.

Temporomandibular Joint Dysfunction

Temporomandibular joint dysfunction following the administration of an anesthetic is quite unusual. Etiologic factors include prolonged mouth opening and forcible advancement of the mandible during airway maneuvers. Subluxation with dislocation has been reported.[59] On awakening, the patient notices the inability to close the mouth. Subluxation and dislocation may occur during intubation when patients are profoundly relaxed. Although the mandible can be manually manipulated, it is painful. Do not hesitate to consult an oral surgeon when the problem arises. The temporomandibular joint is quite complicated and must be handled carefully.

Vocal Cord Injury

Postintubation Croup

Postintubation croup occurs in association with edema of the true vocal cords and is most commonly seen in children. A barking cough is diagnostic. The smaller the child, the greater the concern. It is usually self-limiting, and treatment consists of humidified oxygen, racemic epinephrine, and dexamethasone (2 mg/kg IV). Caution should be used before discharging a child from outpatient facilities when stridor is present; if in doubt, admit the patient overnight for observation. As it progresses, the treatment presents the physician with a real dilemma because the very instrument that caused the problem may also be the one needed to deal with it.

Difficult Extubation

Volumes have been written about the "difficult" intubation; however, it is interesting to note that extubation may also be difficult, for a variety of reasons. Clearly, pathology within the larynx can interfere with your ability to withdraw an endotracheal tube. Occasionally, and not always easily explained, the cuff of an endotracheal tube remains inflated. This complication has occurred with the Laser-Flex tube but may also occur with regular endotracheal tubes. Sometimes an endotracheal tube will become inadvertently fixed to surrounding structures by an unsuspecting surgeon operating in the vicinity of the oropharynx or neck. The inability to deflate the cuff is easily remedied by piercing the balloon under direct vision, or by inserting a needle through the cricothyroid ligament. The number of anecdotes about endotracheal tubes being accidentally fixed in place with Kirschner wires, screws, and sutures increases with time.

Arytenoid Dislocation

Dislocation of an arytenoid cartilage is an unusual injury that can occur following blunt trauma to the neck, or medical instrumentation of the larynx (Fig. 9.7). The symptoms and signs include, hoarseness, aphonia, stridor, sore throat, a "lump in the throat," and unilateral or bilateral vocal cord paresis or paralysis. The condition has been reported in adults, children, and neonates. Older patients and women may be more susceptible, and left-sided dislocation appears to be more common. There are only about 80 cases reported in the anesthesia literature.[60] The problem may become evident immediately upon recovering from anesthesia or later, although the diagnosis is usually made clinically or laryngoscopically, or by CT scan. The dislocation may be corrected by manipulating the arytenoid cartilage with a spatula, which is done under local anesthesia and requires the expertise of an otolaryngologist. Postoperative vocal cord paralysis may be a manifestation. A neurogenic cause must be ruled out. Arytenoid dislocation has been reported in two patients

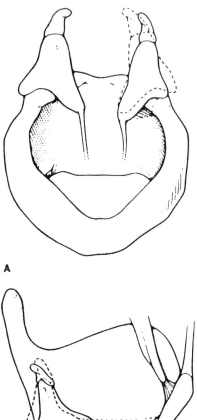

FIGURE 9.7. Position of a displaced arytenoid (*solid line*) compared to normal (*dotted line*). **A.** Anterior view showing the left arytenoid displaced anteriorly, medially, and inferiorly with bowing of the true vocal fold. **B.** Sagittal view showing anteroinferior displacement of the arytenoid with paradoxical posterior displacement of the superior process. (From Close LG, et al. *Head Neck Surg.* 1987;9: 341, with permission.)

A

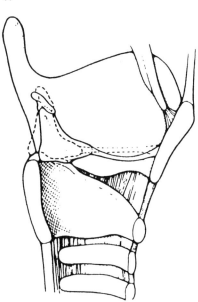

B

following the use of the lighted stylet.[61] Usui et al[62] reported a case following the use of the McCoy laryngoscope. Common sense would suggest that the incidence might be higher following traumatic intubation. For more complete details about this interesting condition, refer to a treatise on the topic published in the *Archives of Otolaryngology* by Quick and Merwin.[63]

Cord Avulsion

Avulsion of the vocal cords is a rare form of traumatic injury associated with endotracheal intubation that occurs in association with unsuccessful blind attempts at intubation using a styletted endotracheal tube. If suspected at any time, an ENT surgeon should be consulted regarding further treatment.

Neural Injury

Recurrent Laryngeal Nerve Injury

Unilateral or bilateral vocal cord paralysis or paresis is a rare occurrence following intubation and the etiology is not well understood.[64–66] It may occur following prolonged intubation or intubation for a brief period.[67] Symptoms may be immediately evident or delayed. Patients usually present with stridor and dyspnea and tracheostomy may be necessary. The etiology is not well understood but it has been suggested that the cuff of the endotracheal tube exerts pressure on one or both recurrent laryngeal nerves. Ellis and Pallister[68] have suggested that the anterior branch of the recurrent laryngeal nerve can be compressed against the lamina of the thyroid cartilage by the inflated cuff of the endotracheal tube. Whited[69] has suggested that traumatic cricoarytenoid joint arthritis is the mechanism of this malady. The prognosis depends upon whether the recurrent laryngeal nerves recover spontaneously or not, which is dependent upon the degree of scarring and fibrosis in the cricoarytenoid joints. Tracheostomy is the initial line treatment for this problem and arytenoidectomy may be necessary later if decannulation cannot be achieved.

The authors recollect one case of vocal cord paralysis in our combined 50 years' experience. The patient developed bilateral vocal cord paresis following a relatively short surgical procedure. The anesthesiologist reported an uneventful laryngoscopy and intubation and even recorded the amount of air that was used to inflate the cuff. Fortunately, this patient did not require a tracheostomy and recovered fully after several days. Ironically, this patient was the wife of a very prominent physician in the community.

Although neuropraxic injury is the most likely explanation, other possibilities must also be considered. The random nature of Bell's palsy, for example, is well known; perhaps some recurrent laryngeal nerve injuries are caused by a viral neuritis. The recurrent laryngeal nerve can be injured during attempts to place a central venous catheter. Surgical trauma during thyroid surgery or thoracotomy should be considered. Hyperextension of the neck may exert traction on the recurrent laryngeal nerve. Vocal cord paralysis has also been linked with nasogastric tube insertion. The mechanism is thought to be due to erosion or ulceration of the posterior cricoid plate followed by diffuse inflammation, eventually involving the recurrent laryngeal nerves.[70,71] In a way, this condition is a bit of a medical curiosity, though not a pleasant experience for the person afflicted. Therefore, be meticulous when performing endotracheal intubation. Select the correct-sized tube and inject only the minimal amount of air into the cuff. Also be aware that nitrous oxide can diffuse into the cuff and add significantly to the pressure applied to the tracheal mucosa. When the cuff pressure on the mucosa exceeds normal capillary pressure (25–30 mm Hg), ischemia may occur.

Lingual, Hypoglossal, and Mental Nerve Damage

Neurological deficits over the distribution of the lingual and hypoglossal nerves have been reported.[72,73] They are probably related to traction during airway management or intubation, and the patient usually recovers with time. Lingual nerve injury is a rare complication of laryngoscopy and airway management that may occur as an isolated event or in association with hypoglossal nerve injury. Although the etiology is not clearly delineated, it is likely due to compression of the nerve during forceful laryngoscopy. A recent report by Venkatesh and Walker[74] describes a case of hypoglossal nerve injury following an unplanned extubation of a patient while the cuff of the endotracheal tube remained inflated. They suggested that the inflated cuff may have compressed the hypoglossal nerve up against the hyoid bone (see Fig. 1.6) and that traction during extubation may have stretched the nerve. Cricoid pressure and vigorous mandibular maneuvers may be contributing factors. As many as eight cases have been reported in the world literature so far. Similar to other neuropraxic injuries, the condition is usually temporary and recovery is complete.

Mental Nerve

Montoya Pelaez et al recently reported a case of mental nerve compression secondary to pressure exerted on the chin by a ring adhere Elwin (RAE) tube.[75]

Complications Arising from Long-Term Intubation

With advances in technology, materials used for endotracheal intubation have become less injurious to the tissues. However, long-term complications still occur.

Ulceration of the Mouth, Pharynx, Larynx, and Trachea

Ulcers are uncommon following endotracheal intubation and heal spontaneously after the offending agent is removed.

Granuloma Formation

Polypoid growths occur on the vocal cords of some patients who have been intubated and are most likely the result of trauma. The incidence varies between 1 per 1,000 and 1 per 20,000 cases and is more common in women. Surgical removal may be required.

Formation of Synechiae and Webs

Trauma to the vocal cords may lead to loss of mucous membrane, causing the vocal cords to adhere to one another. This condition, called synechiae formation, is a rare occurrence. Membrane or web formation may occur in the larynx or trachea following intubation and is also rare, usually an incidental finding at autopsy.

Tracheal Stenosis

Tracheal stenosis occurs because of damage to the mucous membrane and cartilaginous framework of the trachea. It is most often associated with prolonged intubation. In recent years, however, cuffs have been designed to minimize the amount of pressure exerted on the tracheal wall, and the current materials used to manufacture endotracheal tubes are less irritating to tissues.

When the pressure exerted laterally on the tracheal wall exceeds capillary pressure (approximately 25 mm Hg in a healthy patient), ischemia to the mucous membrane may occur. This can be minimized by using more compliant cuffs and injecting the minimal amount of air required. The cuff should be deflated at intervals in any patient undergoing prolonged ventilation to allow perfusion of the mucous membrane at the cuff site.

The length of time an endotracheal tube should be allowed to remain in place before a tracheostomy is a controversial issue. There are two schools of thought. One is the traditional approach; perform tracheostomy after 2 weeks of endotracheal intubation unless the patient is ready to be extubated in the near future. The other is more liberal; allow intubation for several months before a tracheostomy is considered. There are no hard-and-fast rules about which school is correct. Each should be assessed on its own merits. Patients requiring chronic airway care are rarely accepted by chronic care institutions unless a tracheostomy is performed. This is one of the more common indications for tracheostomy in a hospital setting today. More outcome studies are needed to make a decision on this very important issue.

Complications Occurring Specifically in Relation to Nasotracheal Intubation

Epistaxis

Bleeding is common during nasal intubation. Sometimes it occurs as a result of nasal polyps or trauma to Little's area (or Kiesselbach's area). Endotracheal tubes should be well lubricated, and a decongestant should be used whenever possible. When introducing a nasal tube, be sure to run its bevel parallel with the septum lest its tip disrupt the turbinates. On attempting to pass a tube through the nose, direct it at a right angle to the horizontal in a supine patient. The tube selected should be a half to one whole size less than that commonly used for orotracheal intubation.

Submucosal Dissection

Occasionally, an endotracheal tube may be forcibly passed submucosally into the nasopharynx. This complication manifests itself by creating an elongated bulge just above the tonsillar area of the oropharynx on either side. The operator usually complains of not being able to find the tip of the tube in the oropharynx. This complication is self-limiting, unless the tube is hooked to an oxygen source. In that event, massive subcutaneous emphysema and airway obstruction may develop.

Middle Turbinectomy

Middle turbinectomy is a reported complication of nasotracheal intubation. Dislocation of the middle turbinate has also been reported following nasotracheal intubation. These complications can also follow the passage of nasopharyngeal airways. The authors observed an unusual case of airway obstruction following passage of a nasopharyngeal airway. The patient developed complete airway obstruction following passage of a nasopharyngeal airway. Direct laryngoscopy revealed a large polyp completely occluding the airway. The polyp was removed with a McGill forceps and the obstruction was immediately relieved.

Baumann et al[76] recently reported airway obstruction following the passage of a "trumpet" nasopharyngeal airway into the nose that entered the submucosal space and eventually the retropharyngeal space, causing serious airway obstruction.

Trauma to the Posterior Pharyngeal Wall

As with oral intubation, when nasotracheal intubation is being done, the endotracheal tube may encroach on the posterior pharyngeal wall and cause bleeding.

Trauma to the Adenoids

Bleeding during either nasotracheal or orotracheal intubation may occur secondary to trauma to the adenoids, especially in children.

Pressure Necrosis in the Nose

Ischemia of and necrosis within the nose may occur following nasotracheal intubation, but it can be prevented by proper stabilization of the tube and by using a specially designed connector. Necrosis may eventually lead to stricture of a nostril.

Obstruction of the Eustachian Tube

The eustachian tube may become obstructed secondary to prolonged nasotracheal intubation.

Maxillary Sinusitis

Sinusitis[77] is a complication of nasotracheal intubation caused by blockage of the opening into the maxillary sinus. It may be a hidden source of sepsis in a critically ill patient on an intensive care ward.

Complications of Laser Surgery

Laser surgery is now in vogue for the treatment of many conditions, including laryngeal tumors.[78] A number of precautions must be taken when it is performed on the larynx. First, the exposed part of the endotracheal tube must be wrapped with metallic foil lest the tube ignite. Second, nitrous oxide and oxygen both support combustion. Therefore, a combination of oxygen and helium may be preferable in these situations because the mixture is less likely to flare and helium is capable of dissipating the heat at a greater rate. Furthermore, because of its physical characteristics, helium may enhance the flow of gases through the tube. Finally, personnel should wear protective glasses when laser treatment is in progress.

Summary

Although the list of complications associated with endotracheal intubation is lengthy and imposing, most of them can be avoided by paying attention to details. Many are associated with hypoxemia and thus every effort must be made to maintain adequate oxygenation at all times. If difficulties are anticipated, preoxygenate the patient for 2 or 3 minutes. Traumatic complications are quite common and some can be disfiguring and annoying to the patient; others, such as tension pneumothorax, are life-threatening.

Never use force when placing an endotracheal tube. Dental damage, though common, is often avoidable and is a great source of annoyance to patients. Esophageal intubation is a major cause of serious morbidity and mortality. You can never be too sure about placing an endotracheal tube, and there is no guarantee that once placed correctly, it will remain in place. Even experienced clinicians have failed to detect esophageal intubation. Finally, remember: There is no greater responsibility than that of oxygenating the patient who is unable to breathe on his own.

References

1. Griffith HR, Johnson GE. The use of curare in general anesthesia. *Anesthesiology.* 1942;3:418.
2. Caplan RA. The ASA Closed Claims Project: lessons learned. *ASA Refresher Course #265.* 2000;1–7.
3. Domino KB. Office-based anesthesia: lessons learned from the Closed Claims Project. *ASA Newsletter.* 2001;65(6):9–15.
4. Cheney FW. The American Society of Anesthesiologists Closed Claims Project. *Anesthesiology.* 1999;91(2):552–556.

5. Miller CG. Management of the difficult intubation in closed malpractice claims. *ASA Newsl.* 2000;64(6):13–19.

6. Cheney FW. Aspiration: a liability hazard for the anesthesiologist? *ASA Newsletter.* 2000;64(6):5–26.

7. Caplan RA, et al. Adverse anesthetic outcomes arising from gas delivery equipment. *Anesthesiology.* 1997;87(4):741–748.

8. Posner KL. Liability profile of ambulatory anesthesia. *ASA Newsl.* 2000;64(6):5–12.

9. Domino KB, et al. Airway injury during anesthesia. *Anesthesiology.* 1999;91(6):1703–1711.

10. Williamson JA, Webb RK, Szekely S, et al. Difficult intubation: an analysis of 2000 incident reports. *Anaesth Intensive Care.* 1993;21(5).

11. Russell WJ, et al. Problems with ventilation: an analysis of 2000 incident reports. *Anaesth Intensive Care.* 1993;21(5):617–620.

12. Petty WC. Anesthesia critical incidents: ASA and AIMS (part II). *Current Reviews in Clinical Anesthesia* Lesson 23, 2000; Vol 20: (Miami).

13. Webb RK, et al. Equipment failure: an analysis of 2000 incident reports. *Anaesth Intensive Care.* 1993;21(5):673–677.

14. Holland R, et al. Oesophageal intubation: an analysis of 2000 incident reports. *Anaesth Intensive Care.* 1993;21(5):608–610.

15. Szekely SM, et al. Problems related to the endotracheal tube: an analysis of 2000 incident reports. *Anaesth Intensive Care.* 1993;21(5):611–616.

16. Williamson JA, et al. Difficult intubation: an analysis of 2000 incident reports. *Anaesth Intensive Care.* 1993;21(5):602–607.

17. Webb RK, et al. Which monitor? an analysis of 2000 incident reports. *Anaesth Intensive Care.* 1993;21(5):529–542.

18. Runciman WB, et al. The pulse oximeter: applications and limitations—an analysis of 2000 incident reports. *Anaesth Intensive Care.* 1993;21(5):543–550.

19. Williamson JA, et al. The capnograph: applications and limitations—an analysis of 2000 incident reports. *Anaesth Intensive Care.* 1993;21(5):551–557.

20. Sinclair M, et al. Incidents in obstetric anaesthesia and analgesia: an analysis of 5000 incident reports. *Anaesth Intensive Care.* 1999;27(3):275–281.

21. Warden JD, Horan BF. Deaths attributed to anaesthesia in New South Wales, 1984–1990. *Anaesth Intensive Care.* 1996;24(1):66–73.

22. Morray JP, et al. Anesthesia-related cardiac arrest in children. *Anesthesiology.* 2000; 93(1):6–14.

23. Warner ME, et al. Perianesthetic dental injuries. *Anesthesiology.* 1999;90(5):1302–1305.

24. NCEPOD. Executive summary. 2000.

25. Gray AJG, et al. NCEPOD. *Anaesthesia.* 2000:37.

26. NCEPOD. Report summary; recommendations. 1996/1997.

27. *Scottish Audit of Surgical Mortality.* 1999:19–20.

28. Rosenstock C, et al. Complaints related to respiratory events in anaesthesia and intensive care medicine from 1994 to 1998 in Denmark. *Acta Anaesthesiol Scand.* 2001;45:53–58.

29. Pandey K, Badola R, Kumar S. Time course of intraocular hypertension produced by suxamethonium. *Br J Anaesth.* 1972;44:191.

30. Koh THHG, Coleman R. Oropharyngeal burn in a newborn baby: new complication of light-bulb laryngoscopes. *Anesthesiology.* 2000;92:277–279.

31. St Paul Fire & Marine Insurance Company. *Summary Report, 1980–85.*

32. Klokie C, Metcalf I, Holland A. Dental trauma in anaesthesia. *Can J Anaesth.* 1989; 36(6):675–680.

33. Marty-Ane CH, Picard E, Jonquet O, Mary H. Membranous tracheal rupture after endotracheal intubation. *Ann Thorac Surg.* 1995;60(5):1367–1371.

34. Tu HN, Saidi N, Leiutand T, et al. Nitrous oxide increases endotracheal cuff pressure and the incidence of tracheal lesions in anesthetized patients. *Anesth Analg.* 1999; 89(1):187–190.

35. Karasawa F, Mori T, Kawatani Y, Ohshima T, Satoh T. Deflationary phenomenon of the nitrous oxide-filled endotracheal tube cuff after cessation of nitrous oxide administration. *Anes Analg.* 2001;92:145–148.

36. Langer O, Masso E, Huraux C, et al. Prediction of difficult mask ventilation. *Anesthesiology.* 2000;19:209–216.

37. Blitt CD, et al. Silent regurgitation and aspiration during general anesthesia. *Curr Res.* 1970;49:707.

38. Engelhardt T, Webster NR. Pulmonary aspiration of gastric contents in anaesthesia. *Br J Anaesth.* 1999;83(3):453–460.

39. Roberts RB, Shirley MA. Reducing the risk of acid aspiration during cesarean section. *Anesth Analg.* 1974;53(6):859–868.

40. Schwartz DJ, Wynne JW, Gibbs CP, et al. The pulmonary consequences of aspiration of gastric contents at pH values greater than 2.5. *Am Rev Respir Dis.* 1980;121: 119–126.

41. Sellick BA. Cricoid pressure to control regurgitation of stomach contents during induction of anesthesia. *Lancet.* 1961;2:404.

42. Utting J.E. Pitfalls in anaesthetic practice. *Br J Anaesth.* 1987;59:877–890.

43. Keenan RL, Boylan CP. Cardiac arrest due to anesthesia. *JAMA.* 1985;253:2373–2377.

44. Caplan R.A, Posner KL, Ward RJ, Chaney SW. Adverse respiratory events in anaesthesiology: a closed claims analysis. *Anesthesiology.* 1990;72:828–833.

45. Conrardy TA, Goodman LR, Lainge F, Singer MM. Alteration of endotracheal tube position. Flexion and extension of the neck. *Crit Care Med.* 1976;4:7–12.

46. Block EFJ, Cheatham ML, Parrish GA, et al. Ingested endotracheal tube in an adult following intubation attempt for head injury. *Am Surgeon.* 1999;65:1134–1136.

47. Ince Z, Tuğcu D, Çoban A. An unusual complication of endotracheal intubation: ingestion of a laryngoscope bulb. *Ped Emerg Care.* 1998;14(4):275–276.

48. Kumar MS, Pandey SK, Cohen PJ. Tracheal laceration associated with endotracheal anesthesia. *Anesthesiology.* 1977;47:298.

49. Wagener DL, Gamage GW, Wong ML. Tracheal rupture following the insertion of disposable double lumen endotracheal tube. *Anesthesiology.* 1985;63:700.

50. Foster JMG, Lao OJ, Alimo ED. Ruptured bronchus following endobronchial intubation. *Br J Anaesth.* 1983;55:697.

51. Sakuragi T, Kumano K, Yasumoto M, Dan K. Rupture of the left mainstem bronchus by the tracheal portion of a double-lumen endobroncheal tube. *Acta Anaesthesiol Scand.* 1997;41:1218–1220.

52. Fink BR. The etiology and treatment of laryngospasm. *Anesthesiology.* 1956;17:569.

53. Roy WL, Lerman J. Laryngospasm in paediatric anaesthesia. *Can J Anaesth.* 1988; 35(1):93–98.

54. Larson CP. Laryngospasm—the best treatment. *Anesthesiology.* 1998;89:1293–1294.

55. Hartsell CJ, Stevens CR. Incidence of sore throat following endotracheal intubation. *Can Anaesth Soc.* 1964;111:307.

56. Stout D, et al. Correlation of endotracheal tube size with sore throat and hoarseness following general anesthesia. *Anesth Analg.* 1986;65:155.

57. Steward DJ. Experience with an outpatient anesthesia service for children. *Anesth Analg.* 1973;52:877.

58. Monroe MC, Gravenstein N, Saga-Rumley S. Postoperative sore throat: effect of oropharyngeal airway in orotracheally intubated patients. *Anesth Analg.* 1990;70:512–516.

59. Kinbbe MA, Carter JB, Frokjer GM. Postanesthetic temporomandibular joint dysfunction. *Anesth Prog.* 1989;36:21–25.

60. Castella X, Gilabert J, Perez C. Arytenoid dislocation after tracheal intubation: an unusual cause of acute respiratory failure. *Anesthesiology.* 1991;615–618.

61. Szigeti CL, Beauerle JJ, Mongan PD. Arytenoid dislocation with lighted stylet intubation: a case report and retrospective review. *Anesth Analg.* 1994;78:185–186.

62. Usui T, Saito S, Goto F. Arytenoid dislocation while using a McCoy laryngoscope. *Anesth Analg.* 2001;92:1347–1348.

63. Quick CA, Merwin GE. Arytenoid dislocation. *Arch Otolaryngol.* 1978;104:267–270.

64. Hahn FW, et al. Vocal cord paralysis with endotracheal intubation. *Arch Otolaryngol.* 1970;92:226.

65. Holley HS, Gildea JE. Vocal cord paralysis after tracheal intubation. *JAMA.* 1971; 214:281.

66. Lim EK, Schia KS, Ng BK. Recurrent laryngeal nerve palsy following endotracheal intubation. *Anaesth Intensive Care.* 1987;15:342–345.

67. Dalton C. Bilateral vocal cord paralysis following endotracheal intubation. *Anesthesia and Intensive Care.* 1995;23:350–351.

68. Ellis PDM, Pallister WK. Recurrent laryngeal nerve palsy and endotracheal intubation. *J Laryngol Otol.* 1975;89:823–826.

69. Whited RE. Laryngeal dysfunction following prolonged intubation. *Ann Otol.* 1979;88:474–478.

70. Sofferman RA, Hubbell RN. Laryngeal complications of NG tubes. *Ann Otol Rhino Laryngol.* 1981;90:465–468.

71. Friedman M, Baim H, Shelton V, et al. Laryngeal injuries secondary to NG tubes. *Ann Otol Rhino Laryngol.* 1981;90:469–474.

72. Tichner RL. Lingual nerve injury: a complication of oral tracheal intubation. *Br J Anaesth.* 1971;43:413.

73. Silva DA, Colingo KA, Miller R. Lingual nerve injury following laryngoscopy. *Anesthesiology.* 1991;76:650–651.

74. Venkatesh B, Walker D. Hypoglossal neuropraxia following endotracheal intubation. *Anesth Int Care.* 1997;25:699–700.

75. Montoya Pelaez LF, et al. Mental nerve neuropraxia associated with tracheal intubation using a RAE tube. *Br J Anaesth.* 1999;82:650–651.

76. Bauman RC, McGregor DA. Dissection of the posterior pharynx resulting in acute airway obstruction. *Anesthesiology.* 1995;82:1516–1518.

77. Deutschman CS, et al. Paranasal sinusitis associated with nasotracheal intubation: a frequently unrecognized and treatable source of sepsis. *Crit Care Med.* 1986;14: 111–114.

78. Hermens JM, et al. Anesthesia for laser surgery. *Anesth Analg.* 1983;62:218.

Suggested Readings

American Heart Association standards and guidelines for cardiopulmonary resuscitation (CPR) and emergency cardiac care (ECC). *JAMA.* 1986;255:2905.

Blanc VF, Tremblay NAG. The complications of tracheal intubation: a new classification with a review of the literature. *Curr Res Anesth Analg.* 1973;53:202.

Cowley RA, Trump BF, eds. *Pathophysiology of Shock, Anoxia, and Ischemia.* Baltimore: Williams & Wilkins; 1982.

Harrison TR, et al, eds. *Harrison's Principles of Internal Medicine.* 6th ed. New York: McGraw-Hill; 1970.

10
Surgical Approaches to Airway Management

A large body of literature dealing with the surgical approach to airway management has been published. At this juncture, consideration of the topic has evolved along three paths. The first involves the description of equipment designed specifically for surgical airway management. The second pertains to the place and role of percutaneous tracheostomy techniques utilized under **controlled conditions.** Trained surgeons performing elective tracheostomies have published many articles comparing percutaneous tracheostomy with traditional open techniques. Some are critically designed so that differences between techniques can be analyzed with more validity. This body of literature presents **best-case scenarios** concerning surgical airway management. The third avenue of consideration involves management of the **emergency** surgical airway. Much less literature has been published concerning the emergency setting. Many of the techniques to be described in this chapter represent suggestions you can consider if faced with the necessity to establish a surgical airway. Fortunately, much knowledge has been gained by surgeons who have studied percutaneous tracheostomy techniques in the **nonemergency setting.**

The objectives of this chapter are to present the following:

1. An overall consideration of **surgical airway management**
2. A summary of the literature concerning **percutaneous tracheostomy** in the controlled surgical setting
3. A description of various **surgical airway management techniques,** including those for the emergency situation

Overall Surgical Airway Management Considerations

Oxygenation versus Ventilation

In an airway emergency, the patient is faced with irreversible organ damage or death from hypoxia. The primary objective of surgical airway intervention in this setting is to provide **oxygenation.** Although ventilation may be desirable, **in an emergency, oxygenation alone can be lifesaving!**

Protocols and Algorithms

Many devices, techniques, and protocols have been proposed to deal with the "cannot intubate, cannot ventilate" airway emergency.[1] Airway practitioners are indebted to these authors and inventors for the following reasons:

1. They have increased awareness of and preparedness to deal with the critical airway.
2. They have led to the development of new equipment used to deal with the critical airway.
3. They have developed formal protocols designed to organize the approach to deal with the critical airway.

Although the validity of protocols has not been scientifically tested, they should not be ignored. Protocols, algorithms, and guidelines proposed by "airway experts" are logically structured courses of action based on clinical experience, outcome studies (in some cases), wishful thinking, and bias. Each practitioner should establish his own protocol to deal with the critical airway. Define a prescribed approach to the airway, choose and master use of appropriate equipment, establish a means to verify proficiency, and finally, define and recognize endpoints of each planned intervention. Ultimately, you must be able to defend your actions in a logical manner. A protocol or algorithm helps to organize your thinking.

Preparing to Manage the Surgical Airway

Managing the surgical airway demands **psychological, logistical,** and **clinical** preparation. These considerations are summarized below:

1. **Psychological preparation:** You must be mentally prepared to abandon standard familiar airway management techniques in the critical situation and to institute more invasive surgical intervention.
2. **Logistical preparation:** All of the equipment you have decided to use must be immediately available and functional.
3. **Clinical preparation:** Establish a protocol or algorithm dealing with surgical airway management. Learn to recognize potential problems and to recognize critical events. Finally, be trained and proficient in the use of equipment specified in the protocol.

Psychological Preparation

Few situations are more anxiety-provoking or challenging than the one faced by airway managers who recognize that they cannot ventilate or intubate a patient who is not breathing. One is often reluctant to admit that familiar and standard techniques have failed. To be psychologically prepared to establish a surgical airway, consider the following **before** a critical situation is encountered:

1. Admit that a patient **will** present with a life-threatening airway problem that cannot be rectified with standard techniques.
2. Admit that standard techniques can and do fail.
3. Establish, learn, and trust protocols and algorithms dealing with surgical airway intervention.
4. Once it is recognized that standard techniques have failed, be prepared to institute the protocol **immediately.**
5. Recognize that **time** is the most critical variable in the protocol. Do not waste it! If one technique is unsuccessful, proceed to the next step in the protocol. If the clinical situation does not change, do not back up.
6. Expect to assume total responsibility for managing the airway.
7. Accept help from those more proficient and immediately available to help.
8. Realize that some patients will experience a poor outcome or death **despite** one's best effort.

You need to be mentally prepared **before** a difficult airway is encountered, to make decisions, take responsibility, and initiate the protocol to establish a surgical airway.

Logistical Preparation

All of the equipment necessary to establish a surgical airway must be functional and available. It may be stored on a cart or tray that can be brought to the site where it is needed. The equipment should be inspected at regular intervals and documented to be in working order. Practice retrieving, setting up, and using emergency airway equipment to help retain proficiency.

Clinical Preparation

To be clinically prepared, adopt a protocol and/or algorithm designed to guide your actions in managing the surgical airway. The algorithm may be one that is already published (ASA Difficult Airway Algorithm), one that is modified, or one that is uniquely designed for a given practice. The protocol should be logical, practical, and thorough. The practitioner should know, trust, and modify the protocol as indicated by new knowledge and experience. You must be proficient in the use of all equipment specified in the protocol.

Next, learn to recognize pathological conditions or abnormal anatomy that is associated with a difficult airway. If difficult airway management is anticipated, all surgical equipment must be on hand **before** you start to manage the airway, whether mask ventilation or intubation is planned. If time permits and the patient is still breathing, consider instituting awake intubation techniques or a formal tracheostomy to establish the airway.

The most difficult aspect of clinical preparation involves recognizing the critical event that dictates the need to perform a surgical airway. You may be tempted to fall back on familiar techniques, equipment, and skills. But at some point, one must admit that standard techniques have failed. The patient cannot be ventilated or intubated. Worse, the patient is likely to experience hypoxic injury or death **unless** a surgical airway is established. The timing of the decision is critical and depends on experience, skill, and knowledge. If you are **psychologically, logistically,** and **clinically** prepared to establish a surgical airway, you will initiate the protocol, hopefully, with time to spare. Even with the equipment on hand, it will take 2 to 3 minutes to establish and confirm placement of a needle/catheter cricothyrotomy and at least 1 to 2 minutes to perform an emergency surgical cricothyrotomy.

The techniques described in this chapter proceed from the most simple to the more complex. When confronted with a difficult airway, you must weigh the risks and benefits of each technique and choose the one with the highest probability of success. This decision is often difficult to make. You need to be **taught** by an experienced person and to **practice** surgical techniques to establish and maintain **proficiency.**

Techniques

The terms *cricothyrotomy* and *cricothyroidotomy* are used interchangeably in this chapter.

The techniques to be described in this chapter include the following:

1. Needle/catheter cricothyroidotomy
2. Retrograde catheter-guided intubation

3. Minitracheostomy
4. Percutaneous dilatational tracheostomy (PDT)
5. Commercially available cricothyroidotomy kits of unique design
6. Adjunctive equipment and techniques
7. Emergency surgical cricothyrotomy
8. Formal tracheostomy

Needle/Catheter Cricothyroidotomy

Objective of Technique

The objective is to insert a catheter into the trachea through which oxygen can be insufflated or injected with low-pressure or high-pressure systems. This technique is considered to be a temporary intervention utilized until a more formal airway can be established.

Needles and catheters inserted percutaneously into the trachea through the cricothyroid or another tracheal membrane have been used to provide oxygenation and sometimes ventilation in both pediatric and adult patients.[2] Anecdotal reports have appeared in the literature for years. Utility of the technique has been documented in animal[3] and human subjects. Variables such as catheter design, material, diameter, driving pressures,[4,5] lung compliance, ventilatory rates, I:E ratios, and delivery systems have been studied. Many authors[1,6-10] have proposed systems utilizing the needle/catheter, jet injectors,[11] jet stylets,[12,13] jet cannulae,[14] and modified tube changers.[15] The technique is also described in a textbook on the subject of difficult intubation management, edited by Hagberg.[16] The technique is the **first step** in many other surgical airway maneuvers—for example, retrograde catheter-guided intubation and percutaneous dilatational cricothyrotomy.

Equipment

The following equipment is needed to perform a needle/catheter cricothyroidotomy:

1. 14-gauge or 16-gauge intravenous needle/catheter
2. Nonkinking "dilator"-type catheter
3. Commercial kit available: Emergency Transtracheal Airway Catheter (Cook Critical Care, Bloomington, IN) (Fig. 10.1)
4. Guide wire that passes through the 14-g or 16-g catheter and over which the dilator can be passed (size: 0.025 to 0.035 in)
5. Skin prep solution
6. Lidocaine 1%
7. 3-ml syringe with 25-g needle
8. 20-ml syringe
9. Sterile saline solution
10. Scalpel blade (#11)

EMERGENCY TRANSTRACHEAL AIRWAY CATHETERS

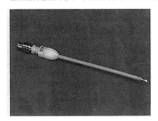

Used for emergency airway access when conventional endotracheal intubation cannot be performed. Supplied sterile in peel-open packages. Intended for one-time use.

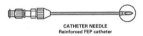

CATHETER NEEDLE
Reinforced FEP catheter

ORDER NUMBER	French Size	CATHETER Inner Diameter	Length	NEEDLE Gage	Quick Reorder Number[1]
C-DTJV-6.0-5.0-BTT	6.0	2 mm	5.0 cm	15	238137
C-DTJV-6.0-7.5-BTT	6.0	2 mm	7.5 cm	15	227593

[1] The Quick Reorder Number is for U.S.A. domestic use only.

FIGURE 10.1. Emergency Transtracheal Airway Catheter (Cook Critical Care, Blooming-ton, IN, with permission).

Technique

Proceed as follows (Fig. 10.2):

1. Administer 100% oxygen to the patient with a face mask (if breathing spon-taneously) or with a resuscitation bag-mask system.
2. Extend the neck (if safe to do so).
3. Prep the skin (if time permits).
4. Palpate the thyroid and cricoid cartilages in the midline. The cricothyroid membrane lies between these structures. (*Note:* To reduce the likelihood of vascular injury or glottic damage, one author[17] suggests using a subcricoid approach [through the cricotracheal ligament], one level down.)
5. Inject lidocaine intradermally and submucosally down to the trachea (if time permits).
6. Put 5 to 10 ml of saline in the 20-ml syringe.
7. Put the needle/catheter device on the 20-ml syringe.
8. Insert the needle through the tracheal membrane with a slight caudal angle. Aspirate on the 20-ml syringe. Air will be aspirated into the syringe when the needle enters the trachea. Advance the device a few millimeters and slide the catheter into the trachea, removing the needle.
9. Aspirate air through the catheter to insure that it is still in the trachea.
10. At this point, one may try to deliver oxygen into the trachea (see below).
11. One may wish to exchange a thin-walled catheter with a rigid dilator to pre-vent kinking. To do this, pass the guide wire through the catheter, remove

the catheter, make a small incision into the trachea by sliding the scalpel blade along the wire, and place the dilator (or rigid catheter) into the trachea. At this point, remove the wire and proceed from Step 6 as described above.

12. The Cook Emergency Transtracheal Airway Catheter (Cook Critical Care, Bloomington, IN) used from the start eliminates the need to switch to a more rigid catheter.

Helpful Comments on Catheter Insertion and Function

Sdrales and Benumof[18] suggested that one may ease insertion of the catheter and lessen the likelihood of kinking if the needle were bent 15°, about 2.5 cm from the distal tip, and if the needle were inserted at a 15° angle to the skin. Southwick[19] wrote in response to the article that at least one manufacturer had already marked a "precurved" transtracheal catheter (VBM Medizintechnik, Germany). Soto and Mesa[20] point out that new needle/catheter systems designed to prevent accidental needle sticks, such as the BD InSyte Autogard catheter (BD, Franklin Lakes, NJ), cannot be attached to a syringe to be used as described above. Finally, Ames and Venn[21] reported a case where the catheter was lacerated near its hub. Although the tip of the catheter was in the trachea, enough oxygen leaked through the laceration to cause subcutaneous emphysema.

At this point, either a 14-gauge or 16-gauge catheter, or a rigid cannula, has been inserted into the trachea. The next step is to **oxygenate** and/or **ventilate** the patient.

Oxygenation through the Catheter

Two methods may be used to oxygenate the patient through a small tracheal catheter. A **low-pressure** system may be the only option available and it may provide oxygenation but not ventilation. A **high-pressure** system has been demonstrated to provide oxygenation and, in some cases, ventilation, and it is the method of preference.

Expiration of Gases

When using any system, observe for expiration of gas from the lungs. This is especially true when using a **high-pressure** oxygenation system. If the glottis is not totally obstructed, gas can escape through the mouth. If the glottis or upper airway is obstructed, a second cannula or a valve (stopcock or other device) will have to be added to the oxygenation system to allow for expiration.

Low-Pressure Oxygenation Systems

Some authors advocate that low-pressure oxygenation systems "should not be considered"[22] when describing acceptable techniques to oxygenate through a tracheal catheter. The authors of this book disagree. A low-pressure system may be the only system available. These systems may be lifesaving until a formal

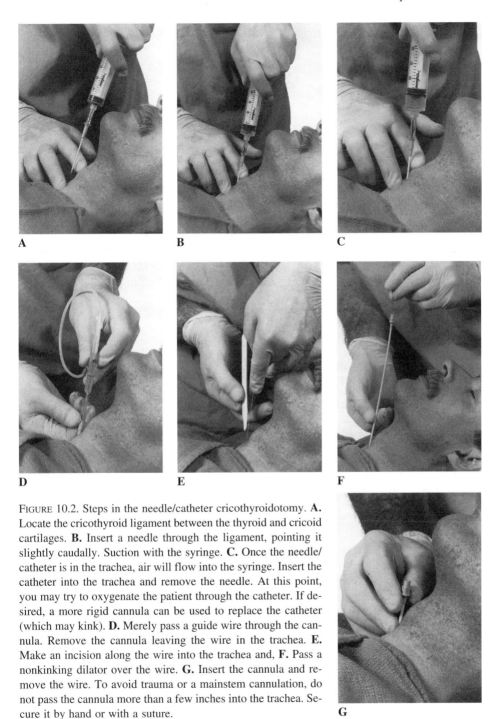

FIGURE 10.2. Steps in the needle/catheter cricothyroidotomy. **A.** Locate the cricothyroid ligament between the thyroid and cricoid cartilages. **B.** Insert a needle through the ligament, pointing it slightly caudally. Suction with the syringe. **C.** Once the needle/catheter is in the trachea, air will flow into the syringe. Insert the catheter into the trachea and remove the needle. At this point, you may try to oxygenate the patient through the catheter. If desired, a more rigid cannula can be used to replace the catheter (which may kink). **D.** Merely pass a guide wire through the cannula. Remove the cannula leaving the wire in the trachea. **E.** Make an incision along the wire into the trachea and, **F.** Pass a nonkinking dilator over the wire. **G.** Insert the cannula and remove the wire. To avoid trauma or a mainstem cannulation, do not pass the cannula more than a few inches into the trachea. Secure it by hand or with a suture.

cricothyroidotomy has been performed or a high-pressure system is substituted. Four low-pressure systems will be described. These include:

1. Spontaneous ventilation
2. Apneic oxygenation
3. Resuscitation bag
4. Anesthesia machine circuit

Spontaneous Ventilation

Successful ventilation and oxygenation through one or two large-bore (12-gauge) intravenous catheters inserted into the trachea of a spontaneously ventilating patient has been documented.[23] However, research on models[24,25] has documented that the work of breathing through 12-gauge to 14-gauge catheters dramatically increased from 250% to 12,000% depending on flow. Two 12-gauge catheters inserted into the trachea of a spontaneously breathing patient may be lifesaving. Oxygen can be supplied to the catheters as shown in Figure 10.3A. Oxygen should also be administered with a face mask–resuscitation bag system, since some gas exchange through the upper airway may occur.

Apneic Oxygenation

Even if the patient is apneic, oxygen may be delivered through a tracheal catheter at relatively low flows (5 to 10 L/min) and low pressures. The oxygen supply hose will have to be fitted with a male Luer-Lok fastener on the distal end to connect to the tracheal catheter. Animal studies have documented the technique's efficacy.[26,27]

You should look for signs of overdistention of the lungs and listen for expiration of gas through the mouth. Although the technique has been used in humans, its use in the emergency setting needs further research.

Resuscitation Bag and Circle System Bag on an Anesthesia Machine

A manual resuscitation bag or the low-pressure component of an **anesthesia machine circuit (bag)** may be interfaced with the tracheal catheter to supply oxygen. Use the highest flow of oxygen available when using these systems. Neither system will provide ventilation, though either may be used in an attempt to deliver oxygen to the patient.

For either system to be used, a 15-mm adapter interface has to be established. Three methods can be used. The following equipment is needed:

1. 3-ml Luer-Lok syringe with plunger removed
2. 10-ml Luer-Lok syringe with plunger removed
3. 15-mm adapter from a 7.5-mm ID endotracheal tube
4. 15-mm adapter from a 3.0-mm ID endotracheal tube
5. 7.0-mm endotracheal tube with a 10-ml syringe attached to the pilot balloon port
6. Resuscitation bag or anesthesia machine circuit
7. Oxygen source and tubing

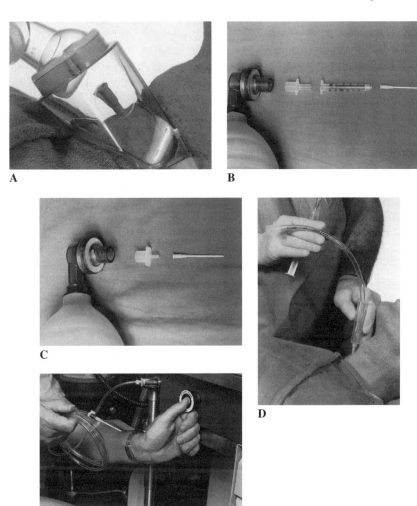

FIGURE 10.3. **A.** Oxygen can be delivered via tracheal collar to a patient breathing spontaneously through two large-bore (12-gauge) tracheal catheters. **B.** An interface may be created between a resuscitation bag and the tracheal catheter using a 3-ml syringe and the 15-mm adapter from a 7.5-mm ID endotracheal tube. **C.** An interface may be created between a resuscitation bag and the tracheal catheter using a 15-mm adapter from a 3.0-mm ID endotracheal tube. **D.** An interface may be created between a resuscitation bag and the tracheal catheter using a 10-ml syringe and a 7.0-mm ID endotracheal tube with the cuff inflated to create a tight seal. **E.** A "jet" ventilator can be made of rigid tubing with a male Luer-Lok interface bonded to its distal end. The proximal end of the system is a 15-mm plastic adapter from an endotracheal tube bonded to the tubing. The 15-mm adapter is inserted into the fresh-gas outlet of an anesthesia machine. The system is activated by pressing the flush valve of the machine.

Three interfaces can be established:

1. Connect the 3-ml syringe to the tracheal catheter. Insert the adapter from the 7.5-mm ID endotracheal tube into the open end of the syringe (Fig. 10.3B).
2. Insert the adapter from a 3.0-mm ID endotracheal tube firmly into the tracheal catheter (Fig. 10.3C).
3. Connect the 10-ml syringe to the tracheal catheter. Insert a 7.0-mm endotracheal tube into the syringe and blow up the cuff until tight (Fig. 10.3D).

After establishing the 15-mm adapter interface, the resuscitation bag or the bag of the anesthesia machine may be used to deliver oxygen to the patient. The bag should be compressed vigorously and the flow of oxygen to the bag should be high. Pressure in the bag will be high due to resistance. The mouth and nose of the patient may need to be held closed if gas escapes during inspiration.

Remember: Low-pressure systems will not ventilate the patient. Convert to a high-pressure system or a more formal airway *as soon as possible!*

High-Pressure Systems

The use of high-pressure (50 psi) "jet" ventilation has been advocated as the optimal modality for oxygenating and ventilating a patient whose trachea has been cannulated.[1] Although true jet ventilation may or may not occur depending upon many factors (e.g., glottic closure above the catheter), a high-pressure ventilating device does deliver large volumes of oxygen (500 ml/s) to the trachea, even through a small catheter (14- or 16-gauge). Two high-pressure systems will be described.

Anesthesia Machine Flush Valve

Compared to a formal jet ventilator, newer anesthesia machines deliver reduced pressures of oxygen when the flush valve is activated (less than 10 psi).[5] However, if a high-pressure jet ventilating system is not immediately available, the anesthesia flush valve system is a convenient substitute and is available in every operating room. Morley and Thorpe[28] reported that a 1-second press of the flush valve delivered 628 ml of oxygen to their test analyzer through a system made of IV tubing.

Equipment Needed. To connect the anesthesia machine to the tracheal catheter, the following equipment is needed:

1. An anesthesia machine
2. 5- to 6-foot length of noncompliant tubing with a 15-mm adapter bonded to its proximal end and a male Luer-Lok needle attachment bonded to its distal end
3. High-flow stopcock bonded in line into the noncompliant tubing

Attach the equipment as follows:

1. Plug the 15-mm adapter into the fresh-gas outlet of the anesthesia machine. (*Note:* A plastic adapter fits more firmly than a metal adapter.)
2. Attach the Luer-Lok to the tracheal catheter.
3. Activate the system by pushing the flush valve of the anesthesia machine. Hold inspiration for 1 second. Observe the patient for chest movement, both inspiration and expiration. If expiration does not occur, relieve pressure by opening the system with the stopcock.
4. Repeat inspirations 8 to 10 times per minute (Fig. 10.3E).

High-Pressure "Jet" Ventilation

To apply high-pressure "jet" ventilation through the tracheal cannula, the following equipment should be available.

Equipment for High-Pressure "Jet" Ventilation

1. A high-pressure oxygen source, 50 psi (wall or portable)
2. A formal "jet" ventilator with appropriate connector to interface with the oxygen source
3. A male Luer-Lok bonded to the distal end of the system with a high-flow stopcock (or another type of valve) bonded in line

To use this equipment, proceed as follows:

1. Attach the "jet" ventilator to the oxygen source.
2. Connect the distal end of the tubing via the Luer-Lok fitting to the tracheal cannula.
3. Activate the jet ventilator for 0.5 to 1.0 seconds and observe the patient for chest movement or signs of barotrauma.
4. Repeat the activation 6 to 10 times per minute
5. If the lungs do not deflate, open the stopcock to relieve pressure (Fig. 10.4).

Cautionary Note: Barotrauma is a significant complication of this technique. Observe the patient carefully to detect whether or not the cannula remains in the trachea and insure that the patient has time to exhale by observing the chest and listening for gas to escape either through the glottis or the stopcock.

Efficacy of the Technique. A study published by Patel[29] documented that percutaneous transtracheal jet ventilation instituted in the **emergency setting** provided safe and effective oxygenation to patients whose oxygenation could not be maintained with bag-mask systems and who had proven to be difficult to intubate. In 23 of 29 patients (79.3%), tracheal cannulation and jet oxygenation was successful. Failure occurred in 6 patients for the following reasons:

1. Poor landmarks because of obesity and short neck (n = 2)
2. Poor landmarks because of previous tracheostomy (n = 1)
3. Catheter kinking (n = 2)
4. Catheter misplacement because of improper technique (n = 1)

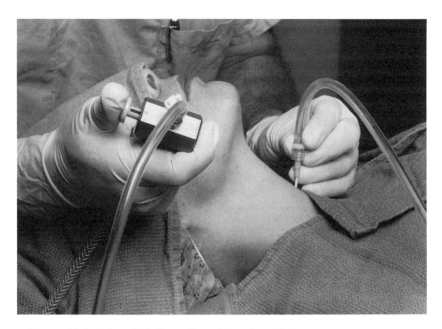

FIGURE 10.4. A formal "jet" ventilator driven by a high-pressure oxygen source.

Two of these 6 patients were intubated over an airway exchange catheter, while 4 of the patients were subsequently intubated after several attempts.

Many anecdotal reports support the technique's clinical efficacy.

Obtaining a Formal Airway

All of the systems described thus far should be considered to be temporary interventions to establish oxygenation. After the patient has stabilized, you must proceed to the next step, that is to **establish a formal airway.** At this point, the following options should be considered.

1. If drugs had been used to facilitate intubation, the patient may be allowed to wake up with the tracheal catheter left in place until he is able to spontaneously ventilate and to protect his airway. (This option implies that there is no airway pathology that would obstruct spontaneous breathing.)
2. Further attempts to intubate with adjunctive equipment (e.g., fiberoptic bronchoscope or retrograde catheter) may be undertaken with the tracheal catheter in place.
3. Emergency cricothyroidotomy may be performed.

Your algorithm or protocol should outline all of the steps necessary to establish a formal airway.

Complications of Needle/Catheter Cricothyroidotomy[1,2,30]

The complications associated with needle/catheter cricothyroidotomy techniques are many. They include the following:

1. **Barotrauma** (subcutaneous emphysema, pneumothorax, pneumomediastinum, pneumopericardium)
2. Breakage or bending of the needle if the patient moves
3. Kinking, dislodgement, or breakage of the catheter
4. Perforation of the esophagus or other structures in the neck or thorax
5. Bleeding at the insertion site or into the trachea, causing obstruction
6. Expiratory obstruction
7. Hypoventilation with hypercapnia and acidosis
8. Sore throat
9. Infection

The complication rate can be expected to be higher in pediatric patients, patients with abnormal anatomy, or patients with coagulopathies. Use of the technique for infants and very small children has been questioned.

Are You Prepared to Perform a Needle/Catheter Cricothyroidotomy?

Needle/catheter cricothyroidotomy techniques have been incorporated into many difficult airway protocols. However, the question remains, *Are you ready to perform a needle cricothyroidotomty?* Davies[31] asked this question to physicians in 184 accident and emergency departments seeing more than 30,000 new patients per year in Great Britain. He reported that "47% of the departments had made provision for immediate use of needle cricothyroidotomy. Forty-five percent of the doctors interviewed were fully conversant in the use of needle cricothyroidotomy." He concluded that provisions to use the technique immediately were generally inadequate and that all departments should provide the necessary equipment and train their physicians on a regular basis to use the equipment properly. If you include needle/catheter cricothyroidotomy techniques in your algorithm or protocol, **make sure the equipment is available and functional, and practice the technique on a regular basis! This can be done with commercially available plastic models.**

Retrograde Catheter-Assisted Intubation

Objective of the Technique

A retrograde wire or catheter passed from the trachea and through the glottis into the upper airway may be used to guide an endotracheal tube between the vocal cords and into the trachea.[17,30,32,33]

This technique may be planned from the onset or if attempts to intubate a patient fail and the glottic opening is not completely obstructed.

The retrograde wire technique has been used in a variety of patients, including infants,[34] adults receiving a double-lumen endobronchial tube,[35] and in those undergoing cardiac surgery.[36] Many suggestions have been made concerning its use.[37–40] A training model using patients scheduled for elective tracheostomy has been described.[41] Transtracheally injected lidocaine and laryngeal nerve blocks have made retrograde intubation more comfortable for the awake patient.[42]

Equipment

1. Oxygen source and insufflation device
2. Skin prep solution
3. Lidocaine 1%
4. 3-ml syringe with 25-gauge needle
5. Laryngoscope
6. Magill forceps
7. 12-gauge intravenous needle/catheter
8. 20-inch self-contained intravenous catheter kit (antecubital or peripheral central venous pressure catheter-through-needle kit)
9. Another plastic (e.g., epidural or angiographic) catheter at least 20 inches long
10. Long (at least 20 inches) guide wire, 0.035-inch diameter
11. Suture needle with 1-0 silk suture attached
12. Various sizes of endotracheal tubes
13. Suction apparatus

Methods

Three methods to perform a retrograde wire or catheter-assisted intubation will be presented.

Method 1: Using the Self-contained Catheter Through Needle Intravenous Kit (Fig. 10.5)

1. Administer oxygen to the patient with oral insufflation and/or nasal prongs.
2. Extend the patient's neck.
3. Palpate the cricothyroid ligament (or the next lower tracheal membrane).
4. Inject local anesthetic into the skin overlying the ligament.
5. Puncture the ligament in the midline with the needle from the kit aiming slightly cephalad.
6. Thread the self-contained catheter through the glottis.
7. Visualize the pharynx with a laryngoscope.
8. With the Magill forceps, direct the catheter out of the mouth, or toward the nasal passage, while gently advancing the catheter from below.
9. Gain control of the catheter as it exits the mouth or nose.
10. Thread an endotracheal tube over the catheter into the trachea. The catheter may pass through the Murphy eye of the endotracheal tube or through the tube's central lumen.[33]
11. Remove the catheter from below.
12. Inflate the cuff of the tube and ventilate the patient.

Method 2: Using a Silk Suture to Guide the Tube into the Trachea

1. Pass the catheter of a self-contained needle/catheter kit out through the mouth as described in Method 1.
2. Suture a silk tie onto the end of the catheter.
3. Pull the needle out of the skin and take hold of the catheter.

4. Pull the catheter through the airway and out of the trachea. Take hold of the silk suture.
5. Tie the end of the suture that exits the upper airway to the endotracheal tube by passing it through the tube's distal end and out the Murphy eye. Tie the knot 2 to 3 inches from the tube so a loop passes through the Murphy eye.
6. Guide the tube into the trachea by pulling the suture from below and advancing the tube from above. When the tip gets to the glottis, you may have to twist the tube to the left or right to facilitate passage through the vocal cords.
7. Pull the suture knot through the skin.
8. Cut and remove the suture.
9. Inflate the cuff and ventilate the patient.

Method 3: 12-Gauge Intravenous Needle/Catheter and Guide Wire

1. Insert the needle/catheter as described in the previous section but direct it slightly cephalad.
2. Remove the needle.
3. Direct the catheter cephalad.
4. Insert the guide wire (or a plastic catheter) through the 12-gauge tracheal catheter and pass it into the pharynx.
5. Proceed as described in Methods 1 and 2.

Parmet and Metz[43] suggest that one way to facilitate passage of the endotracheal tube through the vocal cords is to pass an obturator or guide with a ta-

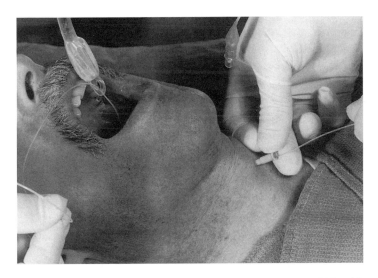

FIGURE 10.5. A retrograde wire passed out of the mouth extends through the side port of an endotracheal tube. The tube passes over the wire into the trachea. When the tip of the tube gets to the glottis, passage into the trachea may be facilitated by twisting the tube to the left or right.

COOK RETROGRADE INTUBATION SET WITH RAPI-FIT® ADAPTERS

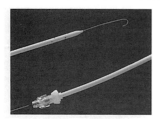

Used to assist in the placement of an endotracheal tube during difficult airway access procedures.

* Initial access utilizing the Seldinger technique via the cricothyroid membrane permits retrograde (cephalad directed) placement of a wire guide exiting orally or nasally.

* Antegrade introduction of a hollow guiding catheter with distal side-ports and Rapi-Fit® Adapters allows patient oxygenation and facilitates placement of an endotracheal tube.

Supplied sterile in peel-open packages. Intended for one-time use.

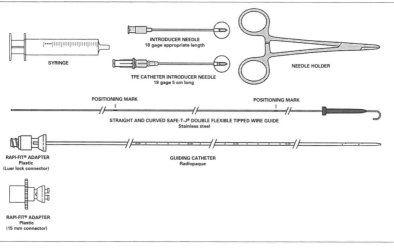

		CATHETER		WIRE GUIDE				
ORDER NUMBER		**French Size**	**Length**	**Diameter**	**Length**	**Tip**	**Use with Endotracheal Tube with Inner Diameter**	**Quick Reorder Number[1]**
SET								
C-RETRO-14.0-70-38J-110-CAE		14.0	70 cm	.038 inch	110 cm	straight and 3 mm "J"	5.0 mm or larger	240407
REPLACEMENT WIRE GUIDE								
C-DOC-38-110-0-3-RETRO				.038 inch	110 cm	straight and 3 mm "J"		202173

[1] The Quick Reorder Number is for U.S.A. domestic use only.

FIGURE 10.6. Cook Retrograde Intubation Set with Rapi-Fit Adapters (Cook Critical Care, Bloomington, IN, with permission).

pered tip over the wire first, then to thread the endotracheal tube over the guide once its tip has passed the vocal cords. Two commercially available kits are marketed by Cook Critical Care (Bloomington, IN). The first kit is supplied with a Rapi-Fit adapter, which allows you to oxygenate through the dilator as well as guide the endotracheal tube (Fig. 10.6). The other kit has a slightly larger obturator with tapered tips at each end (Fig. 10.7). Both kits come with a retrograde wire and the other equipment needed to perform a needle/catheter cricothyroidotomy.

Useful modifications to the retrograde wire techniques using the fiberoptic bronchoscope are presented later in the chapter in the section on adjunctive equipment used to establish a surgical airway.

COOK RETROGRADE INTUBATION SETS

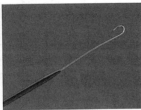

Used to assist in the placement of an endotracheal tube during difficult airway access procedures.

• Initial access utilizing the Seldinger technique via the cricothyroid membrane permits retrograde (cephalad directed) placement of a "J" tipped wire guide exiting orally or nasally.

• Antegrade introduction of a guiding catheter will facilitate placement of an endotracheal tube.

Supplied sterile in peel-open packages. Intended for one-time use.

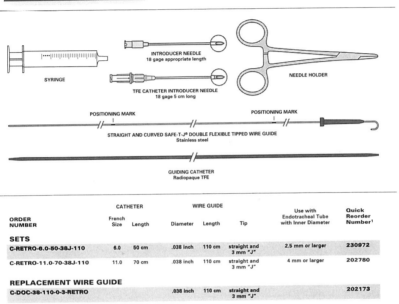

ORDER NUMBER	CATHETER		WIRE GUIDE			Use with Endotracheal Tube with Inner Diameter	Quick Reorder Number[1]
	French Size	Length	Diameter	Length	Tip		
SETS							
C-RETRO-6.0-50-38J-110	6.0	50 cm	.038 inch	110 cm	straight and 3 mm "J"	2.5 mm or larger	230972
C-RETRO-11.0-70-38J-110	11.0	70 cm	.038 inch	110 cm	straight and 3 mm "J"	4 mm or larger	202780
REPLACEMENT WIRE GUIDE							
C-DOC-38-110-0-3-RETRO			.038 inch	110 cm	straight and 3 mm "J"		202173

[1] The Quick Reorder Number is for U.S.A. domestic use only.

FIGURE 10.7. Cook Retrograde Intubation Sets (Cook Critical Care, Bloomington, IN, with permission).

Minitracheostomy

Objective of the Technique

The objective is to establish a small bore (3.5 to 6.0 mm or 6.0 to 9.0 French) percutaneous tracheostomy tube. Two techniques are available. In the first, the tracheostomy tube is passed over a tapered dilator that is guided into the trachea with a wire or catheter. In the second, the tracheostomy tube is passed over a dilator and needle introducer. (See Patil Emergency Cricothyrotomy Catheter Sets [Cook Critical Care, Bloomington, IN] in the following section.)

The minitracheostomy was first described in 1984[44] for use on patients who did not require a formal tracheostomy. Indications included:

1. Pulmonary toilet (suction secretions)
2. Supplemental oxygen delivery directly to the trachea
3. High-frequency jet ventilation to augment respiration

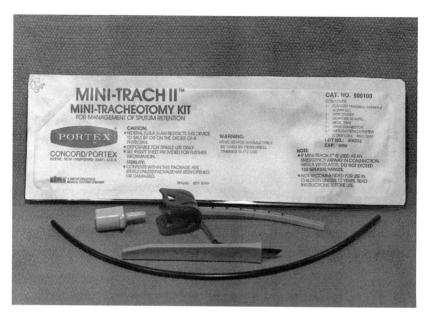

FIGURE 10.8. The Portex Minitrach II Kit (Portex, Keene, NH, with permission).

More recently, authors have proposed that the technique be considered as an option for use in managing the emergency surgical airway.

Various minitracheostomy kits have been marketed. Five kits with different design characteristics are described below.

Mini-Trach II Kit (Portex)

A 4.0-mm flanged tracheostomy tube is inserted through a scalpel incision in the cricothyroid ligament and passed over a plastic introducer.[45] Clinical use of this kit is described in an article by Ala-Kokko, et al (Fig. 10.8).[46]

Melker Emergency Cricothyrotomy Catheter Sets
(Cook Critical Care, Bloomington, IN) (Figs. 10.9 and 10.10)

The Melker kits come with various-sized cricothyrotomy tubes. The tubes are inserted by (1) passing a guide wire into the trachea (as described in the needle/catheter cricothyroidotomy section of this chapter), (2) making a small scalpel incision along the wire into the trachea, and (3) passing the dilator/airway catheter over the wire into the trachea. The dilator and wire are then removed.[47] Once in place, the tracheal cannula's 15-mm distal port can be interfaced with standard airway equipment to provide oxygenation and ventilation. The technique is illustrated in Figure 10.11 from an article by Chan et al.[48]

Successful clinical use of the minitracheostomy is described in an article by Van Heurn et al.[49]

MELKER EMERGENCY CRICOTHYROTOMY CATHETER SETS

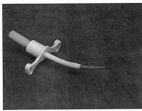

Used for emergency airway access when endotracheal intubation cannot be performed.

• Airway access is achieved utilizing percutaneous entry (Seldinger) technique via the cricothyroid membrane.

• Subsequent dilation of the tract and tracheal entrance site permits passage of the emergency airway.

• Airway catheter has radiopaque stripe.

Supplied sterile in peel-open packages. Intended for one-time use.

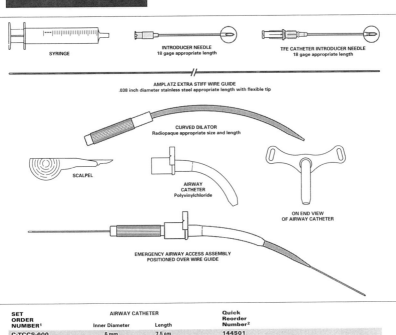

SET ORDER NUMBER[1]	AIRWAY CATHETER		Quick Reorder Number[2]
	Inner Diameter	Length	
C-TCCS-600	6 mm	7.5 cm	144501
C-TCCS-400	4 mm	4.2 cm	175438
C-TCCS-350	3.5 mm	3.8 cm	175437

[1] Sets consist of items shown above and cloth tracheostomy tape strip for fixation of airway catheter.
[2] The Quick Reorder Number is for U.S.A. domestic use only.
Patent Number 4,677,978

FIGURE 10.9. Melker Emergency Cricothyrotomy Catheter Sets (single cannula sets) (Cook Critical Care, Bloomington, IN, with permission).

Arndt Emergency Cricothyrotomy Catheter Set (Cook Critical Care, Bloomington, IN)

The Arndt Emergency Cricothyrotomy Set (Cook Critical Care, Bloomington, IN) has a few unique design features (Fig. 10.12). The wire is placed through an introducer needle that is protected by a sterile sheath. In addition, the distal end of the minitracheostomy tube can be interfaced with a high-pressure jet ventilator or a standard 15-mm adapter interface. Figures 10.13, 10.14, and 10.15 illustrate insertion of the **Arndt cricothyrotomy airway.**

MELKER EMERGENCY CRICOTHYROTOMY CATHETER SET
SPECIAL OPERATIONS

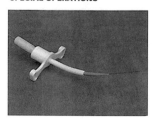

Used for emergency airway access when endotracheal
intubation cannot be performed.

* Airway access is achieved utilizing percutaneous entry
  (Seldinger) technique via the cricothyroid membrane.
* Subsequent dilation of the tract and tracheal entrance
  site permits passage of the emergency airway.
* Airway catheter has radiopaque stripe.
* Custom packaged in slip peel-pouch design for easy transportation.
* Combines 4.0 mm catheter with a 6.0 mm catheter in one
  package thereby reducing the number of kits needed in the field.
* Dilators are pre-inserted into airway catheters.

Supplied sterile in peel-open packages. Intended for one-time use.

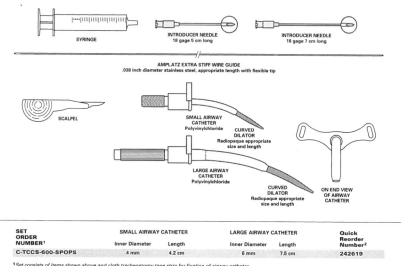

SET ORDER NUMBER[1]	SMALL AIRWAY CATHETER		LARGE AIRWAY CATHETER		Quick Reorder Number[2]
	Inner Diameter	Length	Inner Diameter	Length	
C-TCCS-600-SPOPS	4 mm	4.2 cm	6 mm	7.5 cm	242619

[1] Set consists of items shown above and cloth tracheostomy tape strip for fixation of airway catheter.
[2] The Quick Reorder Number is for U.S.A. domestic use only.
Patent Number 4,677,978

FIGURE 10.10. Melker Emergency Cricothyrotomy Catheter Set (special operations) (Cook Critical Care, Bloomington, IN, with permission).

Patil Emergency Cricothyrotomy Catheter Sets (Cook Critical Care, Bloomington, IN)

With Patil Cricothyrotomy Catheter Sets (Cook Critical Care, Bloomington, IN), an airway is inserted into the trachea over a needle/dilator trocar. No guide wire is used with this technique (Fig. 10.16).

Complications and Problems with Minitracheostomies

Minitracheostomy kits used under controlled conditions appear to be safe and efficacious. Complication rates were reported to range from 10% to 17% (mostly minor and nonfatal).[49–51] Reported complications are listed below:

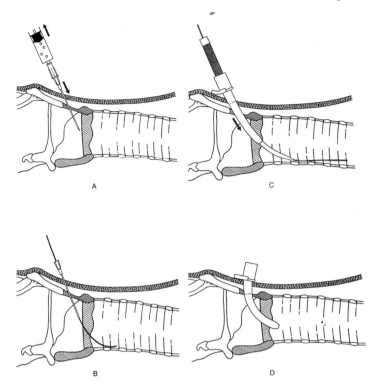

FIGURE 10.11. Insertion of a Melker Cricothyrotomy Airway (Cook Critical Care, Bloomington, IN). (From Chan et al,[49] with permission.)

1. Difficult insertion[52–55]
2. Misleading signs of tracheal positioning[52]
3. Pneumothorax[56]
4. Surgical emphysema[57]
5. Bleeding[45,58,59]
6. Respiratory difficulty—insufficient respiratory support after placement[60]
7. Loss of the introducer into the pleural space[61]
8. Esophageal perforation[62–64]
9. Neck extension during insertion—may be contraindicated if underlying cervical spine injury is suspected[65]
10. Cricothyroid ligament ossification[66]
11. Upper airway CPAP during and after minitracheostomy placement—predisposing to barotrauma[67]
12. Stenosis
13. Laryngeal damage
14. Placement of the catheter into the pretracheal or paratracheal space[49]

Remember: No scientific study documents this technique's degree of efficacy in emergency airway situations.

ARNDT EMERGENCY CRICOTHYROTOMY CATHETER SET

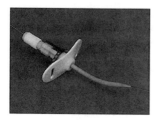

Used for emergency airway access when conventional endotracheal intubation and ventilation cannot be performed. Supplied sterile in peel-open packages. Intended for one-time use.

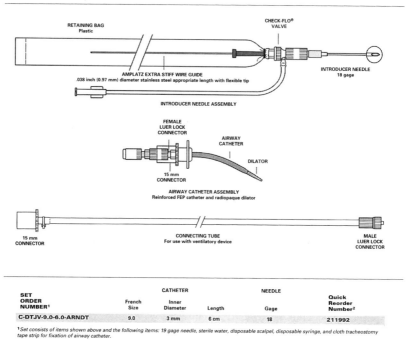

SET ORDER NUMBER[1]	French Size	CATHETER Inner Diameter	Length	NEEDLE Gage	Quick Reorder Number[2]
C-DTJV-9.0-6.0-ARNDT	9.0	3 mm	6 cm	18	211992

[1] Set consists of items shown above and the following items: 19 gage needle, sterile water, disposable scalpel, disposable syringe, and cloth tracheostomy tape strip for fixation of airway catheter.

[2] The Quick Reorder Number is for U.S.A. domestic use only.

Patent Number 4,677,978

FIGURE 10.12. Arndt Emergency Cricothyrotomy Catheter Set (Cook Critical Care, Bloomington, IN, with permission).

Suggestion: Be sure to train with and maintain proficiency with the equipment selected for use in your emergency airway algorithm or protocol.

Contraindications for Use of Minitracheostomy Techniques

Although the minitracheostomy has been used on pediatric patients,[68] its use is not generally endorsed for children. Historically, the absolute and relative contraindications to its use have been the following:

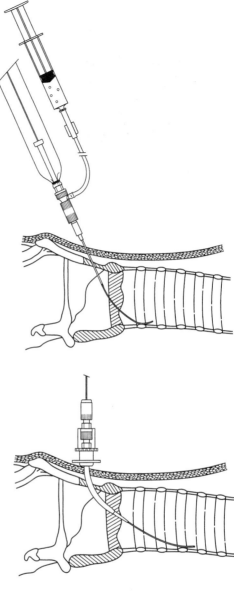

FIGURE 10.13. Inserting the needle and guide wire of an Arndt kit. Air is aspirated through the side port as the needle enters the trachea. The guide wire is left in the trachea.

FIGURE 10.14. Inserting the minitrach of an Arndt kit.

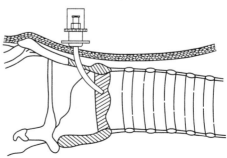

FIGURE 10.15. The Arndt cricothyroidotomy catheter in place.

PATIL EMERGENCY CRICOTHYROTOMY CATHETER SETS

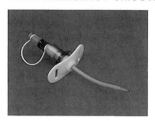

Used for emergency airway access when conventional endotracheal intubation cannot be performed. Supplied sterile in peel-open packages. Intended for one-time use.

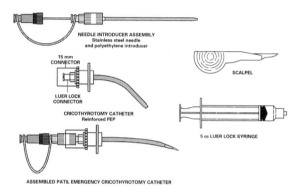

SET ORDER NUMBER[1]	CATHETER			NEEDLE	Quick Reorder Number[2]
	French Size	Inner Diameter	Length	Gage	
C-DTJV-6.0-6.0-PATIL	6.0	2 mm	6 cm	19	221138
C-DTJV-9.0-6.0-PATIL	9.0	3 mm	6 cm	19	205356

[1] Sets consist of items shown above and cloth tracheostomy tape strip for fixation of airway catheter.
[2] The Quick Reorder Number is for U.S.A. domestic use only.
Patent Number 5,380,304

FIGURE 10.16. Patil Emergency Cricothyrotomy Catheter Sets (Cook Critical Care, Bloomington, IN, with permission).

1. Pediatric patients
2. Obesity or obscure airway anatomy
3. Coagulopathies
4. Platelet count less than 100,000
5. Calcified larynx

Relative contraindications may differ when considering the use of minitracheostomy techniques in your difficult airway algorithm or protocol.

Percutaneous Dilational Tracheostomy (PDT)

Objective of the Technique

The objective is to establish a large-bore percutaneous tracheal airway utilizing techniques that require minimal surgical incision and/or dissection. Although originally intended for use in emergency or elective settings, PDT is currently recommended for elective use only.

Numerous articles have been published in the last decade regarding various PDT techniques. Most of these techniques (with modifications) are based on a guide wire used to direct various types of cannulae or dilating forceps into the trachea from the skin surface. Powell et al[69] published a review of the literature on PDT and offered the following historical perspective of the subject:

1. **1969:** Toye and Weinstein described a technique that was based on a single tapered dilator that was advanced into the airway over a guide catheter. The dilator had a recessed blade that was designed to cut tissue as the dilator was forced into the trachea.
2. **1985:** Ciaglia et al described a technique that was based on the Seldinger technique of passing dilators of increasing diameter over a guide wire that had been inserted into the trachea. A formal tracheostomy tube is passed into the trachea over an **appropriately sized** dilator. (More description of this technique will be presented later in this chapter.)
3. **1989:** The Rapitrac (Fresenius, Runcorn, Cheshire, UK), developed by Schachner et al, utilized a cutting-edged dilating forceps device, which was passed under force into the trachea over a guide wire.
4. **1990:** Griggs et al reported a guide wire dilating forceps (GWDF) that did not have a cutting edge like the Rapitrach. This forceps was passed under force into the trachea over a guide wire.

The technique of Fantoni et al[70] can be added to this historical list:

5. **1995:** Fantoni et al described a technique involving a single percutaneous dilatational device that was passed through the trachea and skin from an internal approach.

A large number of studies were undertaken in the 1990s to examine the utility of PDT. At present, many authors are strong proponents of the technique when used to establish an elective tracheostomy in critically ill, long-term ventilator-dependent patients.[71] Other authors, though, have reported that their studies show no great advantage of the technique when compared to traditional surgical tracheostomy. More will be presented later in this chapter regarding this issue.

The recent literature has provided information that enables one to make a more valid evaluation of PDT used in the controlled setting of **elective tracheostomy** for long-term ventilator-dependent patients. Many considerations of PDT had to be evaluated before practitioners could decide rationally whether or not to use the technique. These considerations include the following:

1. Why use PDT?
2. Cost considerations
3. Complication rates associated with PDT techniques
4. Comparison of PDT with traditional open tracheostomy
5. Comparison of various PDT techniques
6. What techniques are available?

The following sections of this chapter will address these considerations.

General Comments

Much of the literature concerning PDT is retrospective, uncontrolled, and anecdotal. Keep in mind the following when reviewing the PDT literature:

1. The vast majority of articles discussing PDT deal with patients who require **elective** tracheostomy.
2. Very few current writers advocate the use of PDT to establish an **emergency airway.** Surgical cricothyroidotomy is considered the preferred interventional method in the emergency setting.
3. Most often, PDT techniques should be applied **only** when immediate surgical backup is available to perform an open tracheostomy should the PDT fail.

Why Use PDT?

Recent writers and clinicians support the development and study of PDT for the following reasons:

1. Lower cost to perform elective tracheostomies.
2. Lower morbidity of PDT compared to open tracheostomy.
3. Less risk of transportation-related injury to the patient if PDT is performed in the ICU.
4. The procedure can be performed by nonsurgeons.
5. PDT can be performed in the ICU so operating room time need not be scheduled.

Not all studies support these claims.

Cost Considerations

PDT performed in the ICU offers a cost/charge savings as compared to open tracheostomy performed in the operating room, in most of the studies reviewed.[69,72–76] One study documented that the cost/charge savings was greatest when open tracheostomy was performed in the ICU. One should be careful when comparing cost and charge data. Was there an anesthesiology charge? Was there a charge for bronchoscopy if used to assist PDT? Are cost/charge statistics from different practices, not to mention different countries, easily comparable? If a death or injury did occur, what were the liability costs?

Complications Associated with PDT

A great deal of information is available concerning the complications associated with PDT. The data concerning complications is published **anecdotally, in review articles, in retrospective studies, and in prospective studies.**

Review Articles

In 1998, Powell et al[69] published a review of the literature up to 1995 that dealt with complications associated with PDT. Their search identified 40 studies containing 1,684 patients. Various PDT techniques were compared. Tables 10.1,

TABLE 10.1. Perioperative complications of four percutaneous tracheostomy methods and standard tracheostomy

Complication (%)	Toye	GWDF	Rapitrach	PDT	Standard tracheostomy
Bleeding	1.0	1.2	1.5	1.7	1.4
Pneumothorax	1.0	—	1.9	0.6	0.9 (0–4)
Desaturation	1.0	—	0.8	0.9	—
Hypotension	—	—	—	0.4	0.3
Tracheostomy tube displacement or damage	—	—	8.8	1.6	—
Peritracheal insertion	6.0	—	3.4	0.8	—
Guide wire misplacement	—	—	—	0.8	—
Arrhythmia	1.0	—	0.8	0.2	0.1
Inability to complete procedure	—	—	5.7	0.7	—
Overall	10.0% (10/100)	1.2% (3/248)	22.9% (60/262)	7.6% (82/1074)	

GWDF = guide wire dilator forceps; PDT = percutaneous dilatational tracheostomy.
Source: Powell,[69] with permission.

10.2, and 10.3 summarize their findings. For comparison, they reported data from two studies of the standard tracheostomy.

Important conclusions from this paper were the following:

1. The Rapitrac had a high perioperative complication rate.
2. Most of the complications associated with PDT occurred earlier in the process of learning the technique. Precautions should be undertaken to prevent complications resulting from inexperience.

TABLE 10.2. Postoperative complications for four percutaneous tracheostomy methods and standard tracheostomy

Complication (%)	Toye	GWDF	Rapitrac	PDT	Standard tracheostomy
Bleeding	—	2.0	1.1	2.1	(1–37)
Tube occlusion	—	—	0.4	0.3	2.7
Tube displacement	—	—	1.5	0.6	1.5 (0–7)
Emphysema, subcutaneous or mediastinal	4.0	—	2.7	0.9	0.9 (0–9)
Wound infection	1.0	—	0.4	1.5	1.0
Tracheoinnominate fistula	—	—	—	0.2	0.4–4.5
Tracheoesophageal fistula	—	—	0.4	—	0.2
Vocal cord paralysis	—	—	—	0.1	0.0
Overall	5.0 (5/100)	2.0 (5/248)	6.5 (17/262)	5.5 (59/1074)	

Source: Powell,[69] with permission.

TABLE 10.3. Late and/or postdecannulation complications for four percutaneous tracheostomy methods and standard tracheostomy

Complication (%)	Toye	GWDF	Rapitrac	PDT	Standard tracheostomy
Tracheal stenosis	—	—	0.8	1.0	0.5
Disfiguring scar	—	—	0.8	0.1	—
Residual stoma	—	—	—	0.2	0.2
Granulation of stoma	—	—	0.4	0.6	0.4
Overall	0.0	—	1.9	1.9	
	(0/100)	(NR)	(5/262)	(20/1074)	
NR = not reported					

Source: Powell,[69] with permission.

3. The Toye and Griggs methods, utilizing dilatational forceps, at first were not studied by many investigators who had not invented the techniques.
4. More follow-up studies were needed to define late and post-cannulation problems associated with PDT.

In 1999, Moe et al.[77] published another literature review in which over 1,500 cases involving various PDT techniques were identified. They also presented a prospective series of 130 cases that they performed using Ciaglia's PDT technique. Tabulation of their findings are presented in Table 10.4.

The methods of PDT utilized were the following:

Method 1: Toye
Method 2: Rapitrac
Method 3: Ciaglia Kit
Method 4: Griggs (dilating forceps)
Method 5: Hazard, modified Ciaglia technique
Method 6: Wang (Shiley Kit)
USZ: University of Zurich Hospital series of 130 patients utilizing Ciaglia, Cook kit
AVE: Average of the seven methods listed above
OT: Open Tracheostomy (five references listed by Moe et al)

Moe et al also listed the following **contraindications to percutaneous tracheostomy:**

1. Pediatric or other small airway
2. Scarring in operative field
3. Obesity obscuring landmarks of palpation
4. Edema in pretracheal region
5. Mass or tumor in or near operative field
6. Patients difficult to intubate for any reason
7. Diseases of urgent or emergent nature
8. Nonintubated patients
9. Any case expected to be technically difficult

TABLE 10.4. Complications of tracheostomy by type and method

	1	2	3	4	5	6	USZ	AVE	OT
No. of procedures	94	150	428	228	79	7	130	1,116	
Total complications (%)	16	19	8	3	16	71	7	10	6–66
Type of complication									
Death	1	0.7	0.2			14		0.4	0–80
Major hemorrhage		0.7	0.2	0.8	4			0.6	0–36
Pneumothorax	1	1.3			3	14	0.7	0.6	0.5–4
Paratracheal insertion	6					14	2	0.8	0.5
Accidental decanulation	1	2	0.5					0.5	3–4
Tracheal perforation					1	14		0.2	
Trach tube occlusion			0.7					0.3	1–11
Inability to complete procedure		4.7	0.2			14	2	1	
Cardiac dysrhythmia		1.3	0.2					0.3	1–4
Wound infection	1		1		3		0.7	0.8	1–36
Tracheal stenosis			0.2		3			0.3	0.4–60
Trach cartilage damage		2						0.3	
Tracheoesoph fistula		0.7						0.09	0.5–2
Tracheomalacia		0.7						0.09	
Subcut. emphysema	4	2	0.7			3	0.7	1.1	1–3
Mild hemorrhage		1.3	3	2			2	2	
Hematoma	1							0.09	
Stomal granulation		2.7	0.7					0.6	
Change of voice			0.7					0.3	
Poor cosmetic result		1.3			1			0.3	

Source: Modified from Moc,[77] with permission.

Important conclusions from this paper include the following:

1. Techniques using sharp instrumentation such as the Toye, Griggs, and Rapi-trac have "poor performance records" when compared to the Ciaglia PDT.
2. Modification to the Ciaglia PDT did not decrease complications.
3. In the emergency setting, cricothyroidotomy is more effective than PDT to **establish a definitive airway.**
4. In their institution, the cost for PDT was slightly higher than that of open tracheostomy.
5. PDT "should be performed only by physicians with detailed knowledge of the anatomy and physiology of the upper airway, with skills in emergent tracheostomy, and preferably by surgeons with extensive experience in airway management and intubation."
6. The Ciaglia Kit (Cook Critical Care, Bloomington, IN) set a "new gold standard for tracheostomy" performed electively in the prospective study portion of the paper.

Billy and Bradrick[78] reviewed 19 studies including 1,012 patients who had undergone PDT. They compared PDT complication and mortality rates with those of 1,925 patients who had undergone traditional tracheostomy (Table 10.5).

TABLE 10.5. Complication and mortality rates

Method	Complication rate	Mortality rate
PDT	11.7%	0.3%
Traditional Tracheostomy	15.8%	1.6%

Source: Billy and Bradrick,[78] with permission.

These authors also warned against the use of PDT in the emergency setting, or for patients with potentially unstable airways.

Finally, Bobo and McKenna[79] reported the overall complication rates compiled from 18 studies (some of which were reviewed in previous papers) and concluded that PDT appeared to be safe and efficient. They warned against using the technique in the emergency setting.

Retrospective Studies

Muhammand et al[80] published a retrospective study of 497 patients who had undergone PDT. Significant hemorrhage occurred in 4.8% of their patients. They concluded that the risk of hemorrhage could be reduced if the PDT were placed above the fourth tracheal ring, that fiberoptic endoscopy should be used to confirm correct placement, that the neck should not be fully extended, and that if one suspects abnormal anatomy, diagnostic tests such as ultrasound could define vascular anatomy in the neck.

Vigliaroli et al[81] presented the results of 304 PDTs with the Ciaglia Kit. Table 10.6 summarizes their findings.

The investigators examined the larynx and trachea of 41 patients up to 1,115 days after extubation. Mucosal findings were similar to those found after standard tracheostomy.

Finally, Gaukroger and Allt-Graham[82] reported the complications associated with the use of the Ciaglia PDT in 50 patients. One patient (who was anticoagulated when the PDT was placed) had a clot in the trachea 4 hours after placement. Another patient dislodged her tracheostomy tube after 3 days and it could not be replaced. She subsequently had a formal surgical tracheostomy. In 3 pa-

TABLE 10.6. Complications of PDT (n = 304 patients)

Complication	Incidence
Pneumothorax	0.3%
Tube displacement	1.0%
Peritracheal insertion improper	0.7%
Tracheoesophageal fistula	0.3%
Tracheocutaneous fistula	0.7%
Tube occlusion	0.7%
Endoluminal tube displacement	1.0%
Wound infection	1.7%

Source: Vigliaroli, et al,[81] with permission.

tients, the guide wire kinked in the final stages of the procedure, resulting in pre-tracheal placement of the tracheostomy tube. In all 3 patients, the complication was recognized immediately and the patients were all successfully percutaneously intubated over a guide wire placed correctly.

Prospective Studies and PDT Complication Rates

The largest single-center prospective study reporting experience with PDT was that of Kearney et al.[71] Over an 8-year period, experienced surgeons performed 827 PDTs on 824 patients using the Ciaglia technique exclusively. For the first half of the study (1990–1996), the investigators used the Ciaglia Percutaneous Tracheostomy Introducer Set (Cook Intensive Care, Bloomington, IN). After 1996, they used the Sims Per-Fit Kit (Sims Inc., Keene, NH), which had a "tracheostomy tube specifically designed for percutaneous placement." They found no differences between kits with respect to outcome. The overall results of the study are summarized in Table 10.7.

Tables 10.7, 10.8, 10.9, and 10.10 summarize the specific complications reported by Kearney et al.

These investigators did not advocate the use of PDT in the emergency setting. They noted that Cook had introduced a simplified PDT kit with "a better tracheostomy tube-dilator interface."

Kearney et al concluded that **"PDT is a technical improvement over the open surgical technique. On the basis of our study, we believe that PDT is the preferred method for intubated critically ill patients who require elective tracheostomy."**

Other prospective studies published between 1996 and 2000, in which the Ciaglia technique was used, documented similar low mortality rates associated with PDT insertion.[83–89] In these studies, the majority of PDTs were inserted by surgeons or surgical residents. In a few, internists and an anesthesiologist inserted the PDT. The fiberoptic bronchoscope was used to facilitate PDT and to confirm correct tube placement by most investigators, though not all. In all of the studies, the PDT was deemed to be safe and efficacious. Many studies also claimed

---

TABLE 10.7. Single-center 8-year experience with percutaneous dilational tracheostomy

1. Type of study: Prospective
2. Personnel performing PDT: Trained Surgeons
3. Number of patients: 824
4. Number of PDTs: 827
5. Mean procedure time: 15 minutes
6. Intraoperative complication rate: 6%
7. Procedure-related death rate: 0.6%
8. (Immediate) postoperative complications: 5%
9. Mean follow-up more than 1 year, tracheal stenosis rate: 1.6%

Source: Kearney, et al,[71] with permission.

TABLE 10.8. Surgical complications (827 procedures)

Complication	Number	%
No complication	778	94.0
Premature extubation	9	1.0
Bleeding/no transfusion	7	0.9
False passage	6	0.7
Tracheostomy tube size	5	0.6
Pneumothorax	4	0.5
Guidewire displacement	4	0.5
Unable to complete procedure	2	0.2
Subcutaneous emphysema	2	0.2
Transient hypotension	2	0.2
Difficult tube placement	2	0.2
Tracheal laceration	2	0.2
Tracheoesophageal fistula	2	0.2
Other*	4	0.5

*Puncture of endotracheal tube balloon, needle insertion at wrong level, puncture of tracheal ring, and bleeding with transfusion.
Source: Kearney, et al,[71] with permission.

TABLE 10.9. Postoperative complications (827 procedures)

Complication	Number	%
No complication	781	95.0
Bleeding without transfusion	13	1.6
Airway obstruction with decanulation	8	1.0
Bleeding with transfusion	5	0.9
Premature extubation	4	0.5
Stomal infection	4	0.5
Excessive granulation tissue	5	0.6
Other*		

*Dysphagia, hoarseness, aspiration, balloon rupture, and subcutaneous emphysema.
Source: Kearney, et al,[71] with permission.

TABLE 10.10. Postdischarge complications

Complication	Number*	%
No complications	522	95.4
Dysphagia	10	1.8
Tracheal stenosis or malacia	5	0.9
Airway obstruction with decannulation	4	0.7
Hoarseness	3	0.5
Other†	4	0.7

*Of 548 (80 of the 628 patients discharged were lost to follow-up).
†Aspiration, excessive granulation tissue, subglottic web, and stomal infection.
Source: Kearney, et al,[71] with permission.

a "cost" savings when PDT was used. **None of the authors advocated use of the PDT in the emergency setting.**

Conclusions Regarding PDT-Related Complications

Many studies document that the Ciaglia PDT technique is safe, efficacious, and possibly cost-effective. The technique is not advocated for emergency use. It should be used by **experienced physicians. Immediate surgical backup should be available.** Fiberoptic bronchoscopic guidance is suggested, at least while the technique is being learned. A description of the traditional Ciaglia technique, and others, will be presented later in the chapter.

The authors of the review articles agreed with Moe et al,[77] warning that techniques requiring the use of dilating instruments with sharp edges had "poor performance records" when compared to Ciaglia PDT.

Comparisons between the Ciaglia PDT and Open Tracheostomy

In 1909, Jackson standardized the open tracheostomy technique used by surgeons today. Many studies over the past decade have compared this "gold standard" to various percutaneous dilational tracheostomy methods (primarily the Ciaglia technique). While some studies support open tracheostomy as the technique of choice to establish an elective surgical airway,[90–92] others found that PDT is also safe and efficacious when performed by a trained surgeon.[93–95] PDT has gained considerable popularity in some areas[96] and has proven superior to open tracheostomy in prospective studies.[48,97]

Debate over the method of choice for establishing an elective surgical airway continues.

Even though many prospective studies compared the various techniques, methodological differences among studies have not allowed experts to agree on conclusions. Investigators have used tests including bronchoscopy, MRI, radiographic studies, pulmonary function testing, and physical examination to define and evaluate long-term complications of PDT and open tracheostomy. Using endoscopy to evaluate the airway, one investigator noted a very high incidence of asymptomatic "airway abnormalities" after PDT in 36 of 41 survivors.[98] Other studies showed much lower rates of long-term PDT-related sequellae.[99–102] This discrepancy remains unresolved due to the unfortunate number of patients lost to follow-up. Norwood et al[103] evaluated long-term complications in 100 of 422 patients who had undergone PDT. Of these 100 patients, 38 agreed to computerized tomography (CT) and fiberoptic airway endoscopy, 10 patients had CT only, while 52 were evaluated by interview alone. The results of the study are summarized in Table 10.11.

Disagreement continues as to the preference of PDT versus open tracheostomy used to establish an elective surgical airway. To read more on this topic, consider the debate between Bernard and Kenady,[104] proponents of conventional surgical tracheostomy, and Griffen and Kearney,[105] proponents of PDT. Excellent reviews by Barba[106] and Pryor et al[107] summarize various surgical techniques commonly undertaken in the ICU setting, including PDT, tracheostomy, and cricothyroidotomy.

TABLE 10.11. Late complications after percutaneous tracheostomy (n = 100 of 422 patients who underwent PDT)

Complication	Number
Voice change	27/100 (27%)
Persistent severe hoarseness	2/100 (2%)
Vocal cord abnormalities	4/38 (11%)
Laryngeal granuloma	1/38 (3%)
Focal tracheal mucosal erythema	2/38 (5%)
Severe tracheomalacia/stenosis	1/38 (3%)
Mild (11–25%) stenosis	10/48 (21%)
Moderate (26–50%) stenosis	4/48 (8.3%)
Severe (greater than 50%) stenosis	1/48 (2%)
Long-term stomal complications	0

Source: Norwood, et al,[103] with permission.

Comparisons of Different PDT Techniques

Recent publications document clinical comparisons of various PDT techniques. Most studies are prospective, though the methodology utilized to collect the data varies.

Byhahn et al.[108] compared the Ciaglia Blue Rhino (CBR) (Cook Critical Care, Bloomington, IN) to standard Ciaglia PDT in 50 patients. The mean procedure time for the Blue Rhino was 165 seconds vs. 386 seconds for standard Ciaglia PDT. Tracheal cartilage rupture occurred in 9 of 25 patients in the Blue Rhino group vs. 2 of 25 in the standard PDT group. The authors noted that the long-term sequellae of tracheal ring fracture needs further study. Other complications with the standard PDT included posterior tracheal wall injury (2/25), pneumothorax (1/25), and bleeding during tracheostomy tube change (1/25). No life-threatening complications were associated with use of the Blue Rhino. The authors concluded that the "new CBR is more practicable than PDT."

Westphal et al.[109] compared the standard Ciaglia PDT and the Fantoni translaryngeal technique (TLT) in 90 patients. They reported that the mean procedure time for the TLT was slightly shorter than for PDT, 9.8 vs. 10.4 minutes. Complications for PDT included severe bleeding (1/45), aspiration of blood (4/45) and lower postoperative PaO_2/FiO_2. The main complications of the TLT technique were difficult retrograde wire placement (14/45) and higher $PaCO_2$ intraoperatively. The authors concluded that both techniques were "safe and attractive" to establish long-term airway access in critically ill patients.

In another study by Byhahn et al,[110] the Griggs Guide Wire Dilating Forceps (GWDF) and Fantoni TLT techniques were compared in 100 patients. The mean procedural time was shorter for the GWDF technique, 4.8 vs. 9.2 minutes. The overall complication rates for both groups was 4%. Complications of the GWDF included moderate to severe bleeding in 2 of 50 patients. Complications of the TLT included tracheal wall rupture in 1 of 50 patients and pretracheal tube placement in 1 of 50 patients. They rated both techniques safe when performed by experienced physicians.

Three studies compared the GWDF technique and the standard Ciaglia PDT. Nates et al,[111] in a study of 100 patients, documented a slightly shorter mean procedural time for PDT than for GWDF, 9.3 vs. 10 minutes. They preferred standard PDT to GWDF because of a lower overall complication rate (2% vs. 25%). The major complication with GWDF was bleeding. Van Heerden et al[112] studied 54 patients and reported equal rates of bleeding between GWDF and PDT patients. The major difference between groups was reported to be more difficulty with tracheostomy tube change at day 7 with the Ciaglia group (4/29) due to a smaller stoma size. The authors regarded both techniques to be safe. Finally, Ambesh and Kaushik[113] compared the techniques in a study that included 80 patients. The mean procedural time was shorter for the GWDF group, 6.5 vs. 14 minutes. The complication rates were similar for both groups with two exceptions. Stomal dilation was more difficult with the PDT technique, while tracheal cannulation was more difficult with the GWDF group. No clinical tracheal stenosis at 9 months post-decannulation was reported in patients from either group. The authors reported that both techniques were safe and easy to use.

In conclusion, the studies reported that the PDT techniques analyzed were safe and efficacious when used by experienced physicians. Fiberoptic bronchoscopic guidance was recommended by all authors. It was reported that TLT could be used with pediatric patients, a claim not made for standard Ciaglia PDT. Finally, no authors endorsed any technique for use in the emergency setting.

Five popular and well-studied techniques to establish percutaneous tracheostomy tube placement will now be described. The techniques include the following:

1. Ciaglia Percutaneous Tracheostomy Introducer Set (Cook Critical Care, Bloomington, IN)
2. Ciaglia Blue Rhino Percutaneous Tracheostomy Introducer Set (Cook Critical Care, Bloomington, IN)
3. Sims Per-Fit Percutaneous Dilatational Tracheostomy Kit (Sims, Inc., Portex, Keene, NH)
4. Griggs Guide Wire Dilating Forceps (Portex, UK)
5. Fantoni Translaryngeal Tracheostomy Kit (Mallinckrodt, Europe)

Additional comments will be offered regarding the NuTrach (Portex, Keene, NH)

Ciaglia Percutaneous Tracheostomy Introducer Set

The Ciaglia PDT technique was first described in 1985[114] and advocated to be a method to establish an **elective** tracheostomy at the bedside. Since then, the original authors and many others have studied the technique's efficacy. Modifications to the technique have been suggested, but the Ciaglia PDT technique is practiced much as it was first described. The major modification to the technique is that most clinicians recommend using the fiberoptic bronchoscope to visually verify that placement of the percutaneous needle and the guiding catheter is positioned properly,[115–117] at least while learning the technique. Most clinicians who describe the technique pull the endotracheal tube back toward the glottis and verify that the tip of the tube is still in the trachea with a fiberoptic bronchoscope. The tube is pulled back to lessen the chance of needle perforation of the cuff or the tube itself. Velmahos et al[87] suggested that the endotracheal tube should be left in place, with the cuff below the level of needle insertion. They claim that there is enough room in the trachea to insert the guiding catheter alongside of the endotracheal tube. The tube is pulled back after dilatator placement and the tip of the tube is felt digitally and verified to be above the dilatational tracheostomy site before the formal tracheostomy tube is placed.

The instructions used to perform Ciaglia PDT are provided with the kit (Fig. 10.17). Quotations from these instructions (with a few modifications) are used to describe the technique.

Technique

1. The PDT is inserted through the first or preferably the second tracheal membrane (Fig. 10.18).
2. After identifying the proper level, inject lidocaine with epinephrine locally

CIAGLIA PERCUTANEOUS TRACHEOSTOMY INTRODUCER SETS AND TRAY

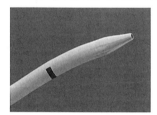

Used for controlled percutaneous introduction of tracheostomy tubes. Sequentially sized dilators advanced over a wire guide/guiding catheter system facilitates gradual dilation of the tracheal entrance site. Tracheostomy tube placement is accomplished by fitting the tracheostomy tube over the appropriate size dilator and advancing into position. **This technique is not recommended for emergency tube placement and those patients with enlarged thyroids.**
NOTE: Refer to product insert prior to use. Supplied sterile in peel-open packages. Intended for one-time use.

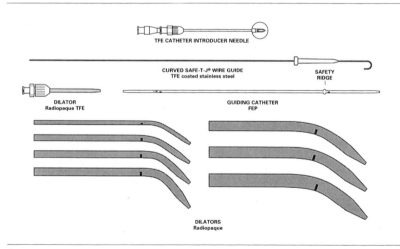

FIGURE 10.17. Ciaglia Percutaneous Tracheostomy Introducer Set (Cook Critical Care, Bloomington, IN, with permission). (*Note:* The black rings on the dilators are skin-level positioning marks.)

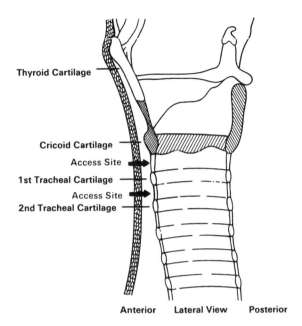

FIGURE 10.18. (Cook Critical Care, Bloomington, IN, with permission).

Thyroid Cartilage

Cricoid Cartilage

Access Site

1st Tracheal Cartilage

Access Site

2nd Tracheal Cartilage

Anterior   Lateral View   Posterior

and make a vertical 1.5-cm incision in the midline from the lower edge of the cricoid cartilage. You may wish to gently dissect the incision with a curved mosquito clamp down to the anterior tracheal wall. Next, use a finger to dissect the front of the trachea and to displace thyroid tissue downward.

3. After deflating the endotracheal tube cuff, pull the tube back 1 cm. (A fiberoptic bronchoscope can verify that the tip of the tube is still in the trachea and guide the operator with the next four steps.)

4. Direct the introducer needle in a posterior/caudad direction into the trachea seeking air aspiration to verify that the tip of the needle has entered the trachea. Inject 1.0 cc of lidocaine into the trachea and remove the needle (Fig. 10.19).

5. Attach a syringe half filled with lidocaine to the needle and reinsert the tip into the trachea. Aspirate on the needle to make sure that the tip is still in the trachea by observing for air. Move the endotracheal tube to make sure that the needle has not impaled the tube or cuff (the needle will move if it has impaled the endotracheal tube).

6. When the needle's position is verified, remove the needle and advance the catheter into the trachea; aspirate for air (Fig. 10.20).

7. Remove the syringe and insert the 0.052-inch "J" wire into the trachea (Fig. 10.21).

8. Hold the guide wire in place and remove the catheter. Dilate the tract by placing the 11 French introducing dilator into the trachea over the wire. Remove the dilator but keep the wire in the trachea. Note the wire's skin-level mark.

9. Following the direction of the arrow on the guiding catheter, advance the

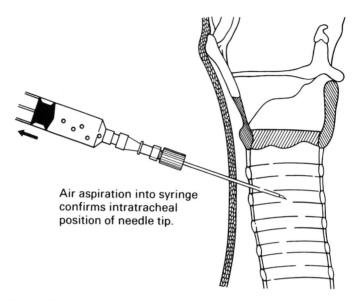

Air aspiration into syringe
confirms intratracheal
position of needle tip.

FIGURE 10.19. (Cook Critical Care, Bloomington, IN, with permission).

8.0 French Teflon guiding catheter over the wire guide to the skin-level mark
on the wire guide. Insert the guiding catheter and wire guide **as a unit** into the
trachea until the safety ridge on the guiding catheter is to the skin level. **The
end of the guiding catheter with the safety ridge should be introduced toward the patient.** Align the proximal end of the Teflon guiding catheter at the

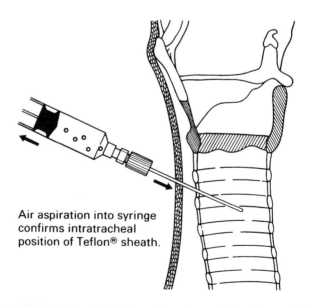

Air aspiration into syringe
confirms intratracheal
position of Teflon® sheath.

FIGURE 10.20. (Cook Critical Care, Bloomington, IN, with permission).

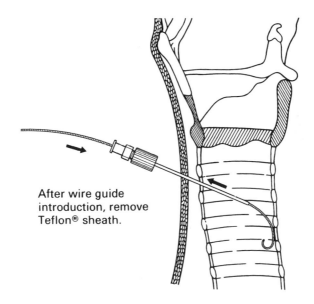

FIGURE 10.21. (Cook Critical Care, Bloomington, IN, with permission).

mark on the proximal portion of the wire guide. This will assure that the distal end of the guiding catheter is properly positioned back on the wire guide, preventing possible trauma to the posterior tracheal wall during subsequent manipulations. Position the guiding catheter and wire guide **as a unit** so that the safety ridge on the guiding catheter is at the skin level (Fig. 10.22).

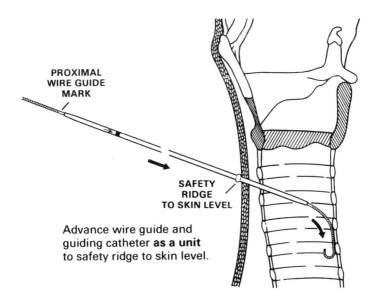

FIGURE 10.22. (Cook Critical Care, Bloomington, IN, with permission).

10. Begin to serially dilate the access site into the trachea. This is accomplished by first advancing the 12 French blue dilator over the wire guide/guiding catheter assembly. **To properly align the dilator on the wire guide/guiding catheter assembly, position the proximal end of the dilator at the single positioning mark on the guiding catheter. This will assure that the distal tip of the dilator is properly positioned at the safety ridge on the guiding catheter to prevent possible trauma to the posterior tracheal wall during introduction.** While maintaining the visual reference points and positioning relationships of the wire guide, guiding catheter, and dilator, advance them **as a unit,** with a twisting motion, to the skin-level mark on the blue dilator. Advance and pull back the dilating assembly several times, while twisting, to perform effective dilatation of the tracheal entrance site. Remove the blue dilator leaving the wire guide/guiding catheter assembly in position (Fig. 10.23).

11. Continue the dilatation procedure by advancing the sizing-sequence (small to large) dilators. **Positioning of the dilators on the wire guide/guiding catheter assembly and dilatation of the tracheal entrance site should be done as described in Step 10.**

12. Slightly overdilate the tracheal entrance site to a size appropriate for passage of the tracheostomy tube of choice; overdilate to allow easy passage of the balloon portion of the tracheostomy tube into the trachea.

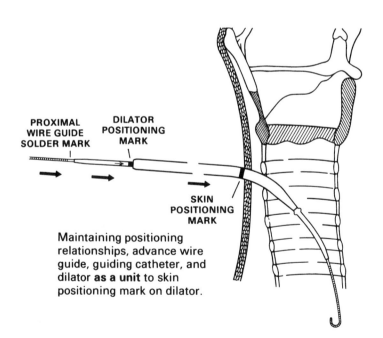

PROXIMAL WIRE GUIDE SOLDER MARK

DILATOR POSITIONING MARK

SKIN POSITIONING MARK

Maintaining positioning relationships, advance wire guide, guiding catheter, and dilator **as a unit** to skin positioning mark on dilator.

FIGURE 10.23. (Cook Critical Care, Bloomington, IN, with permission).

Tracheostomy tube inner diameter	Appropriate dilator for initial overdilation
6 mm	24 French
7 mm	28 French
8 mm	32 French
9 mm	36 French

13. Preload the flexible tracheostomy tube to be inserted on the appropriate-size blue dilator by first generously lubricating the surface of the dilator. Position the tracheostomy tube onto the dilator so that its tip is approximately 2 cm back from the distal tip of the dilator. Make sure the balloon is totally deflated. Thoroughly lubricate the tracheostomy tube assembly prior to insertion. The sizing chart below should be used as a guide to assure correct fit (Fig. 10.24).

Tracheostomy tube inner diameter	Appropriate dilator for introduction
6 mm	18 French
7 mm	21 French
8 mm	24 French
9 mm	28 French

Note: Dual cannula tracheostomy tubes may also be placed using this technique. The inner cannula must be removed for introduction. Always check fit of dilator to tracheostomy tube prior to insertion. **Follow tracheostomy tube manufacturer's instructions for testing of balloon cuff and inflation system prior to insertion.**

14. Advance preloaded tracheostomy tube over wire guide/guiding catheter assembly to the safety ridge and then advance as a unit into the trachea. As soon as the deflated balloon enters the trachea, withdraw the blue dilator, guiding catheter, and wire guide (Fig. 10.25).

15. Advance the tracheostomy tube to its flange. *Note:* If using a dual cannula tracheostomy tube, insert the inner cannula at this point.

16. Connect the tracheostomy tube to the ventilator, inflate the balloon cuff, and remove the endotracheal tube. *Note:* Prior to complete removal of the endotracheal tube, test ventilation through the tracheostomy tube.

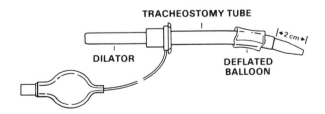

FIGURE 10.24. (Cook Critical Care, Bloomington, IN, with permission).

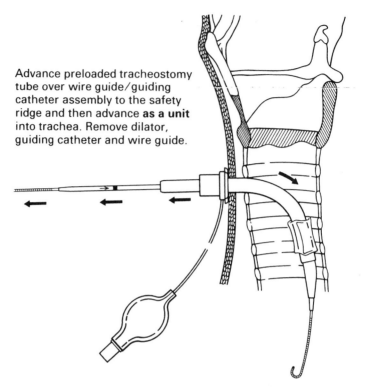

Advance preloaded tracheostomy
tube over wire guide/guiding
catheter assembly to the safety
ridge and then advance **as a unit**
into trachea. Remove dilator,
guiding catheter and wire guide.

FIGURE 10.25. (Cook Critical Care, Bloomington, IN, with permission).

17. Perform suction to determine if any significant bleeding or possible obstruction exists that has not been noted to this point.
18. If necessary, one suture may be taken at the bottom of the initial incision.

Postplacement. Apply neosporin dressing to the stoma site three times per day (TID) for three days. Elevate the head of the patient's bed 30 to 40 degrees for one hour after insertion.

Precautions

1. Always confirm access into trachea by air bubble aspiration.
2. Maintain safety positioning marks of wire guide, guiding catheter, and dilators during dilating procedure to prevent trauma to posterior wall of the trachea.
3. Tracheostomy tube should fit snugly to dilator for insertion. Generous lubrication to the surface of the dilator will enhance fit and placement of the tracheostomy tube.

Ciaglia Blue Rhino Percutaneous Tracheostomy Introducer Set with
EZ-Pass Hydrophilic Coating (Cook Critical Care, Bloomington, IN)

The Blue Rhino kit contains a single, tapered, hydrophilic dilating catheter. The contents of the kit are shown in Figure 10.26.

CIAGLIA BLUE RHINO™ PERCUTANEOUS TRACHEOSTOMY
INTRODUCER SET WITH EZ-PASS™ HYDROPHILIC COATING

Used for controlled percutaneous introduction of tracheostomy tubes. The Ciaglia Blue Rhino™ dilator advanced over a wire guide/guiding catheter system facilitates dilation of the tracheal entrance site. Tracheostomy tube placement is accomplished by fitting the tracheostomy tube over the appropriate size loading dilator and advancing into position. This technique is not recommended for emergency tube placement and those patients with enlarged thyroids. Refer to product insert prior to use. Supplied sterile in peel-open packages. Intended for one-time use.

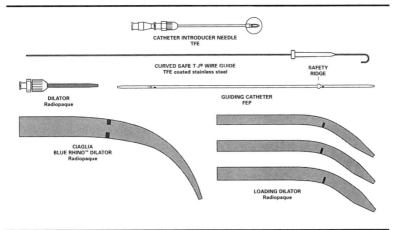

ORDER NUMBER	Remarks	Quick Reorder Number[1]
SETS		
C-PTIS-100-HC	SET consists of 17 gage TFE catheter introducer needle 7 cm long, .052 inch (1.32 mm) diameter TFE coated stainless steel wire guide 55 cm long with 3 mm Safe-T-J® tip, 8.0 French FEP guiding catheter 29 cm long tapered on both ends to .052 inch diameter wire guide, 14.0 French dilator 4.5 cm long tapered to .052 inch diameter wire guide, one Ciaglia Blue Rhino™ dilator and three loading dilators (24.0, 26.0, 28.0 French) 20 cm long tapered to fit the 8.0 French FEP guiding catheter, disposable syringe, disposable scalpel, lubricating jelly and gauze sponges.	253159
C-PTIS-100-A-HC	SET consists of 17 gage TFE catheter introducer needle 7 cm long, .052 inch (1.32 mm) diameter TFE coated stainless steel wire guide 55 cm long with 3 mm Safe-T-J® tip, 8.0 French FEP guiding catheter 29 cm long tapered on both ends to .052 inch diameter wire guide, 14.0 French dilator 4.5 cm long tapered to .052 inch diameter wire guide, one Ciaglia Blue Rhino™ dilator and one 28 French loading dilator 20 cm long tapered to fit the 8.0 French FEP guiding catheter, disposable syringe, disposable scalpel, lubricating jelly and gauze sponges.	256566
TRAYS		
C-PTISY-100-HC	TRAY consists of all items listed above for C-PTIS-100-HC and the following items: 25 gage needle, 22 gage needle, 19 gage needle, lidocaine (1.5% with epinephrine), double swivel connector, iodophor PVP swabs, fenestrated drape, suture with needle, needle holder, CSR wrap and prep tray.	258562
C-PTISY-100-A-HC	TRAY consists of all items listed above for C-PTIS-100-A-HC and the following items: 25 gage needle, 22 gage needle, 19 gage needle, lidocaine (1.5% with epinephrine), double swivel connector, iodophor PVP swabs, fenestrated drape, suture with needle, needle holder, CSR wrap and prep tray.	258563

[1]The Quick Reorder Number is for U.S.A. domestic use only.

Additional product configurations are available upon request. Contact Cook Customer Service or your local sales representative for availability and pricing.

Use of the Shiley PERC tracheostomy tube with a tapered distal tip (Mallinckrodt Medical, Inc., St. Louis, MO, 1-888-744-1414) is recommended.

FIGURE 10.26. Contents of the Blue Rhino Tracheostomy Kit (Cook Critical Care, Bloomington, IN, with permission).

To use the Blue Rhino kit, perform Steps 1 through 8 as described above. At this point, the guide wire is in the trachea. Proceed as follows.

1. Activate the EZ-Pass hydrophilic coating by immersing the distal end of the Ciaglia Blue Rhino dilator in sterile water or saline.
2. Advance the Ciaglia Blue Rhino dilator and the guiding catheter as a unit over the wire guide while maintaining the wire guide position. Align the proximal end of the guiding catheter at the mark on the proximal portion of the wire guide. This will assure that the distal end of the guiding catheter is properly positioned back on the wire guide, preventing possible trauma to the posterior tracheal wall during subsequent manipulations.

3. Begin to dilate the access site by advancing the guiding catheter and Ciaglia Blue Rhino dilator as a unit over the wire guide into the trachea. **To properly align the dilator on the wire guide/guiding catheter assembly, position the proximal end of the dilator at the single positioning mark on the guiding catheter. This will assure that the distal tip of the dilator is properly positioned at the safety ridge on the guiding catheter to prevent possible trauma to the posterior tracheal wall during introduction.** While maintaining the visual reference points and positioning relationships of the wire guide, guiding catheter, and dilator, advance them **as a unit** to the skin-level mark on the Ciaglia Blue Rhino dilator. Care **must** be taken not to advance the Blue Rhino dilator beyond the black skin-level mark. Advance and pull back the dilating assembly several times to perform effective dilation of the tracheal entrance site (Fig. 10.27).

4. Remove the Ciaglia Blue Rhino dilator, leaving the wire guide/guiding catheter assembly in position.

5. *Note:* The wire guide must always lead the dilator and the guiding catheter assembly to prevent possible trauma to the posterior tracheal wall during dilation. Care must be taken to keep the guiding catheter assembly properly aligned with the mark on the proximal portion of the wire guide.

6. Slightly overdilate the tracheal entrance.

7. Proceed from Step 13 in the previous section.

Clinical use of the Ciaglia Blue Rhino kit has been described by Byhahn et al and Bewsher et al.[118,119]

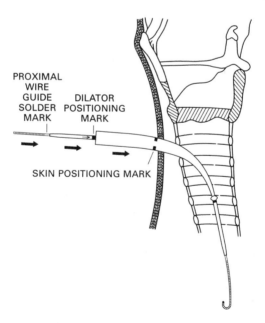

FIGURE 10.27. (Cook Critical Care, Bloomington, IN, with permission).

Sims Per-Fit Percutaneous Dilational Tracheostomy Kit
(Sims, Inc., Portex, Keene, NH)

The technique used to insert a tracheostomy tube using the Sims Per-Fit Kit is similar to that used with the Ciaglia Kit as described above. The Sims Kit has straight rather than curved dilators. Some clinicians who had used the Ciaglia Kit switched to the Sims Kit because the latter kit included a tracheostomy tube with a tapered tip, which they claimed facilitated tube placement. Recent anecdotal reports, though, speculate that the tapered tip may, in some cases, collapse and obstruct the trachea.[120,121] A personal communication from a product consultant confirmed that Portex is redesigning many of the components of its percutaneous tracheostomy kit. Therefore, no further description of the Portex product will be presented, as a totally new kit will be available by the time this book is published. Let it suffice to say that many investigators have found the current Sims-Portex product to be very efficacious and safe to use. Both manufacturers will introduce new and safer equipment as more is learned about percutaneous dilational tracheostomy in the future.[122]

Griggs Guide Wire Dilating Forceps (GWDF) (Portex, Hythe, Kent, UK)

The Portex GWDF Tracheostomy Kit is not yet available in the United States. However, it has been used extensively in other countries.[110,112,123–125] The principal instrument in the kit is a modified Howard Kelly forceps with a curved tip. The blades of the tip have a guide wire groove that, when the forceps is closed, will allow the wire to pass through the forceps' blades (Fig. 10.28).

To perform the GWDF technique, the following steps are undertaken.[110,112,126]

1. A 2-cm horizontal incision is made through the skin at the desired tracheal level (between the second and third thyroid ring).
2. A guide wire is inserted as described in the Ciaglia PDT technique. Fiberoptic guidance is recommended to insure that the wire is placed in the midline.
3. The GWDF is closed over the wire and passed through the dilated tract to the pretracheal wall. The forceps can be opened to dilate the tract.
4. The GWDF is then passed into the trachea (with fiberoptic guidance).
5. The forceps are then opened (using both hands) to the diameter desired (the diameter of the stoma tract).
6. The forceps are removed with the blades "open" to dilate the tract.[112]
7. An appropriately sized tracheostomy tube with obturator is inserted over the wire.
8. The wire and obturator are removed, the cuff inflated, and ventilation begun.

Clinicians using the Griggs GWDF warn that the procedure is not for emergency tracheostomy use and should be performed with fiberoptic guidance.

Fantoni Translaryngeal Tracheostomy Kit (Mallinckrodt, Europe)

Translaryngeal tracheostomy (TLT) was described by Fantoni and Ripamonti in 1995.[70] Since then, the technique has been utilized in Europe, Canada, and Australia. A clinical kit is not yet available in the United States. The technique is

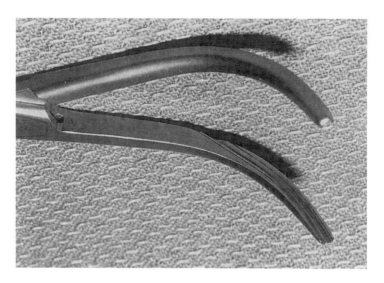

FIGURE 10.28. The modified Howard Kelly forceps used in the Portex Percutaneous Dilational Tracheostomy Kit (Portex; Hythe, Kent, UK). Note the guide-wire grooves in the forceps blades. The forceps are used when performing a Griggs (GWDF) tracheotomy. (From Van Heerden,[112] with permission.)

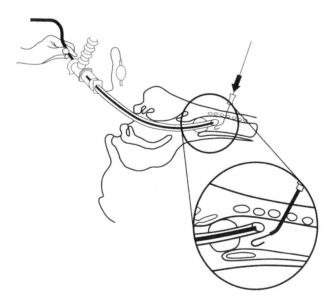

FIGURE 10.29. The Fantoni translaryngeal tracheostomy (TLT). After bronchoscopically guided puncture of the trachea, the guide wire is introduced and advanced retrograde parallel to the endotracheal tube. (From Westphal, et al,[131] with permission.)

unique in that the tracheostomy tube is passed from within the trachea outward through the skin. The technique has been studied by many authors[127–130] and is deemed an acceptable approach to percutaneous tracheostomy. Westphal et al[130] used TLT to perform 120 elective percutaneous tracheostomies. They concluded that the technique, as performed in the intensive care unit, was "safe and cost effective." The following figures, 10.29 to 10.33 (borrowed from Westphal et al), illustrate the TLT technique.

Other percutaneous tracheostomy techniques are described below.

Nu-Trake (Portex, Keene, NH)

The Nu-Trake was introduced as a device to be used in emergent airway situations.[131] No studies of the technique were identified in the recent literature. A brief description of the technique follows.

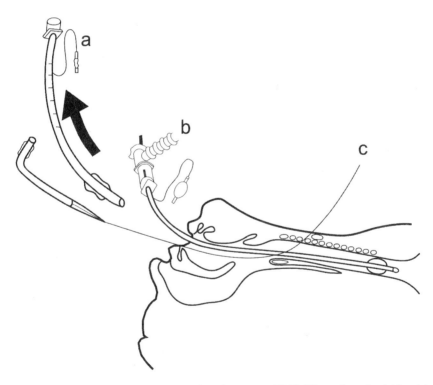

FIGURE 10.30. The Fantoni translaryngeal tracheostomy (TLT). The endotracheal tube, (a) was replaced under direct laryngoscopy with the thin tube of the set (b), the tracheostomy tube is connected to the guide wire and, (c), by pulling the wire's distal end, is advanced to the trachea. (From Westphal, et al,[130] with permission.)

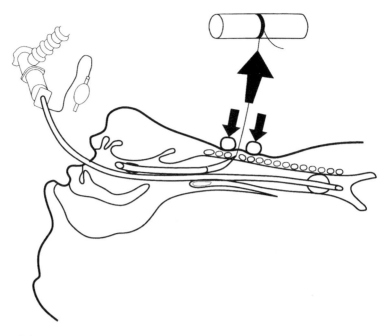

FIGURE 10.31. The Fantoni translaryngeal tracheostomy (TLT). By pulling the wire and by using digital counterpressure, the tracheostomy tube is advanced through the anterior tracheal wall and the soft tissues of the neck. (From Westphal, et al,[131] with permission.)

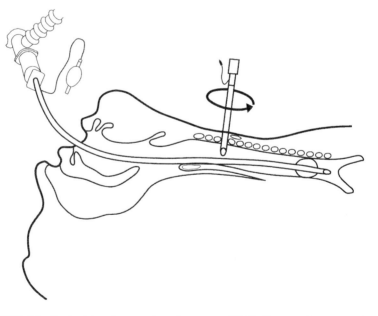

FIGURE 10.32. The Fantoni translaryngeal tracheostomy (TLT). Correct placement of the tracheostomy tube is achieved with 180° rotation by means of an obturator. Intratracheal rotation of the tracheal cannula can be done either with the thin endotracheal tube in place or after removal. (From Westphal, et al,[131] with permission.)

1. The cannula housing, 13-gauge needle stylet, and syringe are locked together into one unit.
2. A 1 to 2 cm skin incision is made in the midline over the "lower third of the cricothyroid membrane."[16(p199)]
3. The cannula housing–stylet unit is inserted through the incision into the trachea in a slight caudad approach.
4. Confirmation of tracheal position is made by aspirating air.
5. The stylet is removed.
6. The metal cannula–obturator assemblies are inserted through the housing from the smallest obturator to the largest (dependent on tracheal size).
7. Once the largest obturator has been inserted, the position is confirmed and the housing is secured with cloth tape. The 15-mm adapter on the housing is attached to airway equipment (ventilating bag).

Quicktrach Emergency Cricothyrotomy Device
(Life-Assist, Inc., Sacramento, CA)[132]

The Quicktrach device is a tracheal cannula-over-trochar device that comes in two sizes, 4-mm I.D. for adult use, and 2-mm I.D. for pediatric use. Insertion of the tracheostomy cannula is accomplished as follows. First, firmly grasp the device and puncture the cricothyroid membrane at an angle 90 degrees to the skin. Second, after aspirating air, tilt device caudally to a 60-degree orientation to the

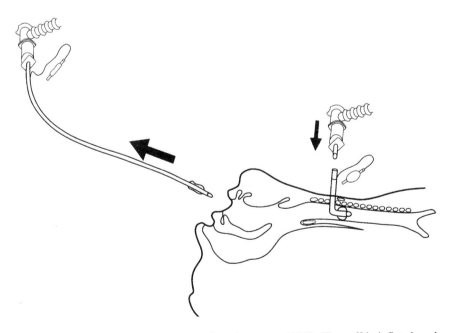

FIGURE 10.33. The Fantoni translaryngeal tracheostomy (TLT). The cuff is inflated, and the tube is connected to the respirator. (From Westphal, et al,[131] with permission.)

skin and advance the device to the stopper. Finally, remove the stopper, advance the cannula, and remove the trochar. The cannula is secured and ventilation can begin.

Rapitrach Kit (Fresenius, Runcom, Cheshire, UK)[126]

The principal component of the Rapitrach Kit is a percutaneous tracheostomy dilator (tracheostome). The developers of the technique made the following claim in a 1989 publication:

> The procedure is safe and rapid and can be carried out, after initial training, by a surgeon or a surgical resident at the scene of trauma, or in an ICU or ED [emergency department]. As the method is easily learned, physicians working in anesthesia, ICU, ED, and/or CPR ambulances and helicopters should be able to perform this procedure with ease.[133]

Most of the articles describing the Rapitrach were published before 1992. When comparisons were made, the Rapitrach was viewed less favorably than other percutaneous tracheostomy techniques discussed earlier. The major criticism of the technique concerned the sharp edges of the tracheostome used to incise and dilate the trachea.

Figure 10.34 illustrates the components of the Rapitrach kit.

Bliznikas[126] describes the technique used to perform a percutaneous tracheostomy with the Rapitrach.

1. Anesthetize the skin below the cricoid cartilage with 1% lidocaine
2. Make a 1.5- to 2-cm incision at the level of the first or second tracheal ring
3. Bluntly dissect the subcutaneous tissues with a forceps
4. Bluntly dissect down to the trachea with a finger

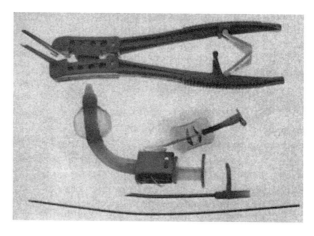

FIGURE 10.34. The Rapitrach kit. (From Bodenham A, et al. *Anaesthesia.* 1992;47:332, with permission.)

5. Insert a 12-gauge needle into the trachea through the first or second tracheal membrane
6. Insert a flexible guide wire into the trachea and remove the needle
7. The Rapitrach dilator is inserted over the wire and introduced into the trachea
8. Open the dilator to dissect an opening into the trachea
9. A tracheostomy tube with obturator is introduced into the trachea between the jaws of the obturator.
10. Remove the wire and obturator.
11. Inflate the cuff of the tube, remove the obturator, ventilate the patient.

You may wish to use the fiberoptic scope to guide wire and for dilator placement.

Adjunctive Equipment and Techniques

Many authors have published letters and studies suggesting that various percutaneous tracheostomy procedures could be more safely or efficiently performed if a variety of adjunctive equipment and techniques were used by the airway manager. This section of the chapter will review some of these suggestions.

Fiberoptic Bronchoscope

As has been mentioned in previous sections, many investigators and clinicians advocate using the fiberoptic bronchoscope when performing most elective percutaneous tracheostomy interventions. The fiberoptic scope is used to visually guide the operator when the following maneuvers are undertaken:

1. To verify that the tip of the endotracheal tube is below the cords and above the level of proposed tracheostomy site after the tube has been pulled back.
2. To confirm that the level of the proposed tracheostomy is correct (usually the first or second tracheal membrane) and in the midline.
3. To guide initial needle-thyroidotomy to help prevent posterior tracheal wall or endotracheal tube perforation.
4. To direct and confirm proper placement and direction of the catheter, guide wire, and/or guiding cannula into the distal trachea.
5. To monitor formal tracheostomy tube placement.
6. To inspect and/or suction the trachea and bronchi after formal tracheostomy tube placement.

Bouvette and Fuhrman,[135] though, remind us that use of the fiberoptic bronchoscope "does not guarantee 100% success of elimination of all complications" associated with PDT. Furthermore, Mphanza and Jacobs[135] comment that use of the fiberoptic bronchoscope may not improve safety, and in some cases may make ventilation more difficult while performing PDT. This could cause an increase in $PaCO_2$ that could lead to deleterious consequences if the patient had increased intracranial pressure. Perhaps the use of end-tidal CO_2 monitoring in selected patients could be used to guide the operator's adjustment of ventilator parameters during PDT placement.

At the present time most, though not all, clinicians and investigators advocate the routine use of the fiberoptic bronchoscope while performing a variety of elective percutaneous tracheostomy techniques.

Video-Assisted Endoscopy

Ciaglia[136] suggested that a video-assisted bronchoscope could be used when a PDT is performed. The advantage of this technique is that the video picture is viewed by the clinician who is performing the PDT, allowing "the operator [to] see the field and be guided in management." Ciaglia writes that "in this way, PDT could become a minimally invasive procedure with maximally increased visibility." The equipment to perform video-assisted endoscopy is marketed by many manufacturers of fiberoptic equipment. Video-assisted endoscopy equipment can be moved easily into the ICU or operating room for routine use during elective PDT.

Laryngeal Mask Airway (LMA)

Dexter[137] first reported performing PDT in patients ventilated with an LMA in 1994. He used a fiberoptic bronchoscope to guide PDT placement. Others have reported performing PDT using the LMA as an adjunctive aid.[138–141] Quinio et al.[142] published a case report of Fantoni TLT placement in a patient whose airway was managed with an LMA. These authors claimed that the technique's main advantages included easier and safer fiberoptic bronchoscopic manipulation, since they did not have to pass the scope through an endotracheal tube. They further pointed out that there was no risk of endotracheal tube displacement or cuff or tube perforation with the tracheostomy needle. They warned, though, that the technique involved a risk of aspiration and that it might be contraindicated if the patient had upper airway pathology or "stiff" lungs.

Lightwand (Trachlight, Laerdal Medical Inc., Wappingers Falls, NY)

Addas et al[143] published a case series of 11 patients in which they used a Trachlight as an adjunctive aid to performing Ciaglia PDT. All of the patients studied were intubated at the time of PDT. Following is a summary of their methods.

1. Mark a reference point on the patient's neck (the level of the first and second tracheal ring or between the cricoid cartilage and the first tracheal ring).
2. Cut the endotracheal tube so the lightwand's tip is at the end of the tube when the lightwand is inserted. (The lightwand has centimeter markings along its shaft.)
3. Remove the stiff retractable stylet from the lightwand.
4. Place the lightwand in the endotracheal tube.
5. Deflate the endotracheal tube's cuff.

6. Withdraw the endotracheal tube and lightwand as a unit until the transillumination of the wand can be seen 1 cm above the marked site of insertion of the needle.
7. Secure the tube.
8. Remove the lightwand.
9. Reinflate the cuff and ventilate the patient
10. Proceed with the Ciaglia PDT technique. The authors dissected down to the trachea, displacing the soft tissue and thyroid gland, and punctured the trachea between the second and third tracheal ring.

The authors reported that PDT was successful in all of their patients. The mean time to perform the technique was 17.8 minutes. They reported no complications caused by the Trachlight.

The authors commented that the technique described was "blind" and that it should be used in caution in patients with a coagulopathy. They also warned that the technique should be avoided in patients in which transillumination might be compromised, such as those who have a short or "thick" neck or those who are obese.

It is postulated that the Trachlight might be an inexpensive adjunctive aid to those who routinely perform PDT "blindly".

Endotracheal Tube Exchangers

Hollow endotracheal tube exchangers have been used as adjunctive aids during PDT. Cooper et al[144] described the use of a tube exchanger (Endotracheal Ventilation Catheter; CardioMed Supplies, Inc.; Gormley, Ontario, Canada) and a manually cycled jet ventilator during PDT placement. The tube exchanger was placed in the trachea with its end at the same level as the end of the endotracheal tube. Ventilation and oxygenation was provided via jet ventilation during PDT placement. Deblieux et al[145] published a case series in which they placed a 4.7-mm O.D., perforated disposable tube exchanger (C-CAE-14.0-83, Cook Critical Care, Bloomington, IN) through the endotracheal tube and advanced it blindly 5 to 8 cm into the trachea past the endotracheal tube's tip. These authors did not ventilate their patients through the tube exchanger. The exchanger was left in place during PDT. They implied that the tube exchanger could have been used to jet-ventilate the patient or as a guide for reintubation if the endotracheal tube was inadvertently pulled out during PDT placement. While both techniques have merit, neither was reported to be routinely used in the clinical studies reported earlier in this chapter. Further research would need to be undertaken to define potential complications that could result from use of either technique.

Ultrasound Guidance of PDT

In 1999, Muhammad et al[146] published a paper in which diagnostic ultrasound was used to assess the suitability of 4 patients to undergo PDT in the ICU. They postulated that ultrasonic evaluation of the pretracheal region could identify patients in whom aberrant anatomy would make PDT more difficult. Anatomic anomalies such as an aberrant blood vessel, deviated trachea, or a very short neck could be identified and evaluated by ultrasonic examination. The findings of the examination could then direct the operators to modify the PDT technique or choose to perform a formal operative tracheostomy. They presented 2 patients, one with a large pretracheal vein crossing anterior to the thyroid isthmus and one with a very short cricoid-sternal distance in whom they opted to perform operative tracheostomy. In the other 2 patients, both exhibiting short cricoid-sternal distances, the ultrasound was used to guide correct needle placement for the PDT. The authors did not specify details of the ultrasonic "guidance." They also discussed technical limitations of the ultrasonic equipment at their disposal. They predicted that technological developments would make ultrasonic guidance of PDT more practicable in the future.

Rigid Bronchoscope

Brimacombe and Clarke[147] published a case report and the findings from a series of 6 additional patients in whom a rigid bronchoscope was used to assist PDT. They found that the view through the rigid scope was excellent and that suctioning a large clot from the distal airway was easily accomplished.

Ventilation and oxygenation could also be maintained through the rigid scope. They reported that the scope's position was easy to maintain. They felt that the two main limitations of the technique were the risk of aspiration during performance of PDT and lack of training in rigid bronchoscopic techniques for most nonsurgical clinicians who perform PDT in the ICU. They concluded that use of the rigid bronchoscope as an adjunct to performing PDT merited further research.

Chest Radiographs After PDT

Many clinicians who perform PDT obtain routine, **immediate** (within 1 hour) postprocedural chest radiographs to document the presence or absence of complications. The cost-benefit aspects of this practice have come under scrutiny. Donaldson et al[148] published a prospective case series of 54 patients who underwent PDT, 18 of whom received **immediate** (less than 1 hour) postprocedural chest radiographs, while 35 received a **delayed** (2 to 12 hour) postprocedural chest radiograph. One patient died immediately after PDT and was not included in the study. They found "no incidents of pneumothorax, pneumomediastinum, or tracheostomy tube malposition in any patient." They concluded that obtaining a routine, **immediate** post-PDT chest radiograph was not cost-effective. They recommended that an **immediate** post-PDT should be obtained if the procedure was difficult, if the PDT was performed for urgent or emergency indications, if the anatomy was abnormal or altered, or if the patient required high levels of positive-pressure ventilation. They opined that significant pneumothorax, the most critical post-PDT radiographic finding, could be diagnosed clinically. Whether or not a chest radiograph should be routine after uneventful PDT placement has been challenged by other clinicians concerned with cost containment.

Capnography during Transtracheal Needle Cricothyrotomy

Tobias and Higgins[149] studied capnography traces obtained during needle cricothyrotomy in dogs. They documented that the capnograph rapidly detected CO_2 when the needle entered the trachea. They also documented that the CO_2 trace was lost when the tip of the needle was passed through the posterior tracheal wall. They recorded capnographic traces of dogs breathing spontaneously and of dogs that were apneic. Finally, they demonstrated that the plunger of the syringe to which the needle was attached did not need to be pulled back for CO_2 to be detected by the capnograph. They concluded by writing, **"Regardless of the reason for the needle cricothyrotomy, the monitoring of CO_2 from the needle during advancement serves as an additional safety measure to ensure the intratracheal location of the needle or catheter."** Use of this adjunctive aid should be studied in human subjects.

Use of the Fiberoptic Bronchoscope to Aid Retrograde Wire–Directed Intubation

The placement of a retrograde wire from the trachea through the upper airway (mouth or nose) used to direct endotracheal tube placement has already been discussed. Several authors have suggested modifying the technique by using the fiberoptic bronchoscope to facilitate intubation. Bissinger et al[150] reported passing a bronchoscope (loaded with a reinforced 6.5- to 8.5-mm I.D. endotracheal tube) over a retrograde wire that had been passed through the cricothyroid membrane. They successfully intubated 89 of 93 patients. They reported a problem with "hanging up" of the endotracheal tube as it was passed over the scope through the glottis in 5 of 93 patients, a phenomenon that was overcome by simple maneuvers such as jaw thrust or rotation of the endotracheal tube. The technique was abandoned in 4 patients who were fiberoptically intubated with conventional techniques. Commenting on this article, Eidelman and Pizov[152] suggested that the technique be modified—first, by placing a rigid plastic guide over the retrograde wire; second, by passing an endotracheal tube (with a pediatric bronchoscope in its lumen but not over the wire) into the trachea as far as the guide wire entry point; third, at this point, passing the bronchoscope into the distal trachea; fourth, removing the guide wire; and finally, passing the endotracheal tube into the trachea over the bronchoscope. In response, Bissinger et al[152] stated that the Eidelman-Pizov modifications did not necessarily prevent "hanging up" of the endotracheal tube. They suggested that the retrograde wire could be passed through the side hole of the endotracheal tube so it could be passed further into the trachea before the guide wire is removed. Roberts and Solgonik[153] reported a successful retrograde intubation with a technique similar to that described by Eidelman and Pizov.[151] Finally, Rosenblatt et al[154] reported a case in which a fiberoptic bronchoscope was passed in retrograde fashion through a surgical cricothyroidotomy into the upper airway of a patient with severe upper airway edema. Attempts to intubate the patient with a laryngoscope and conventional fiberoptic techniques had been unsuccessful. Before passing the retrograde bronchoscope, the patient had already been intubated with a 6.0-mm I.D. tube that had been surgically placed through the cricothyroid membrane. A guide wire was passed through the scope and then a 7.5/5.0-mm double endotracheal tube setup was advanced over the scope and wire until its tip could be seen through the tracheal stoma. The scope was removed, as was the 5.0-mm extender tube, leaving the 7.5-mm endotracheal tube in the trachea, over the wire. The bronchoscope was then passed through the endotracheal tube, alongside of the wire, and positioned in the distal trachea. The wire was removed and the endotracheal tube was passed into the trachea using the bronchoscope as a stylet.

If you consider using the fiberoptic bronchoscope to assist retrograde wire–directed intubation, you have the option of choosing a technique in which the wire is passed through the scope or a technique in which the scope is passed alongside the wire. Both have been used successfully to intubate patients with difficult airway anatomy.

Learning Percutaneous Tracheostomy

It is logical to assume that a learning curve would be associated with the adoption of any new surgical procedure. As experience is gained, the complication rate would be expected to drop. Donaldson et al[155] cited references to this phenomenon by earlier investigators (before 1995). In their study, resident otolaryngologists were taught to perform elective Ciaglia PDT under the supervision of "an attending otolaryngologist experienced in PDT" who was present throughout the procedure. Bronchoscopic guidance was utilized in all cases. They concluded that no learning curve was demonstrated and that PDT could be taught safely to resident physicians who were appropriately supervised.

In another study, Massick et al[156] demonstrated that when a **single** operator was learning Ciaglia PDT, in their case the senior attending surgeon involved with the study, a "steep" learning curve was demonstrated. Their prospective cohort study of 100 patients, 20 patients in each group, revealed that the perioperative and postoperative complication rate was higher in the first group than in any other group. They also noted that the late complication rate was higher in the last 50 patients as compared to the first 50. They did not use bronchoscopic guidance to aid the PDT. They noted also that patients with abnormal cervical anatomy had a higher complication rate when compared to patients with normal anatomy. The late complication rate did not depend on the operator's experience level.

Future studies will establish the learning curve for practitioners of other specialities (general surgery, intensive care physicians, anesthesiologists) who learn various PDT techniques.

Teaching Surgical Airway Techniques

Physicians and other medical personnel who include surgical airway techniques in their difficult airway protocols are obligated to learn the techniques and to maintain proficiency. Many organizations sponsor meetings at which the techniques are taught. Any medical specialty that has adopted standards with regard to managing the difficult airway *must* insure that physicians-in-training learn, practice, and prove that they are proficient practitioners of every technique specified by that specialty's standards. Two ways to teach airway techniques are to use anatomical models, either synthetic or animal,[157] and to develop protocols allowing students (at any level) to use interventional airway equipment in the course of daily practice[158] to gain experience while under the close supervision of experienced physicians.

Contraindications to Performing Percutaneous Tracheostomy

The contraindications to performing percutaneous tracheostomy vary depending on technique. Contraindications are **relative** or **absolute** depending on many factors such as the experience of the operator, institutional standards, availability of ancillary help, time constraints, and the stage of technical development and knowledge concerning a particular intervention. The following list includes conditions and situations constituting **traditional contraindications** to performing percutaneous tracheostomy techniques.

1. Emergency situations
2. Inability to establish a surgical airway **immediately** should the technique fail
3. Abnormal cervical or pretracheal anatomy
    a. Morbid obesity
    b. Thyroid tissue at the level of proposed tracheostomy
    c. Aberrant blood vessels
    d. Short neck
    e. Previous neck/tracheal surgery
4. Infection at the proposed tracheostomy site
5. Burns
6. Pregnancy
7. Cervical spine instability
8. Uncontrolled coagulopathy
9. Pediatric patient
10. Previous sternotomy

The list of contraindications has been modified as more experience performing and knowledge concerning various percutaneous tracheostomy techniques have been gained.

Emergency Percutaneous Tracheostomy

Unfortunately, there is a paucity of scientific information concerning the application of percutaneous tracheostomy techniques in the setting of emergency airway management. Many anecdotal reports have been published. Airway management algorithms suggest consideration of various techniques. Physicians of one specialty differ with those of others when it comes to recommending one technique over another. More study needs to address this important issue. Eisenburger et al[159] reported that in a simulated "emergency" setting, the success rate for performing a surgical cricothyrotomy was 70% as compared to a success rate of 60% for percutaneous dilational cricothyrotomy (Arndt Emergency Cricothyrotomy Catheter Set, Cook Critical Care, Bloomington, IN) for a group of inexperienced clinicians. Many more studies need to be conducted to compare various techniques under controlled conditions. The authors of studies concerning PDT almost unanimously caution against use of the technique in the emergency setting. **If a practitioner assumes the responsibility to perform a surgical airway intervention in the emergency setting, he must select techniques that he is willing to learn and practice, and he must maintain clinical proficiency.**

Emergency Surgical Cricothyrotomy

An emergency cricothyrotomy may be performed when a patient presents with critical airway obstruction or anomaly. A critical airway can be caused by tissue swelling, bleeding or emesis, trauma, infection, burns, hematoma, tumor, foreign body lodgment, cervical spine instability, or congenital malformation. Emergency surgical cricothyrotomy is often lifesaving and can be used before or after conventional attempts to secure the airway fail or are deemed likely to fail. **In all circumstances, an experienced physician, most likely a surgeon, should perform this procedure.**

Anatomy of the Cricothyroid Space

The cricothyroid membrane is located in the anterior midline between the lower border of the thyroid cartilage and the upper border of the cricoid cartilage (Fig. 10.35).

The average size of the cricothyroid cartilage is 9×30 mm.[160] To perform a cricothyrotomy, a midline approach is used. Bleeding is a major complication of the procedure. Goumas et al[161] performed an autopsy study of 107 cadavers to define the vascular anatomy of the cricothyroid space. They considered veins greater than 2 mm in diameter to be "important," implying that this size vein had the potential to cause significant perioperative bleeding. The findings of their anatomic investigation are summarized in Table 10.12.

Since the fewest vascular structures were found in the midline, these investigators recommended that the midline of the cricothyroid space be identified "every time" a cricothyrotomy is performed.

General Comments

Schroeder,[161] reviewing the topic of cricothyroidotomy from the otolaryngologist's point of view, cited evidence that in the **emergency** situation, airway intervention at the cricothyroid level should be considered as reasonable an option as tracheostomy at a lower level. The advantages of the cricothyroidotomy over a lower tracheostomy were reported to be (1) similar complication rates; (2) landmarks are easier to identify; (3) cricothyroidotomy is faster to perform, especially

FIGURE 10.35. The cricothyroid membrane lies between the thyroid and cricoid cartilages. The *cricothyroid space,* which lies between the membrane and the skin, contains many anatomic structures as defined by Goumas et al.[161] These structures are listed in Table 10.12.

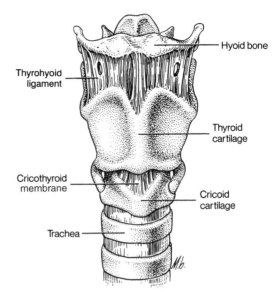

Hyoid bone

Thyrohyoid ligament

Thyroid cartilage

Cricothyroid membrane

Cricoid cartilage

Trachea

in the hands of a nonsurgeon; (4) less risk of pneumothorax; (5) less bleeding; (6) less risk of tracheoinnominate artery fistula; (7) less risk of tracheoesophageal fistula; (8) less cervical hyperextension is required; (9) a dislodged tube is easier to reinsert; (10) the surgical site is higher, perhaps of importance if lower neck surgery or a sternotomy had been or will be performed after the cricothyroidotomy. In more **elective** situations, she cited references that favored a lower tracheostomy level, such as with (1) pediatric patients; (2) patients who had been previously intubated; (3) patients with laryngeal infection or trauma; (4) patients who used their voices professionally (perhaps to lessen the incidence of vocal changes post-tracheostomy). Three other important comments made by the author are the following: In order to avoid vocal cord damage, as the cords lie 0.5 to 2 cm above the cricothyroid membrane, the scalpel blade should incise the

TABLE 10.12. Anatomy of the cricothyroid space (107 cadavers studied)

Structure	Located in the midline	Located within 1 cm of the midline
Veins greater than 2 mm diameter (all veins were superficial)	11 (10.2%)	30 (30.8%)
Artery (1 mm)	4 (3.7%)	
Network of small veins		27 (25%)
Dense network of veins		1 (1%)
Lymph node	1 (1%)	
Pyramidal lobe of thyroid		7 (6.5%)
Two pyramidal lobes		1 (1%)

Source: Goumas, et al, 1997,[161] with permission.

membrane with its tip pointed inferiorly. She warned against damaging the thyroid or cricoid cartilages to lessen the incidence of postoperative stenotic complications. Finally, she stated that because the average size of the cricothyroid membrane was 9 × 30 mm, she recommended use of a tracheostomy tube with an 8.5-mm O.D.

Outcome Studies

The results of retrospective outcome studies published in the 1990s are summarized in Tables 10.13 and 10.14. In most cases, a trained surgeon performed the cricothyroidotomy or tracheostomy. In 28 of 29 cases, in which the surgical airway was established outside of the emergency room or operating room, the specialty of the operator was not specified.

These studies indicate that trained medical personnel have a high rate of success performing emergency cricothyroidotomy. The importance of training programs such as the Advanced Trauma Life Support program outlined by the American College of Surgeons was noted.

Prehospital Airway Management including Cricothyroidotomy

There are many reports of emergency responders using cricothyrotomy to establish a definitive airway in the prehospital setting. Most papers describe retrospective series. It is not possible to compare reported outcomes because many variables are not controlled. For example, some emergency response teams have physicians trained in airway management attending to all patients. Some do not. Some intubation protocols call for the use of paralytic agents, others do not. Different drugs are used to "sedate" patients prior to intubation, some of which may not be appropriately administered. Blind nasotracheal intubation is used by some responders, others do not utilize the technique. The indications to perform emergency cricothyrotomy in the field are not uniform. The level of training and proficiency to perform cricothyrotomy is not the same for all emergency personnel.

Despite these variables, the published reports offer interesting findings. Leibovici et al[165] reported on 29 cricothyroidotomies performed in the field in Israel, a country in which all cases were reported to a national trauma registry. Teams of responders always contained a physician. Group 1 teams included physicians who were surgeons, anesthesiologists, otolaryngologists, thoracic surgeons, plastic surgeons, obstetricians, or intensive care specialists. Group 2 teams

TABLE 10.13. Cricothyroidotomy outcome studies

Study	# of patients	Success rate	# Prehospital patients	# In-hospital patients	Complication rate
Hawkins et al.[162]	66	98.5%	8	58	3%
Isaacs[163]	65	95.4	20	45	Early: 15.4%
					Late: 7.4% (2/27)
Literature review[163]	320	96%			Early: 14.3%

TABLE 10.14. Emergency cricothyroidotomy vs. tracheostomy

Number of patients		Success rate		Complications	
Crico	Tracheo	Crico	Tracheo	Crico	Tracheo
20	14	87%	100%	20%	21%

a. Two patients were successfully converted from cricothyroidotomy to tracheotomy.
b. All patients were managed surgically except 1, who had a successful orotracheal intubation.
c. Needle cricothyroidotomy–jet ventilation was attempted in 3 patients. The technique failed in all 3 cases secondary to misplacement of catheter placement.

Source: Gillespie and Eiselc, 1999,[164] with permission.

included physicians who were general practitioners, internists, cardiologists, and pediatricians. All of the physicians in both groups had ATLS training, while only 3 had prior experience with cricothyroidotomy. The primary indication to perform an emergency cricothyroidotomy was failure to intubate despite no apparent anatomic distortion (n = 13) and trauma to the anatomic landmarks of the pharynx and larynx (n = 12). The results of the study indicate an overall success rate of 89.6%. Two of 13 cricothyroidotomies using the Seldinger method (Cook Cricothyroidotomy Set, Cook Critical Care, Bloomington, IN) and 1 of 16 standard surgical cricothyroidotomies failed. All three patients made it to the hospital. The investigators found no statistical differences between groups, although all failures were reported by Group 2 teams. The only significant acute complication reported was failure to establish an airway.

Gerich et al,[166] in a prospective study designed to evaluate the efficacy of a rapid sequence (no paralytic agent) intubation protocol, analyzed the findings reported on 383 acutely injured patients in the field who required airway control. The response team included a physician surgical resident and a paramedic with more than 10 years' experience. The resident had at least 3 years of postgraduate training, 6 months' training in intensive or critical care medicine, and 24 months in general or trauma surgery. The teams successfully intubated 373 of 383 patients (97%). Cricothyroidotomy was performed successfully in all 8 cases in which it was attempted. The indications for cricothyroidotomy included failure to intubate (n = 2), patient trapped in the vehicle (n = 2), facial fractures or trauma (n = 3), and clenched teeth (n = 1). This group accounted for approximately 2% of the trauma patients. All but one of these patients subsequently died from their injuries. The authors concluded that trained EMS personnel should be able to successfully intubate patients in the field and that the rate of emergency cricothyroidotomy can be kept low. In response to this report, Brohi et al[167] reported that their EMS protocol called for use of suxamethonium. They reported that only 3 of 37 patients who received a cricothyroidotomy did so after failed intubation (0.2%). Their cricothyroidotomy rate was 2.5%.

Jacobson et al[168] reported that over a 5-year period, nonphysician ambulance teams under study in Indianapolis, Indiana, established 509 "definitive" airways. The majority of patients were intubated, while 50 surgical cricothyroidotomies were performed (9.8%). Indications to perform cricothyroidotomy were masseter spasm (n = 23), upper airway visualization problems from blood or vomit despite suctioning (n = 18), facial fractures that posed a contraindication to nasal intubation (n = 16), and entrapment of the patient in the vehicle (n = 5). Fifteen patients had more than one indication. The paramedics performed successful emergency cricothyroidotomy 94% of the time. The authors cited 4 other references in which nonphysician EMS teams performed emergency cricothyroidotomy, reporting success rates ranging from 88% to 99%.

In conclusion, trained physicians and nonphysicians, who *voluntarily* publish accounts of their experiences with emergency cricothyroidotomy, report very good success rates with the technique, generally about 95%. Large-scale, prospective studies are needed to define optimal protocols regarding use of emergency cricothyroidotomy in the prehospital setting. The technique, though, has merit and must be learned by anyone including it in his difficult airway protocol.

Emergency Cricothyroidotomy Techniques

Three cricothyroidotomy techniques will be presented. The first two techniques are described in a paper by Holmes et al.[169] In this paper, two groups were randomly selected from 27 emergency medicine interns, 1 junior medicine resident, and 4 senior medical students. None of the subjects had experience with surgical cricothyroidotomy. One group was taught the **standard technique** and the other was taught the **rapid 4-step technique** in a 15-minute training session. Each subject then performed a cricothyroidotomy on an adult cadaver and was allowed one attempt to insert a No. 6 Shiley tracheostomy tube. The groups were then taught the alternative technique and were tested on their performance of that technique. The necks of the cadavers were dissected and complications were noted.

Standard Technique

Instruments

Scalpel with no. 11 blade
Trousseau dilator
Hemostats
Tracheal hook
No. 6 Shiley tracheostomy tube

Position. Standing at the patient's right side.

Steps

1. Midline vertical incision, 4 cm long, over the cricoid membrane
2. Identification of the cricothyroid membrane by means of blunt dissection
3. Short horizontal stab incision in the lower part of the cricothyroid membrane
4. Stabilization of the larynx with a tracheal hook at the inferior aspect of the thyroid cartilage
5. Dilatation of the ostomy with curved hemostats

6. Placement of the Trousseau dilator in the incision, with dilatation of the ostomy
7. Placement of the Shiley tube in the trachea

Rapid 4-Step Technique[170]

Instruments

Scalpel with no. 20 blade
Tracheal hook
No. 6 Shiley tracheostomy tube

Position. Standing at the patient's left side.

Steps

1. Identification of the cricothyroid membrane by palpation (a vertical incision through the skin to allow palpation of the cricothyroid membrane is recommended if the cricothyroid membrane cannot be initially identified on palpation)
2. Horizontal stab incision through the skin and cricothyroid membrane with the scalpel
3. Stabilization of the larynx with the tracheal hook at the inferior aspect of the ostomy (on the cricoid cartilage), providing caudal traction
4. Placement of the Shiley tube in the trachea

The results of the study are summarized in Table 10.15.

Major complications included complete transection of the cricoid cartilage and posterior tracheal/esophageal perforation.

Alternative Techniques

Wong and Bradrick,[16(p206)] in Hagberg's *Handbook of Difficult Airway Management*, describe two modifications to the techniques described above. They state that a horizontal, rather than a vertical, incision at the level of the cricothyroid membrane is acceptable (Figs. 10.36 and 10.37). They also comment that the surgical opening can be dilated with the handle of the scalpel by inserting it into the stoma and rotating it.

TABLE 10.15. Comparison of two cricothyroidotomy techniques

Parameters	4-step technique	Standard technique
Successful airway (%)	28/32 (88%)	30/32 (94%)
Complications (%)		
Inadvertent tracheotomy	4/32 (13%)	7/32 (22%)
Other complications	8/32 (25%)	5/32 (16%)
Major complications	3/32 (9%)	1/32 (3%)
Time (seconds)		
Mean ± SD	43.2 ± 44.6	138.8 ± 93.4
Median (25th-75th percentiles)	32 (24–42)	114 (74–154)

Source: Holmes, et al,[169] 1998, with permission.

Complications of Emergency Cricothyroidotomy[16(p206),171]

1. Failure to obtain an airway
2. Tracheostomy tube displacement or misplacement
3. Injury to laryngeal structures
4. Pneumothorax, pneumomediastinum
5. Damage to other structures in the neck (esophagus, blood vessels)
6. Vocal cord damage
7. Voice changes (hoarseness, change of pitch)
8. Subglottic stenosis, especially in children
9. Eating/swallowing problems
10. Posterior/lateral tracheal damage
11. Cellulitis
12. Aspiration
13. Shortness of breath
14. Unsightly scar

Isaacs[171] reported that in a series of 27 patients followed for 37 months, most of the late-term complications associated with emergency cricothyroidotomy were considered to be minor. In fact, some of the reported complications could have been caused by the primary trauma and not the cricothyroidotomy.

Contraindications to Emergency Cricothyrotomy

In the setting of the emergency airway, the contraindications to performing a cricothyroidotomy are few. Most authors, though, warn that the technique is not suitable for "young children" or infants.

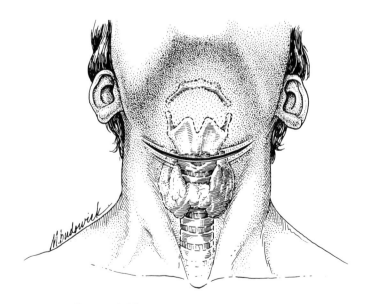

FIGURE 10.36. The cricothyroidotomy incision.

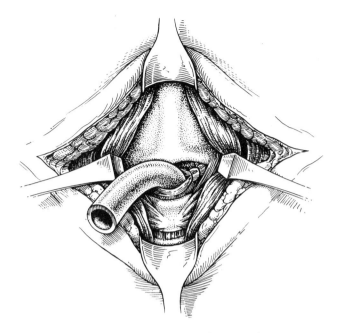

FIGURE 10.37. Inserting the tube into a tracheostomy.

Cricothyrotomy and the Unstable Cervical Spine

Cricothyrotomy has been advocated by some authors to be the method of choice to establish an emergency airway in a patient with known or suspected unstable cervical spine. Gerling et al[171] studied the magnitude of cervical movement associated with the performance of cricothyrotomy on 13 surgically induced unstable cervical spine cadaveric preparations. They reported that the cervical movement associated with the procedure was "less than the threshold for clinical significance." Anterior-posterior displacement was 1 to 2 mm, while less than 1 mm of axial compression was demonstrated.

They concluded by stating that "these results support the safety of cricothyrotomy in the presence of an unstable c-spine." Management of the airway in patients with unstable cervical spine is dealt with in other sections of the book.

Formal Tracheostomy

The technique of formal tracheostomy is not described in this book, since it should only be performed by a trained surgeon. The indications for and complications of the technique will be described.

Most tracheostomies are performed on ventilator-dependent patients, or on patients with impaired airway defensive reflexes. When to perform the tracheostomy is controversial. An endotracheal tube may cause upper airway, laryngeal, or tracheal damage that could lead to long-term complications. However, tracheostomy is not without risk.

The indications and advantages to performing a tracheostomy include the following.

Indications and Advantages of Tracheostomy[172]

1. Long-term secure airway
2. Enhances patient comfort
3. Might make pulmonary suctioning easier
4. Allows the patient to speak
5. Patients can take oral nutrition
6. Might decrease the likelihood of long-term swallowing dysfunction
7. Diminishes the likelihood of laryngeal injury
8. May be needed to establish an airway for head/neck surgical procedures

Complications of Tracheostomy

Goldenberg et al.[173] reported the incidence of tracheostomy-related complications in a retrospective study of 1,130 consecutive patients.

1. Tracheal stenosis (1.85%)
2. Hemorrhage (0.8%)
3. Tracheocutaneous fistula (0.53%)
4. Infection (0.44%)
5. Tube decannulation/obstruction (0.35%)
6. Subcutaneous emphysema (0.08%)
7. Pneumothorax (0.26%)
8. Tracheoesophageal fistula (0.08%)

Other complications include:[172,174]

 9. Laryngeal nerve damage
10. Mediastinal sepsis
11. Air embolism during operation
12. Laryngeal incoordination (phonation or breathing difficulty)
13. Unsightly scar

The complications associated with tracheostomy are similar for adult and pediatric patient populations. Tracheostomy-related mortality is reportedly 0.5% to 5%[175] in the pediatric population.

Submental Orotracheal Intubation

The distal end (ventilator connector) of an endotracheal tube can be exposed through a submental tract, leaving the proximal end in the trachea (Fig. 10.38). This method of tube placement is described for use during maxillofacial surgery in patients with extensive traumatic damage.[176] Placement of the tube must be done by a surgeon. The tube may be useful if a nasal intubation is contraindicated (basilar skull fracture), an oral tube would get in the way of surgery, and a tracheostomy is not desired.[177]

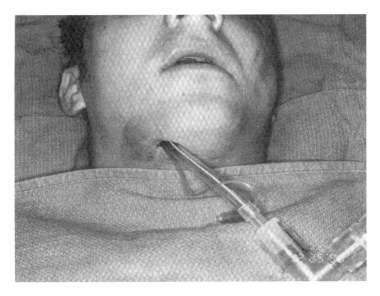

FIGURE 10.38. Submental orotracheal tube. (From Paetkau DJ, et al,[176] with permission.)

Rigid Bronchoscopy

A rigid bronchoscope may be inserted to provide an airway during surgery involving the trachea, mediastinum, vascular rings, aberrant innominate artery, or the removal of foreign bodies. In most circumstances, an experienced surgeon will insert the bronchoscope. The airway operator must be ready to assist the surgeon and to interface the bronchoscope with the anesthesia machine or a ventilating system to provide oxygen, ventilation, and/or anesthesia gases to the patient.

Summary

This chapter has presented a description of surgical equipment and techniques used to manage the airway. Any of these techniques can be considered when managing a difficult airway, if time permits. Time is limited if the patient faces hypoxic injury. It is difficult to decide which techniques are most applicable in the emergency situation. If you decide to include any of the equipment or techniques herein described in your **difficult airway algorithm or protocol,** then you must familiarize yourself with the equipment, learn the technique, practice the technique, and maintain proficiency.

Percutaneous tracheostomy techniques were discussed in detail in the chapter. The reasons for this are (1) the techniques represent the next most invasive surgical airway intervention beyond needle/catheter cricothyrotomy and minitracheostomy; (2) percutaneous tracheostomy techniques received widespread consideration in the literature over the last seven years; and (3) practitioners aggressively sought to define the place of percutaneous tracheostomy in the field of airway management (elective or emergency use). The techniques were compared with one another and with formal open tracheostomy in an effort to determine the utility and efficacy of each. At present, Ciaglia PDT techniques are used the most. The Fantoni TLT is gaining in popularity. The Griggs GWDF has also received much consideration. The techniques are advocated for **elective tracheostomy use only.**

Unfortunately, the literature does not offer convincing evidence that one surgical airway management technique is better than another in the **emergency setting.** Since most clinicians are familiar with the Seldinger technique to insert intravenous catheters, surgical airway equipment and techniques based on the technique have been developed. **The emergency airway practitioner should select and master one needle/rigid catheter technique (be prepared to deliver high-pressure oxygen via jet ventilator) and one minitracheostomy technique. In addition, one must be prepared to immediately perform an emergency cricothyrotomy before the patient experiences hypoxic injury.** These recommendations are not scientifically supported. They represent the considered opinion of the author of this chapter.

Many educational courses offer useful instruction in surgical airway management. Consult an academic anesthesiology, intensive care medicine, or surgery department and ask for information concerning continuing educational programs. Or contact the American Society of Anesthesiologists (Park Ridge, IL) or the Society for Airway Management (Chicago, IL) and ask for information concerning their educational programs and publications.

References

1. Benumof JL, Scheller MS. The importance of transtracheal jet ventilation in the management of the difficult airway. *Anesthesiology.* 1989;71:769.
2. Smith RB, et al. Percutaneous transtracheal ventilation for anesthesia and resuscitation: a review and report of complications. *Can J Anaesth.* 1975;22:607.
3. Zornow MH, et al. The efficacy of three different methods of transtracheal ventilation. *Can J Anaesth.* 1989;36:624.
4. Gaughan SD, et al. A comparison in a lung model of low- and high-flow regulators for transtracheal jet ventilation. *Anesthesiology.* 1992;77:189.
5. Gaughan SD, et al. Can an anesthesia machine flush valve provide for effective jet ventilation? *Anesth Analg.* 1993;76:800.
6. Klein DS, Lees DE. Emergency cricothyroidotomy: a flexible device in the operating room. *South Med J.* 1989;82:661.
7. Kross, et al. A contingency plan for tracheal intubation. *Anesthesiology.* 1990;72:577.
8. Delaney WA, Kaiser RE. Percutaneous transtracheal jet ventilation made easy. *Anesthesiology.* 1991;74:952.
9. Ho AM. A simple anesthesia machine-driven transtracheal jet ventilation system [letter]. *Anesth Analg.* 1994;78:405.
10. Meyer PD. Emergency transtracheal jet ventilation system. *Anesthesiology.* 1990; 73:787.

11. Benumof JL, Gaughan S. Connecting a jet stylet to a jet injector. *Anesthesiology.* 1991;74:963.

12. Gaughan SD, et al. Quantification of the jet function of a jet stylet. *Anesth Analg.* 1992;74:580.

13. Schapera A, et al. A pressurized injection/suction system for ventilation in the presence of complete airway obstruction. *Crit Care Med.* 1994;22:326.

14. McLellan I, et al. Percutaneous transtracheal high frequency jet ventilation as an aid to difficult intubation. *Can J Anaesth.* 1988;35:404.

15. Chipley PS, et al. Prolonged use of an endotracheal tube changer in a pediatric patient with a potentially compromised airway. *Chest.* 1994;105:961.

16. Hagberg CA. *Handbook of Difficult Airway Management.* Philadelphia: Churchill Livingstone; 2000:194.

17. Shantha TR. Retrograde intubation using the subcricoid region. *Br J Anaesth.* 1992; 68:109.

18. Sdrales L, Benumof JL. Prevention of kinking of a percutaneous transtracheal intravenous catheter. *Anesthesiology.* 1995;82:288.

19. Southwick JP. Precurved transtracheal catheters [letter]. *Anesthesiology.* 1995;82(5): 1302.

20. Soto R, Mesa A. New intravenous catheter not suitable for trans-tracheal jet ventilation [letter]. *Anesth Analg.* 2001;92:1074.

21. Ames W, Venn P. Complication of the transtracheal catheter [letter]. *Br J Anaesth.* 1998;81(5):825.

22. Peak DA, Roy S. Needle cricothyroidotomy revisited. *Ped Emerg Care.* 1999;15(3): 224.

23. Dallen LT, et al. Spontaneous ventilation via transtracheal large-bore intravenous catheters is possible. *Anesthesiology.* 1991;75:531.

24. Fawcett W, et al. The work of breathing through large-bore intravascular catheters. *Anesthesiology.* 1992;76:323.

25. Banner MJ, et al. Excessive work imposed during spontaneous breathing through transtracheal catheters. *Anesthesiology.* 1992;77:A1231.

26. Mingus ML, et al. Transtracheal oxygenation using simple equipment and low pressure oxygen delivery. *Anesthesiology.* 1988;69:A835.

27. MacKenzie CF, et al. Tracheal insufflation of oxygen at low flow: capabilities and limitations. *Anesth Analg.* 1990;71:684.

28. Morley D, Thorpe CM. Apparatus for emergency transtracheal ventilation. *Anaesth Intens Care.* 1997;25:675.

29. Patel RG. Percutaneous transtracheal jet ventilation. *Chest.* 1999;116(6):1689.

30. Poon YK. Case history number 89: a life-threatening complication of cricothyroid membrane puncture. *Anesth Analg.* 1976;55:298.

31. Davies P. A stab in the dark! Are you ready to perform needle cricothyroidotomy? *Injury, Int J Care Injured.* 1999;30:659.

32. Hwa-Kou K. Translaryngeal guided intubation using a sheath stylet. *Anesthesiology.* 1985;63:567.

33. Bourke D, Levesque PR. Modification of retrograde guide for endotracheal intubation. *Anesth Analg.* 1974;53:1013.

34. Schwartz D, Singh J. Retrograde wire-guided direct laryngoscopy in a 1-month-old infant. *Anesthesiology.* 1992;77:607.

35. Alfrey DD. Double-lumen endobronchial tube intubation using a retrograde wire technique. *Anesth Analg.* 1993;76:1374.

36. Nicholson SC, et al. Management of a difficult airway in a patient with Hurler-Scheie syndrome during cardiac surgery. *Anesth Analg.* 1992;75:830.
37. Abou-Madi MN, Trop D. Pulling vs guiding: a modification of retrograde guided intubation. *Can J Anaesth.* 1989;6:336.
38. King HK, et al. Soft and firm introducers for translaryngeal guided intubation. *Anesth Analg.* 1989;68:826.
39. Dhara SS. Retrograde intubation: a facilitated approach. *Br J Anaesth.* 1992;69:631.
40. Sanchez AF, Morrison DE. In: Hagberg CA. *Handbook of Difficult Airway Management.* Philadelphia: Churchill Livingstone; 2000:chapter 6.
41. Guggenberger J, Lenz G. Training in retrograde intubation. *Anesthesiology.* 1988;69: 292.
42. Mahiou P, et al. Retrograde tracheal intubation combined with laryngeal nerve block in conscious trauma patients. *Anesthesiology.* 1988;71:A199.
43. Parmet JL, Metz S. Retrograde endotracheal intubation: an underutilized tool for management of the difficult airway. *Contemporary Surgery.* 1996;49(5).
44. Mathews HR, Hopkinson RB. Treatment of sputum retention by minitracheostomy. *Br J Surg.* 1984;71:147.
45. Hutchinson J, Hopkinson RB. How to insert a minitrach. *Br J Hosp Med.* 1989;42: 112.
46. Ala-Kokko TI, et al. Management of upper airway obstruction using a Seldinger minitracheostomy kit. *Acta Anaesth Scand.* 1996;40:385.
47. Corke C, Cranswick P. A Seldinger technique for minitracheostomy insertion. *Anaesth Intensive Care.* 1988;16:206.
48. Chan TC, et al. Comparison of wire-guided cricothyrotomy versus standard surgical cricothyrotomy technique. *J Emerg Med.* 1999;17(6):957.
49. Van Heurn, LWE, et al. Percutaneous subcricoid minitracheostomy: report of 50 procedures. *Ann Thorac Surg.* 1995;59:707.
50. Wain JC, et al. Clinical experience with minitracheostomy. *Ann Thorac Surg.* 1990; 49:881.
51. Pedersen J, et al. Is minitracheostomy a simple and safe procedure? A prospective investigation in the ICU. *Intens Care Med.* 1991;177:333.
52. Randell T, et al. Minitracheostomy: complications and follow-up with fiberoptic tracheoscopy. *Anaesthesia.* 1990;45:875.
53. Randell T, Lindgren L. Inadvertent submucosal penetration with a minitracheostomy cannula inserted by the Seldinger technique. *Anaesthesia.* 1991;46:801.
54. Hammond J, Bray B. A serious complication of minitracheostomy. *Anaesthesia.* 1992;47:538.
55. Combes P, et al. Minitracheostomy: impossible cannulation. *Br J Anaesth.* 1991;66: 275.
56. Silk JM, Marsh AM. Pneumothorax caused by minitracheostomy. *Anaesthesia.* 1989;44:663.
57. Fisher JB. Surgical emphysema, minitracheostomy, and HFJV. *Intensive Care Med.* 1992;18:317.
58. Campbell AM, O'Leary A. Acute airway obstruction as a result of minitracheostomy. *Anaesthesia.* 1991;46:854.
59. Daborn AK, Harris NE. Minitracheostomy: a life-threatening complication. *Anaesthesia.* 1989;44:839.
60. Russell WC. Complications and inappropriate use of minitracheostomy. *Anaesth Intensive Care.* 1989;17:513.

61. McEwan A, et al. A serious complication of minitracheostomy. *Anaesthesia.* 1991;46:1041.

62. Allen PW, Thornton M. Oesophageal perforation with minitracheostomy. *Intensive Care Med.* 1989;15:543.

63. Claffey LP, Phelan DM. A complication of cricothyroid "minitracheostomy": oesophageal perforation. *Intensive Care Med.* 1989;15:140.

64. Ryan DW, et al. Intra-oesophageal placement of minitracheostomy tube. *Intensive Care Med.* 1989;15:538.

65. Brathwaite CEM. Rapid percutaneous tracheostomy. *Chest.* 1991;100:1475.

66. Pedersen J, et al. Ossification of the cricothyroid membrane following minitracheostomy. *Intensive Care Med.* 1989;15:272.

67. Woodcock T. Mask CPAP and minitracheostomy: a cautionary tale. *Intensive Care Med.* 1991;17:436.

68. Allen PW, Hart SM. Minitracheostomy in children. *Anaesthesia.* 1988;43:760.

69. Powell DM, et al. Review of percutaneous tracheostomy. *Laryngoscope.* 1998;108:170.

70. Fantoni A, Ripamonti D. A breakthrough in tracheostomy techniques: translaryngeal tracheostomy. 8th European Congress of Intensive Care Medicine; 1995; Athens, Greece: 1031–1034.

71. Kearney, PA, et al. A single-center 8-year experience with percutaneous dilational tracheostomy. *Ann Surg.* 2000;231(5):701.

72. Schwann NM. Percutaneous dilational tracheostomy: anesthetic consideration for a growing trend. *Anesth Analg.* 1997;84(4):907.

73. Fernandez L, et al. Bedside percutaneous tracheostomy with bronchoscopic guidance in critically ill patients. *Arch Surg.* 1996;131:129.

74. Cobean R, et al. Percutaneous dilational tracheostomy: a safe, cost-effective bedside procedure. *Arch Surg.* 1966;131:265.

75. Chendrasekhar A, et al. Percutaneous dilatational tracheostomy: an alternative approach to surgical tracheostomy. *Southern Med J.* 1995;88(10):1062.

76. McHenry CR, et al. Percutaneous tracheostomy: a cost-effective alternative to standard open tracheostomy. *Amer Surgeon.* 1997;63:646.

77. Moe KS, et al. Percutaneous tracheostomy: a comprehensive evaluation. *Ann Otol Rhinol Laryngol.* 1999;108:384.

78. Billy ML, Bradrick JP. Percutaneous dilatational subcricoid tracheostomy. *J Oral Maxillofac Surg.* 1997;55:981.

79. Bobo ML, McKenna SJ. The current status of percutaneous dilational tracheostomy: an alternative to open tracheostomy. *J Oral Maxillofac Surg.* 1998;56:681.

80. Muhammad JK, et al. Percutaneous dilatational tracheostomy: haemorrhagic complications and the vascular anatomy of the anterior neck: a review based on 497 cases. *Int J Oral Maxillofac Surg.* 2000;29:217.

81. Vigliaroli, et al. Clinical experience with Ciaglia's percutaneous tracheostomy. *Eur Arch Otorhinolaryngol.* 1999;256:426.

82. Gaukroger MC, Allt-Graham JA. Percutaneous dilatational tracheostomy. *Br J Oral and Maxillofac Surg.* 1994;32(6):375.

83. Barrachina F, et al. Percutaneous dilatational cricothyroidotomy: outcome with 44 consecutive patients. *Intensive Care Med.* 1996;22:937.

84. Petros S, Engelmann L. Percutaneous dilatational tracheostomy in a medical ICU. *Intensive Care Med.* 1997;23:630.

85. Carrillo EH, et al. Percutaneous dilational tracheostomy for airway control. *Am J Surgery.* 1997;174:469.

86. Suh RH, et al. Percutaneous dilatational tracheostomy: still a surgical procedure. *Am Surgeon.* 1999;65:928.

87. Velmahos GC, et al. Bedside percutaneous tracheostomy: prospective evaluation of a modification of the current technique in 100 patients. *World J Surg.* 2000;24:1109.

88. Marx WH, et al. Some important details in the technique of percutaneous dilatational tracheostomy via the modified Seldinger technique. *Chest.* 1996;110(3):762.

89. Walz MK, et al. Percutaneous dilatational tracheostomy—early results and long-term outcome of 326 critically ill patients. *Intensive Care Med.* 1998;24:685.

90. Porter JM, Ivatury RR. Preferred route of tracheostomy—percutaneous versus open at the bedside: a randomized, prospective study in the surgical intensive care unit. *Am Surgeon.* 1999;65:142.

91. Massick DD, et al. Bedside tracheostomy in the ICU: a prospective randomized trial comparing open surgical tracheostomy with endoscopically guided percutaneous dilational tracheostomy. *Laryngoscope.* 2001;111:494.

92. Grover A, et al. Open versus percutaneous dilatational tracheostomy: efficacy and cost analysis. *Am Surgeon.* 2001;67:297.

93. Friedman M, et al. Experience with percutaneous dilational tracheostomy. *Ann Otol Rhinol Laryngol.* 2000;109:791.

94. Gysin C, et al. Percutaneous versus surgical tracheostomy: a double-blind randomized trial. *Ann Surg.* 1999;230(5):708.

95. Stoeckli SJ, et al. A clinical and histologic comparison of percutaneous dilational versus conventional surgical tracheostomy. *Laryngoscope.* 1997;107:1643.

96. Street MK, Boyd O. Tracheostomy: the change in practice in a region over a decade. *Br J Anaesth.* 2000;84(5):689P.

97. Friedman Y, et al. Comparison of percutaneous and surgical tracheostomies. *Chest.* 1996;110(2):480.

98. Carney AS. The use of MRI to assess tracheal stenosis following percutaneous dilatational tracheostomy [letter]. *J Laryngol Otol.* 1998;112:599.

99. MP Fischler, et al. Late outcome of percutaneous dilatational tracheostomy in intensive care patients. *Intensive Care Med.* 1995;21:475

100. Callanan V, et al. The use of MRI to assess tracheal stenosis following percutaneous dilatational tracheostomy. *J Laryngol Otol.* 1997;111:953.

101. Rosenbower TJ, et al. The long-term complications of percutaneous dilatational tracheostomy. *Am Surgeon.* 1998;64:82.

102. Leonard RC, et al. Late outcome from percutaneous tracheostomy using the Portex kit. *Chest.* 1999;115(4):1070.

103. Norwood S, et al. Incidence if tracheal stenosis and other late complications after percutaneous tracheostomy. *Ann Surg.* 2000;232(2):233.

104. Bernard AC, Kenady DE. Conventional surgical tracheostomy as the preferred method of airway management. *J Oral Maxillofac Surg.* 1999;57:310.

105. Griffen MM, Kearney PA. Percutaneous dilational tracheostomy as the preferred method of airway management. *J Oral Maxillofac Surg.* 1999;57:316.

106. Barba CA. The intensive care unit as an operating room. *Surg Clin North Am.* 2000;80(3):957.

107. Pryor JP, et al. Surgical airway management in the ICU. *Crit Care Clin.* 2000; 16(3):473.

108. Byhahn C, et al. Percutaneous tracheostomy: Ciaglia blue rhino versus the basic Ciaglia technique of percutaneous dilational tracheostomy. *Anesth Analg.* 2000;91: 882.

109. Westphal K, et al. Percutaneous tracheostomy: a clinical comparison of dilatational (Ciaglia) and translaryngeal (Fantoni) techniques. *Anesth Analg.* 1999;89:938.

110. Byhahn C, et al. Bedside percutaneous tracheostomy: clinical comparison of Griggs and Fantoni techniques. *World J Surg.* 2001;25:296.

111. Nates JL, et al. Percutaneous tracheostomy in critically ill patients: a prospective, randomized comparison of two techniques. *Crit Care Med.* 2000;28(11):3734.

112. Van Heerden PV, et al. Percutaneous dilational tracheostomy—a clinical study evaluating two systems. *Anaesth Intens Care.* 1996;24:56.

113. Ambesh SP, Kaushik S: Percutaneous dilational tracheostomy: the Ciaglia method versus the Rapitrach method. *Anesth Analg.* 1998;87:556.

114. Ciaglia P, et al. Elective percutaneous dilatational tracheostomy: a new simple bedside procedure [preliminary report]. *Chest.* 1985;87:715.

115. Winkler WB, et al. Bedside percutaneous dilational tracheostomy with endoscopic guidance: experience with 71 ICU patients. *Inten Care Med.* 1994;20(7):476.

116. Barba CA, et al. Bronchoscopic guidance makes percutaneous tracheostomy a safe, cost-effective, and easy-to-teach procedure. *Surgery.* 1995;118(5):879.

117. Berrouschot J, et al. Perioperative complications of percutaneous dilational tracheostomy. *Laryngoscope.* 1997;107:1538.

118. Byhahn C, et al. Percutaneous tracheostomy "Ciaglia blue rhino": experiences in 120 critically ill adults [Poster presentation B16]. *Anesthesiology.* 2001;October(suppl).

119. Bewsher MS, et al. Evaluation of a new percutaneous dilatational tracheostomy set. *Anaesthesia.* 2001;56:859.

120. Sakabu SA, et al. Airway obstruction with percutaneous tracheostomy. *Chest.* 1997; 111(5):1468.

121. Ciaglia P. Airway obstruction with percutaneous tracheostomy. *Chest.* 1998;113(3):849.

122. Rumbak MK. More on airway obstruction with percutaneous tracheostomy. *Chest.* 1998;113(3):850.

123. Steele APH, et al. Long-term follow-up of Griggs percutaneous tracheostomy with spiral CT and questionnaire. *Chest.* 2000;117(5):1430.

124. Raine RI, et al. Late outcome after guide-wire forceps percutaneous tracheostomy— a prospective, randomized comparison with open surgical tracheostomy. *Br J Anaesth.* 1999;82(suppl 1):168.

125. Watters MPR, et al. Tracheal rupture during percutaneous tracheostomy: safety aspects of the Griggs method. *Br J Anaesth.* 2000;84(5):671P.

126. Bliznikas D: Percutaneous tracheostomy, *eMedicine Journal.* 2001. 2(11). www.emedicine.com.

127. MacCallum PL, et al. Comparison of open, percutaneous, and translaryngeal tracheostomies. *Otolaryngol Head Neck Surg.* 2000;122(5):686.

128. Karnik A, Freeman JW. Translaryngeal tracheostomy technique (TLT): prospective evaluation of 164 cases. *Br J Anaesth.* 1999;82(suppl 1):169.

129. Vecchiarelli P, et al. Fantoni's trans-laryngeal tracheostomy: two years of experience. *Br J Anaesth.* 1999;82(suppl 1):167.

130. Westphal K, et al. Tracheostomy in cardiosurgical patients: surgical tracheostomy versus Ciaglia and Fantoni methods. *Ann Thor Surg.* 1999;68:486.

131. Weiss S. Letter to the editor. *J Emerg Med.* 1992;10:764.

132. Quicktrach Cricothrotomy Device, Life-Assist, Inc., Sacramento, CA. www.life-assist.com.

133. Schachner A, et al. Percutaneous tracheostomy: a new method. *Crit Care Med.* 1989; 17:1052.

134. Bouvette M, Fuhrman TM. Preventing complications during percutaneous tracheostomy [letter]. *Anesthesiology.* 1999;90(3):918.

135. Mphanza T, Jacobs S. Letter in reply to reference 142. *Anesthesiology.* 1999;90(3): 918.

136. Ciaglia P: Video-assisted endoscopy, not just endoscopy, for percutaneous dilatational tracheostomy. *Chest.* 1999;115(4):915.

137. Dexter T: The laryngeal mask airway: a method to improve visualization of the trachea and larynx during fiberoptic assisted percutaneous tracheostomy. *Anaesth Intensive Care.* 1994;22:35.

138. Lyons BJ, et al. The LMA simplifies airway management during percutaneous dilational tracheostomy. *Acta Anaesthesiol Scand.* 1995;39:414.

139. Brimacombe J. Letter. *Anaesthesia.* 1994;49:358.

140. Verghese C, et al. Airway control during percutaneous dilatational tracheostomy: pilot study with the intubating LMA. *Br J Anaesth.* 1998;81(4):608.

141. Zuleika M, et al. The use of the LMA in suitable ICU patients undergoing percutaneous dilational tracheostomy. *Inten Care Med.* 1997;23(1):129.

142. Quinio P, et al. Translaryngeal tracheostomy through the intubating LMA in a patient with difficult tracheal intubation. *Inten Care Med.* 2000;26(6):820.

143. Addas BM, et al. Light-guided tracheal puncture for percutaneous tracheostomy. *Can J Anesth.* 2000;47(9):919.

144. Cooper RM, et al. Facilitation of percutaneous dilational tracheostomy by use of a perforated endotracheal tube exchanger. *Chest.* 1996;109(4):1131.

145. Deblieux P, et al. Facilitation of percutaneous dilational tracheostomy by use of a perforated endotracheal tube exchanger. *Chest.* 1995;108(2):572.

146. Muhammad JK, et al. Percutaneous dilatational tracheostomy under ultrasound guidance. *Br J Oral Maxillofacial Surg.* 1999;37(4):309.

147. Brimacombe J, Clarke G. Rigid bronchoscope: a possible new option for percutaneous dilational tracheostomy. *Anesthesiology.* 1995;83(3):646.

148. Donaldson DR, et al. Chest radiographs after dilatational percutaneous tracheostomy: are they necessary? *Otolaryngol Head Neck Surg* 2000;123(3):236.

149. Tobias JD, Higgins M. Capnography during transtracheal needle cricothyrotomy. *Anesth Analg.* 1995;81:1077.

150. Bissinger U, et al. Retrograde-guided fiberoptic intubation in patients with laryngeal carcinoma. *Anesth Analg.* 1995;81:408.

151. Eidelman LA, Pizov R. A safer approach to retrograde-guided fiberoptic intubation [letter]. *Anesth Analg.* 1996;82:1107.

152. Bissinger U, et al. Letter in reply to reference 159. *Anesth Analg.* 1996;82:1108.

153. Roberts KW, Solgonick RM. A modification of retrograde wire-guided, fiberoptic-assisted endotracheal intubation in a patient with ankylosing spondylitis. *Anesth Analg.* 1996;82:1290.

154. Rosenblatt WH, et al. Retrograde fiberoptic intubation. *Anesth Analg.* 1997;84:1142.

155. Donaldson DR, et al. Endoscopically monitored percutaneous dilational tracheostomy in a residency program. *Laryngoscope.* 2000;110:1142.

156. Massick DD, et al. Quantification of the learning curve for percutaneous dilatational tracheostomy. *Laryngoscope.* 2000;110:222.

157. Gardiner Q, et al. Technique training: endoscopic percutaneous tracheostomy. *Br J Anaesth.* 1998;81(3):401.

158. Gerig HJ, et al. Fiberoptically-guided insertion of transtracheal catheters. *Anesth Analg.* 2001;93:663.

159. Eisenburger P, et al. Comparison of conventional surgical versus Seldinger technique emergency cricothyrotomy performed by inexperienced clinicians. *Anesthesiology.* 2000;92(3):687.

160. Goumas P, et al. Cricothyroidotomy and the anatomy of the cricothyroid space: an autopsy study. *J Laryngol Otol.* 1997;11:354.

161. Schroeder AA. Cricothroidotomy: when, why, and why not? *Am J Otolaryngol.* 2000; 21(3):195.

162. Hawkins ML, et al. Emergency cricothyrotomy: a reassessment. *Am Surgeon.* 1995; 61:52.

163. Isaacs JH Jr. Emergency cricothyrotomy: long term results. *Ann Surg.* 2001; 67:346–349.

164. Gillespie MB, Eisele DW. Outcomes of emergency surgical airway procedures in a hospital-wide setting. *Laryngoscope.* 1999;109:1766.

165. Liebovici D, et al. Prehospital cricothyroidotomy by physicians. *Am J Emerg Med.* 1997;15(1):91.

166. Gerich TG, et al. Prehospital airway management in the acutely injured patient: the role of surgical cricothyrotomy revisited. *J Trauma: Injury, Infection, Crit Care.* 1998;45(2):312.

167. Brohi K, et al. Letter to editor. *J Trauma.* 1999;46(4):745.

168. Jacobson LE, et al. Surgical cricothyroidotomy in trauma patients: analysis of its use by paramedics in the field. *J Trauma: Injury, Infection, Crit Care.* 1996;41(1):15.

169. Holmes JF, et al. Comparison of 2 cricothyrotomy techniques: standard method versus rapid 4-step technique. *Ann Emerg Med.* 1998;32(4):442.

170. Brofeldt BT, et al. An easy cricothyrotomy approach: the rapid four-step technique. *Acad Emerg Med.* 1996;3:1060.

171. Gerling MC, et al. Effect of surgical cricothyrotomy on the unstable cervical spine in a cadaver model of intubation. *J Emergency Med.* 2001;20(1):1.

172. Spaite DW, Joseph M. Prehospital cricothyrotomy. *Ann Emerg Med.* 1990;19:279.

173. Goldenberg D, et al. Tracheostomy complications: a retrospective study of 1130 cases. *Otolaryngol Head Neck Surg.* 2000;123(4):495.

174. Johnson DR, et al. Cricothyrotomy performed by prehospital personnel: a comparison of two techniques in a human cadaver model. *Am J Emergency Med.* 1993;19:207.

175. Wetmore RF, et al. Pediatric tracheostomy: a changing procedure? *Ann Otol Rhinol Laryngol.* 1999;108:695.

176. Paetkau DJ, et al. Submental orotracheal intubation for maxillofacial surgery. *Anesthesiology.* 2000;92(3):912.

177. Drolet P, et al. Facilitating submental endotracheal intubation with an endotracheal tube exchanger. *Anesth Analg.* 2000;90:222.

11
The Pediatric Airway

Pediatric airway problems are among the most challenging you will face in medicine throughout a lifetime career. Clinicians unaccustomed to dealing with children tend to approach pediatric airway problems with a disproportionate amount of fear—which, often engendered by inexperience, can interfere with performance. This chapter provides you with the knowledge necessary to deal with common airway problems occurring in children.

The anatomical differences between the infant, child, and adult airways have been described in Chapter 1. The salient differences between the adult and pediatric airways are worth repeating at this juncture (see Fig. 1.22). The infant's tongue is proportionally larger than the adult's and is more likely to obstruct a relatively smaller airway during unconsciousness. Infants are compulsive nose breathers during the early months of life, and when the nose becomes obstructed airway obstruction can occur. The epiglottis is larger and stiffer and has a much more horizontal lie in infants and readily causes airway obstruction when it becomes swollen. The larynx is situated at a higher level in relation to the cervical spine than in adults. The cricoid cartilage is the narrowest part of the infant and child larynx, whereas the rima glottidis is the narrowest part of the adult's airway. Even modest edema of the mucous membrane at the level of the cricoid cartilage of an infant causes serious airway obstruction. There are also a number of physiological differences between adults and children, the greatest being between adults and neonates[1] (Table 11.1).

Basic Airway Management and CPR in Infants and Children

The principles of airway management in infants and children are similar to those in adults, with some exceptions. Extension of the infant cervical spine during the head-tilt maneuver tends to flatten the airway, causing some degree of obstruction. Extension of the cervical spine should always be done gently, especially in children with Downs or Hurler syndrome (in which significant instability of the atlantoaxial joint has been reported).[2] Finally, inflation pressures required to ven-

TABLE 11.1. Normal pulmonary function mean values in infants

Variable	Neonate	Adult
Body weight (kg)	3	70
Tidal volume (ml/kg)	6	6
Respiratory rate (breaths/min)	35	15
Volume expired (ml/kg/min)	210	90
Alveolar gas volume (ml/kg/min)	130	60
Anatomical dead space (ml/kg)	2.5	2.0
Physiological dead space/tidal volume ratio	0.30	0.33
O_2 consumption (ml/kg/min)	6.4	3.5
CO_2 production (ml/kg/min)	6.0	3.0
Calories (kg/hr)	2	1
Total lung capacity (ml/kg)	63	86
Functional residual capacity (ml/kg)	30	34
Thoracic gas volume (ml/kg)	36	34
Vital capacity (ml/kg)	35	70
Residual volume (ml/kg)	23	16
Closing volume (ml/kg)	12	7
Closing capacity (ml/kg)	35	23
Tidal volume/functional residual capacity ratio	0.20	0.20
Functional residual capacity/total lung capacity ratio	0.47	0.40
Tracheal length (mm)	57	120
Tracheal diameter (mm)	4	16

Source: Godinez RI, 1985,[1] with permission.

tilate an infant or child satisfactorily are much less than those required in an adult. Thus, much smaller breaths should be used during mouth-to-mouth respiration or positive-pressure ventilation (PPV) of any type, lest pulmonary barotrauma occur. Cardiac arrest in an infant or child is usually secondary to respiratory insufficiency. Following are the most common causes of respiratory insufficiency in otherwise healthy children:

Trauma
Accidental poisoning
Foreign-body aspiration
Drowning
Airway infections
Unexplained (e.g., sudden infant death syndrome)
Burns

The International Guidelines on Pediatric Basic and Advanced Life Support have once again been updated and can be found in Circulation.[3] The guidelines from 1992 have not changed much in principle, but some refinements and qualifications have been added.[4]

The chain of survival in pediatrics includes:

Education in prevention of cardiopulmonary arrest
Basic CPR
Early access to EMS

Early, effective pediatric acute life support (ALS)
Effective pediatric post-resuscitation and rehabilitative care.

"Phone fast" for infants and children under 8 years of age, and "phone first" for children over 8 years old and adults was retained as a guideline and emphasized.

Basic Life Support Sequence

Recommended Sequence

The recommended CPR sequence[3] for use in an infant or child is as follows:

Ensure safety of rescuer and victim.
Assess responsiveness.
Call for help. Activate the emergency medical system (EMS). (The AHA recommends one minute of CPR on a child before calling EMS if a single rescuer is present.)
Position the patient horizontally on a hard flat surface.

Airway

  Open the airway.
    Slight head tilt/chin lift
    Slight head tilt/jaw thrust
    Jaw thrust alone if suspected cervical spine injury

Breathing

  Look, listen, and feel for breathing.
  If there is no spontaneous breathing, give two initial breaths.
    Infant and small child: mouth-to-mouth/mouth-to-nose (Fig. 11.1).
    Larger child: mouth-to-mouth.
  Check for rise and fall of the chest with each ventilation.
  If not successful, reposition the victim's head and attempt to ventilate. (Improper head position is the most common cause of inability to ventilate.)
  If rescue breathing is still unsatisfactory, suspect foreign-body airway obstruction.

Circulation

  Assess the circulation (no pulse check for lay rescuers).
  Lay rescuers should look, listen, and feel for breathing or coughing and look for movement. If none of these signs are present, they should begin compressions. Healthcare (HC) workers should assess the circulation by looking for a pulse (brachial in infants and carotid in children aged 1 to 8 years). HC workers should spend no more than 10 seconds looking for a pulse. If you do not detect a pulse or if the pulse rate is less than 60 beats per minute (bpm) and perfusion seems inadequate, start compressions. (See Table 11.2.)

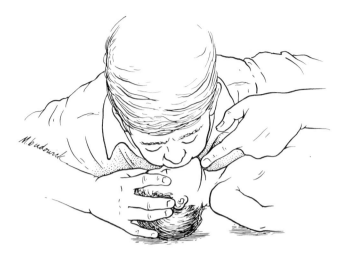

FIGURE 11.1. Mouth-to-mouth/mouth-to-nose ventilation in an infant.

Airway Equipment

Most of the airway equipment used in adults is also available in pediatrics. The routine equipment is very similar to that used in adults except it is proportionally smaller. The laryngeal mask airway (LMA) is used routinely in pediatric practice now and is being incorporated into pediatric difficult airway algorithms. The cuffed oropharyngeal airway (COPA) is also available in pediatric sizes and adds a new dimension to the oropharyngeal airway. Fiberoptic-assisted intubation (FAI) is being used more frequently in pediatric practice now that smaller-gauge fiberscopes (2.1 mm) have become available. Lighted stylets are now being used in difficult airway cases in pediatrics. A Bullard laryngoscope, adapted for pediatric use, is now available for challenging airways.

TABLE 11.2. CPR in infants and children*

	Compression rate (per min)	Ventilation rate (breaths per min)	Compression-to-ventilation ratio	Depth of compressions (in)	Hand position
Infant	At least 100	20	5:1	0.5 to 1.0	1 finger-breadth below nipples
Child	100	20	5:1	1.0 to 1.5	2 finger-breadths above xiphoid
Adult (for comparison)	100	12	15:2	1.5 to 2.0	2 finger-breadths above xiphoid

*This resuscitation sequence is to be used **outside** the hospital, where there is little if any equipment at your disposal.

Mask Ventilation

Self-inflating bags of suitably reduced size are used in infants and children. To the novice, mask ventilation in a child can be quite challenging. The best results are obtained by placing the head in a neutral position (i.e., neither flexion nor extension of the neck) and using one hand to maintain the airway. Excessive pressure should not be exerted in the submental area, because this tends to force the tongue backward toward the posterior pharyngeal wall and creates additional obstruction. Occasionally, both hands will be required to pull the mandible forward. In this situation you may need an assistant, especially if the child is apneic.

If you are still unable to maintain adequate gas exchange despite these maneuvers, an oral or nasal airway should be inserted to hold the tongue forward and relieve obstruction by the lips, teeth, and nose. If the oral airway is too large, however, it may actually cause obstruction by forcing the epiglottis down over the glottis; and if too small, it may cause obstruction by pushing the tongue backward. Furthermore, a poorly positioned airway can induce pressure necrosis of the tongue.

The T-Piece

To avoid confusion, we will consider only one anesthesia circuit, the T-piece. Introduced in 1937 by Ayre,[5] this device can deliver oxygen or anesthetic gases to an infant or child in such a way that carbon dioxide retention is virtually eliminated. There have been a number of modifications, the most notable being the addition of a bag (the Jackson-Rees modification[6]). The T-piece is quite versatile in that it can be used to administer anesthesia to an infant or child in the operating room or during transport to the ward or ICU, for neonatal resuscitation, or whenever the patient needs respiratory assistance for any reason. To prevent rebreathing of carbon dioxide, a flow $2^{1}/_{2}$ times the minute volume should be used. Therefore, from a practical and economic standpoint, the system should not be applied to children weighing more than 20 kg (44 lb).

The modified Ayre T-piece (Mapleson D) consists of a small piece of corrugated tubing about 18 inches long to which a 1-liter reservoir bag is attached (Fig. 11.2). The volume of this tube should be at least 75% of the predicted tidal volume. A valve may be placed at the distal end of the tube, or, alternatively, a deliberate leak may be left in the bag to vent any excessive buildup of gases in the system. A right-angle outlet or plastic adapter is attached to the corrugated tubing at its proximal end. Gas enters the right-angle connector via a hollow adapter. The proximal end of the right-angle adapter fits onto any 15-mm connector (mask or endotracheal) tube. The right-angle connector should also have a fitting that allows the attachment of a manometer for monitoring airway pressures. The T-piece, with minor variations, is one of the most common circuits used for manual ventilation of pediatric patients.

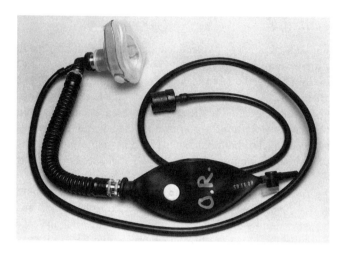

FIGURE 11.2. The Jackson-Rees modification of an Ayre T-piece.

Resuscitation of the Neonate

Neonatal resuscitation is one of the most important tasks in a medical practitioner's career. The consequences of inadequately performed resuscitation not only are devastating to the newborn and family, they place a huge financial burden on the health system. Thus, the task should be delegated only to highly responsible and well-trained individuals. The differential diagnosis of neonatal asphyxiation is presented in Box 11.1.

Asphyxiation of the neonate has been carefully studied in animal models and is characterized by a brief period of vigorous respiratory effort during which the heart rate and blood pressure rise and the PaO_2 falls. Then a primary apnea occurs that lasts for 1 to 5 minutes. If active resuscitation is not performed during

---

Box 11.1. Differential Diagnosis of the Asphyxiated Newborn Infant

1. Hypoxia/ischemia
2. Drug depression
3. Perinatal trauma
4. Anemia
5. Intrauterine infection
6. Congenital malformation
7. Extreme prematurity

Source: Roy and Betheras,[7] with permission.

TABLE 11.3. Features of primary and secondary apnea

Sign	Normal	Primary apnea	Secondary apnea
Color	Pink	Blue	Pale or gray
Heart rate	> 100/min	40 to 100/min	< 40/min
Muscle tone	Good	May be some	Absent
Resuscitation required	Nil	Simple	Vigorous/urgent
Response to resuscitation	—	Gasps before pink	Pink before gasps

Source: Roy and Betheras,[7] with permission.

this phase, the infant enters a gasping phase that eventually results in secondary apnea characterized by profound asphyxiation ($PaO_2 < 50$ and $PaCO_2 \sim 100$ mm Hg, pH < 7.0) and quickly leads to the death of the infant unless there is some intervention. Signs of primary and secondary apnea[7] are included in Table 11.3.

About 6% of all neonates require resuscitation at birth. The Apgar scoring system[8] was devised to assess the immediate outcome of neonatal resuscitation (Table 11.4). The neonatal resuscitation program (NRP)[9] is a structured workshop sponsored by the Canadian Heart and Stroke Foundation and the American Heart Association to assist individuals who are actively involved in resuscitation of newborn infants. It is divided into six educational modules:

1. Preparation for delivery
2. Initial stabilization
3. Ventilation (bag/mask)
4. Chest compressions
5. Tracheal intubation
6. Medications

Stabilization

Figure 11.3 outlines how to handle the initial stabilization period.

Ventilation

Bag/mask ventilation is indicated if after 15 to 20 seconds the infant is apneic, gasping, or cyanotic despite 100% oxygen and has a heart rate of less than 100 bpm. Intubation is indicated if there is no detectable heartbeat. The algorithm for ventilation is presented in Figure 11.4. Positive-pressure ventilation should be instituted at

TABLE 11.4. APGAR scores

Parameter	0	1	2
Heart rate	Absent	< 100	> 100
Respiration	Absent	Slow	Crying
Muscle tone	Limp	Some tension	Active
Reflex activity	Absent	Grimace	Cough
Color	Blue or gray	Mostly pink	All pink

Flow Chart: Initial Stabilization

*The steps in this section should
take no longer than 20 seconds.*

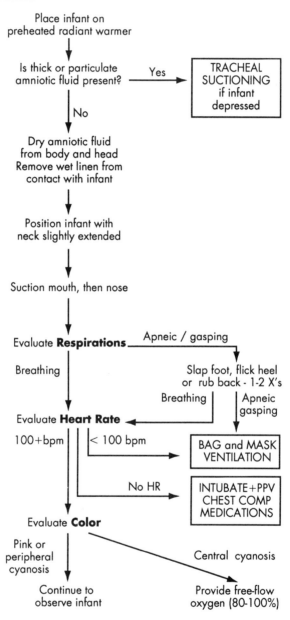

FIGURE 11.3. An algorithm for initial stabilization. (From Elliott,[9] with permission.)

Flow Chart: Ventilation

Equipment check:
- ✔ Resus Bag connected to O_2 - delivers 90-100%
- ✔ Resus Bag pressure tested - gauge working
- ✔ Appropriate size face mask selected

Adequate ventilation is established for 15-30 seconds, before the heart rate is assessed again.

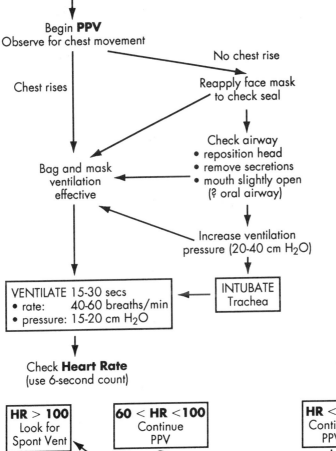

Infant's head extended slightly (± head down tilt)
Mask covers chin, mouth & nose

Begin **PPV**
Observe for chest movement

No chest rise

Chest rises

Reapply face mask to check seal

Check airway
- reposition head
- remove secretions
- mouth slightly open (? oral airway)

Bag and mask ventilation effective

Increase ventilation pressure (20-40 cm H_2O)

VENTILATE 15-30 secs
- rate: 40-60 breaths/min
- pressure: 15-20 cm H_2O

INTUBATE Trachea

Check **Heart Rate**
(use 6-second count)

HR > 100 Look for Spont Vent

60 < HR <100 Continue PPV

HR < 60 Continue PPV

HR rising

HR < 80 not rising

Withdraw PPV
Free-flow O_2
Tactile Stimuli
Monitor

Begin CHEST COMPRESSIONS

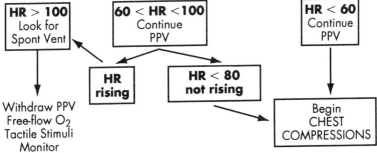

FIGURE 11.4. An algorithm for ventilation. (From Elliott,[9] with permission.)

a rate of 40 to 60 breaths per minute. The initial peak inspiratory pressure should be in the range of 30 to 40 cm H_2O, and subsequent pressures should be in the 15 to 20 cm H_2O range. If chest expansion is inadequate, consider the following:

Reevaluate head position
Suction
Oral airway
Increase ventilating pressure to 20 to 40 cm H_2O
Intubate trachea

Bag/mask ventilation requires considerable practice before competency is achieved. Neonatal resuscitation is frequently done by individuals who are not exposed to bag/mask ventilation often enough to maintain their skills. Paterson et al[10] have suggested an alternative method of PPV using the laryngeal mask. Initial results are quite promising, but further studies are needed to test the hypothesis.

Chest Compressions

Chest compressions are required if after 15 to 20 seconds of PPV with 100% oxygen the heart rate is less than 60 bpm or between 60 and 80 but not increasing. The rate of compressions should be 90 per minute and the depth 1.5 cm. The combined compression and ventilation rate should be 120 per minute (90 compressions with 30 ventilations, or 3:1).

The algorithm for chest compression is included in Figure 11.5. Two methods are acceptable—thumb and two-finger.

Thumb Method

The chest is encircled by both hands and the thumbs are applied side by side on the sternum on an imaginary line between the nipples. The fingers of both hands support the back. Only the **tips** of the thumbs should be used for compression lest rib fractures occur. In premature babies the thumbs may be superimposed upon one another.

Two-Finger Method

This may be used if the resuscitator's hands are too small or if access to the umbilicus is required. The tips of the index and middle fingers are applied to the sternum on an imaginary line between the nipples. The other hand supports the back (Fig. 11.6).

Tracheal Intubation

The indications for intubation in a pediatric population are not that much different from those in adults and generally include:

Prolonged PPV
Ineffective bag/mask ventilation

Flow Chart: Chest Compressions

 The need for Chest Compressions should be recognized and acted upon within 45-50 seconds of birth. Use Medications within 90 secs.

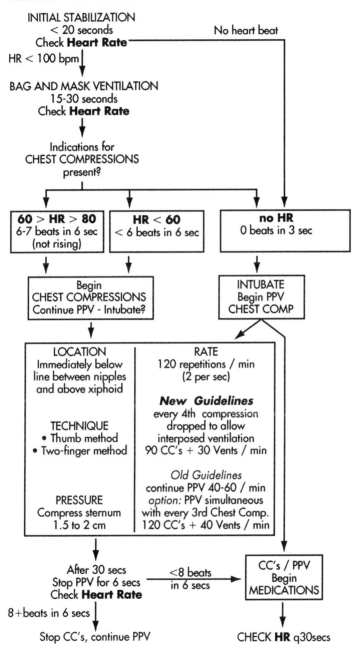

INITIAL STABILIZATION
< 20 seconds
Check **Heart Rate** ─────────────── No heart beat

HR < 100 bpm

BAG AND MASK VENTILATION
15-30 seconds
Check **Heart Rate**

Indications for
CHEST COMPRESSIONS
present?

| **60 > HR > 80**
6-7 beats in 6 sec
(not rising) | **HR < 60**
< 6 beats in 6 sec | **no HR**
0 beats in 3 sec |

Begin
CHEST COMPRESSIONS
Continue PPV - Intubate?

INTUBATE
Begin PPV
CHEST COMP

| LOCATION
Immediately below line between nipples and above xiphoid

TECHNIQUE
• Thumb method
• Two-finger method

PRESSURE
Compress sternum
1.5 to 2 cm | RATE
120 repetitions / min
(2 per sec)

New Guidelines
every 4th compression dropped to allow interposed ventilation
90 CC's + 30 Vents / min

Old Guidelines
continue PPV 40-60 / min
option: PPV simultaneous with every 3rd Chest Comp.
120 CC's + 40 Vents / min |

After 30 secs
Stop PPV for 6 secs
Check **Heart Rate** ──── <8 beats in 6 secs ────▶ CC's / PPV
Begin
MEDICATIONS

8+beats in 6 secs

Stop CC's, continue PPV

CHECK **HR** q30secs

FIGURE 11.5. An algorithm for chest compressions. (From Elliott,[9] with permission.)

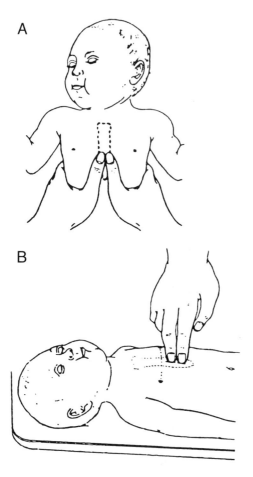

FIGURE 11.6. Chest compressions. **A.** The thumb method; **B.** the two-finger method. (From American Heart Association. *Textbook of Neonatal Resuscitation.* Dallas: American Heart Association; 1990, with permission.)

Suctioning required
Suspected diaphragmatic hernia
Absent heart rate

Specifically, when an infant presents with any of the conditions listed in Box 11.2, endotracheal intubation should be performed if not already in place.

Meconium Aspiration

This is a controversial topic. Endotracheal suctioning is indicated in the following circumstances:

Thick particulate meconium
Depressed infant with meconium

Reintubation and suctioning may be repeated as often as necessary (usually twice). A special meconium aspiration device is recommended (Fig. 11.7). The

Box 11.2. Indications for Intubation

1. $PaO_2 < 60$ mmHg with $FiO_2 \geq 0.6$ (in absence of cyanotic congenital heart disease)
2. $PaCO_2 > 50$ mmHg (acute and unresponsive to other intervention)
3. Upper airway obstruction, actual or impending
4. Neuromuscular weakness (maximum negative inspiratory pressure > -20 cm H_2O; vital capacity (<12 to 15 ml/kg)
5. Absent protective airway reflexes (cough, gag)
6. Hemodynamic instability (CPR, shock)
7. Therapeutic hyperventilation (intracranial hypertension; pulmonary hypertension; metabolic acidosis)
8. Pulmonary toilet
9. Emergency drug administration

Source: Fuhrman B, Zimmerman J. *Pediatric Critical Care.* St Louis: Mosby; 1991:115, with permission.

Canadian experience with meconium aspiration differs from the American. The new Canadian guidelines recommend that an infant with meconium (thick or thin) who is vigorous and breathing well should not be intubated because the risk of morbidity from multiple attempts at tracheal intubation may be greater than the risk of developing the meconium aspiration syndrome.

Medications

Medications may be administered to an infant via the endotracheal tube or intravenously (via the umbilical vein).

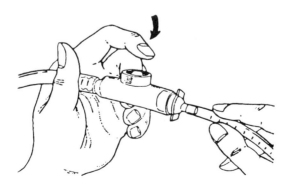

FIGURE 11.7. A meconium aspirator device. (From American Heart Association. *Textbook of Neonatal Resuscitation.* Dallas: American Heart Association; 1990, with permission.)

Epinephrine

Epinephrine is indicated when there is no heartbeat or when the heart rate is less than 80 bpm despite effective ventilation and chest compressions for at least 30 seconds. The dosage (1:10,000 epi) is 0.01 to 0.03mg/kg IV or may be administered endotracheally.

Volume Expanders

Fluid replacement may be given when a neonate presents with any of the following:

Persistent pallor
Weak pulse
Decreased blood pressure (e.g., 50/30)
Poor response to resuscitation

In an infant with O-negative blood, the following solutions should be administered over a 5- to 10-minute period, 10 ml/kg:

NaCl/Ringer's lactate
5% Albumin (in saline)

Naloxone

This narcotic antagonist is given for the reversal of respiratory depressions secondary to maternally administered narcotics. It may be given by IV or endotracheally (dose 0.1 mg/kg).

Other

Sodium bicarbonate and dopamine may be administered when a neonate does not respond to resuscitative efforts.

Techniques of Endotracheal Intubation in Infants and Children

The equipment required for intubation in infants is basically the same as that for children and adults, except that a greater variety of endotracheal tube sizes and laryngoscope blades should be available when dealing with children. You should always have three endotracheal tubes immediately available—the predicted size, one size larger, and one size smaller. When difficulties arise, crucial time may be lost searching for the correct-sized tube, and technical difficulties often do arise from selecting the inappropriate equipment.

Blade Selection

To help you select the proper laryngoscope blade, a list of blades appropriate in children up to age 6 appears in Table 11.5. You should always have 2 working

TABLE 11.5. Blade and tube sizes

Age (yr)	Blade	Endotracheal tube ID (mm)	Suction
Premature	Miller 0	2.5 to 3.0	5
Neonate	Miller 0	3.0 to 3.5	6
Neonate to $1^1/_2$	Miller 1	3.5 to 4.5	8
1 to 2	Miller $1^1/_2$	4.0 to 4.5	8
2 to 6	Macintosh 2	4.5 to 6.0	10

Source: Roy and Betheras,[7] with permission.

laryngoscopes. Straight blades are preferred in children, since the larynx is located more superiorly and the epiglottis lies at an angle of 45°.

Tube Selection

Tube site (internal diameter in mm) is usually selected on the basis of the child's age in years (Table 11.6). Following is a useful formula for most circumstances:

$$\frac{18 + Age}{4} = ID\ (in\ mm)$$

Two other formulas are used to determine how far the tube should be advanced into the trachea:

Oral: $12 + \dfrac{Age}{2}$ = tube length (in cm) **Nasal:** $15 + \dfrac{Age}{2}$ = Tube length (in cm)

Intubation Technique

The indications and techniques of endotracheal intubation in children are much the same as those already discussed in adults.

TABLE 11.6. Guidelines for endotracheal tube diameter in infants and children*

Age	Internal diameter (ID)	Orotracheal length (cm)	Nasotracheal length (cm)
Premature	2.0 to 3.0	6 to 8	7 to 9
Newborn	3.0 to 3.5	9 to 10	10 to 11
3 to 9 mo	3.5 to 4.0	11 to 12	11 to 13
9 to 18 mo	4.0 to 4.5	12 to 13	14 to 15
1.5 to 3 yr	4.5 to 5.0	12 to 14	16 to 17
4 to 5 yr	5.0 to 5.5	14 to 16	18 to 19
6 to 7 yr	5.5 to 6.0	16 to 18	19 to 20
8 to 10 yr	6.0 to 6.5†	17 to 19	21 to 23
11 to 13 yr	6.0 to 7.0†	18 to 21	22 to 25
14 to 16 yr	7.0 to 7.5†	20 to 22	24 to 25

*The ideal tube size will vary according to age, height, weight, specific airway anatomy, and ventilatory requirements of the child. In general, an air leak around the tube at 15 to 30 cm H_2O pressure is desirable.
†Cuffed tube.
Source: Modified from Motoyama EK, Davis PJ, eds. *Smith's Anesthesia for Infants and Children.* St. Louis; Mosby; 1990:659, with permission.

Awake intubation was frequently used in infants up to about 6 weeks who presented with pyloric stenosis or intestinal obstruction. Most pediatric anesthesiologists prefer to administer general anesthesia in these cases today.

Position

Place the infant supine with the head resting on a donut-shaped foam pad. Before proceeding, deliver oxygen for 1 to 2 minutes. The infant's neck is then slightly extended by an assistant. Overextension may lead to airway obstruction by flattening the trachea. To further stabilize the head, the assistant should hold it between the palms of both hands. The shoulders can be stabilized by having the assistant press down on them with the ulnar borders of both hands.

Exposure

Open the infant's mouth using the fingers of your right hand and extend the atlantooccipital joint.

Visualization

Hold the laryngoscope in the left hand and introduce the straight blade at the right side of the mouth and advance slowly. Make an effort to recognize anatomic structures as you advance the laryngoscope blade. When you see the epiglottis, advance the blade beyond the inferior surface and pull the blade forward as you withdraw it slowly. The arytenoids first come into view and then the glottis becomes visible. Occasionally, the epiglottis will drop down beneath the tip of the blade. If this happens, advance the blade again, applying slight manual pressure over the hyoid bone with the little finger of your left hand (Fig. 11.8).

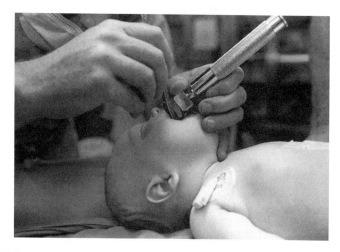

FIGURE 11.8. Manual pressure with the little finger may improve visualization of the airway.

Tube Placement

Insert the endotracheal tube and advance it to the midtracheal region.

Confirmation

The same methods for confirming tube placement in adults apply in children.

Stabilization

The tube should be carefully stabilized as previously described.

Summary

Tracheal intubation is quite an easy procedure in infants and children. Difficult intubation is not as prevalent as in adults. It is important to conduct a proper evaluation and to have all of the necessary and appropriate-sized equipment available. Infants and children desaturate more quickly than adults, so it is important to be well prepared and to have a contingency plan if you encounter difficulties with mask ventilation or intubation.

Upper Airway Obstruction in the Child

Clinical Presentation

The most common cause of death in children is accidental trauma. Asphyxia was the most common cause of infant death in the United States in 1997 (Fig. 11.9).[11]

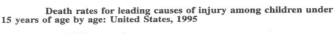

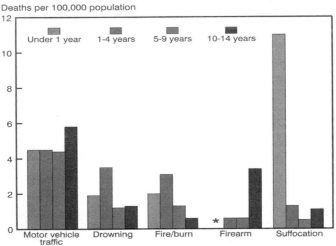

FIGURE 11.9. Death rates for leading causes of injury among children under 15 years of age by age: United States, 1995. (From *Injury Chart Book*,[11] with permission.)

TABLE 11.7. Symptoms and signs of airway obstruction

Symptoms	Signs
Dyspnea	Snoring
Cough	Snorting
Orthopnea	Gurgling
Hoarseness	Stridor
Weakness	Choking
Dysphagia	Chest retraction
Hemoptysis	Nasal flaring
Sore throat	Cyanosis
Exhaustion	Drooling
Nausea	Tachypnea
Vomiting	Unconsciousness

Upper airway obstruction in a child must be taken very seriously. The symptoms and signs are extremely variable and depend upon the etiology and the site of obstruction. Some of the more common symptoms and signs appear in Table 11.7. Obtaining a detailed history is vital for elucidating the cause of upper airway obstruction in a child.

The site of an obstruction can, to some degree, be approximated by pinpointing the phase of respiration at which stridor occurs (Table 11.8). Generally, supraglottic lesions cause inspiratory stridor whereas subglottic lesions cause inspiratory and expiratory stridor. Additional information can be obtained about the nature of the obstruction by studying flow volume loops (which provide a graphic analysis of flow at various lung volumes during continuous inspiration and expiration). These will allow you to determine if an obstruction is fixed or variable and also whether it is intrathoracic or extrathoracic.

The etiology of upper airway obstruction in a child is usually determined clinically. In less urgent situations the radiologist can provide useful information. If radiological studies are deemed necessary, an individual who is capable of dealing with upper airway obstruction must remain with the child at all times. Mag-

TABLE 11.8. Stridor

Stridor: A harsh high-pitched respiratory sound occurring in one or all phases of respiration; usually indicative of upper airway obstruction, the level of obstruction being to some degree determined by the level of the stridor

Level of obstruction	Character
Nose (nasal flaring)	Snoring, snorting
Pharyngeal	Gurgling
Laryngeal, subglottic	Inspiratory
Bronchial	Expiratory

netic resonance imaging (MRI) techniques have a new role in diagnosing complicated airway problems in pediatric patients.[12]

Etiology

Congenital

Laryngomalacia

Laryngomalacia, with flaccidity of the epiglottis and aryepiglottic folds, is responsible for up to 75% of all congenital laryngeal anomalies. The onset of symptoms occurs shortly after birth or within the first few months of life. Classically, the infant presents with a high-pitched crowing inspiratory stridor, often associated with feeding problems, respiratory distress, or upper respiratory tract infections. The stridor is thought to be caused by loose redundant supraglottic mucosa drawn into the airway during inspiration. Symptoms usually disappear within 12 to 24 months, and airway intervention is rarely required. The diagnosis is confirmed by laryngoscopy and bronchoscopy.

Congenital Vocal Cord Paralysis

Vocal cord paralysis is the second most common congenital laryngeal anomaly detected in the neonatal period. It may be unilateral or bilateral. In most cases its etiology remains unknown, although increased intracranial pressure may explain it in some cases. Unless there is an obvious precipitating factor, the condition is self-limiting and shows improvement over a period of weeks or months. The diagnosis is confirmed by direct laryngoscopy and/or bronchoscopy. Tracheostomy may be necessary in some cases.

Congenital Subglottic Stenosis

Congenital subglottic stenosis accounts for a third of all congenital laryngeal defects. Thought to be due to an overabundance of mucosa in the subglottic area, it is the second most common cause of upper airway obstruction in infants under 1 year requiring tracheostomy. (The most common cause is tracheal stenosis secondary to endotracheal intubation.) The definitive treatment includes laser excision of the stenosis and laryngotracheal reconstruction.

Miscellaneous

Other, less common congenital anomalies include aortic arch defects—hemangioma, cystic hygroma, laryngeal atresia, web cyst, and laryngocele.

Acquired

Foreign Body Airway Obstruction

Each year, about 400 children 5 years of age or younger die in the United States from foreign body airway obstruction.[13] Approximately 75% of foreign-body airway obstructions (FBAO) occur in children under 3 years of age. Fortunately, for reasons not well understood, its incidence is declining, although this is of little consolation to the parents of a child who becomes a statistic. Food is one of the more common offending agents, particularly hot dogs, peanuts, and spherically shaped candies or fruits. Small plastic toys are also often implicated.[14] Foreign-body airway obstruction commonly occurs when a child is eating while exercising. Small children (3 years and under) tend to put small objects in their mouth or up their nose that can be swallowed or inhaled during episodes of crying, laughing, or exercise. Most foreign bodies involving the airway lodge in the mainstem bronchi. Life-threatening obstruction occurs when they lodge in the larynx or trachea. Large round objects or cylindrical-shaped objects are most dangerous and have the worst prognosis.[15]

The approach to FBAO depends upon the degree of obstruction, the state of consciousness, and whether the incident was witnessed or not. The majority of FBAOs (88%) are heralded by a choking episode; therefore it is important to ask any present witnesses whether choking occurred.[16] Management in children has many similarities to that in adults, so emphasis will be placed on the differences that pertain to children.

In an **infant** back blows and chest thrusts are recommended to relieve complete airway obstruction. The baby is placed prone, head down, on the rescuer's arm (Fig. 11.10), which in turn rests on the rescuer's thigh. Five back blows are delivered. The infant is then turned supine, head down, and five chest thrusts are

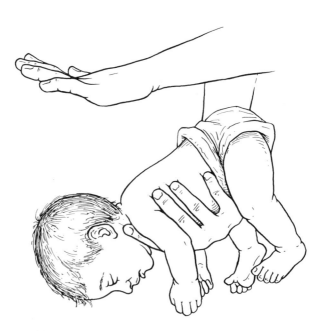

Figure 11.10. Back blows for infant resuscitation.

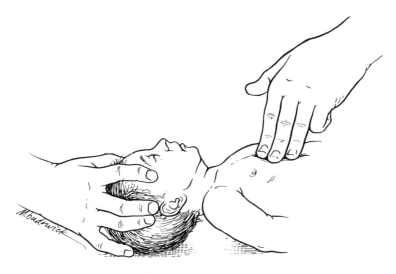

FIGURE 11.11. Chest compressions in an infant.

delivered (Fig. 11.11). The oropharynx should be inspected following these maneuvers to see if a foreign body is visible. Figure 11.12 presents guidelines for the initial and definitive hospital treatment of this emergency.

When dealing with children older than one year, a series of Heimlich maneuvers is performed, in either the upright or supine position. The oropharynx should

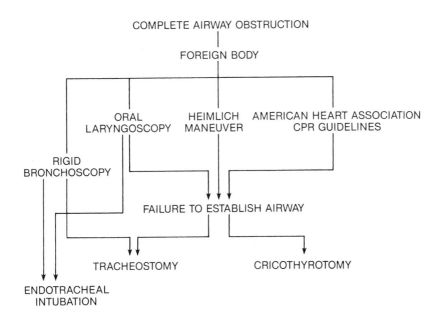

FIGURE 11.12. The management of complete airway obstruction. (Modified from Badgwell JM, et al. *Can J Anaesth.* 1987;34:90, with permission.)

be inspected in between series. Blind finger sweeps are not recommended at any time. If after 2 series of age-specific maneuvers in a prehospital setting airway obstruction persists, one should inspect the airway, and if a foreign body is seen efforts should be made to remove it with a Magill forceps. If the foreign body is in the airway but out of reach, intubation may serve to move the foreign body into one or other mainstem bronchi, thereby relieving complete obstruction. If all of these maneuvers fail, a surgical airway is your only choice. See Figure 11.13[17] for out-of-hospital management of FBAO. In a **child** with incomplete airway obstruction the parent(s) may describe an acute episode of coughing, wheezing, and respiratory distress followed by a symptomless interval, or a history of persistent wheezing may be given. If the problem goes undetected for some time, the child may develop pneumonia, atelectasis, a lung abscess, bronchiectasis, bronchial perforation, or pulmonary hemorrhage. Symptoms include coughing, gagging, cyanosis, and stridor. When they occur in any child, foreign-body aspiration should be high on the list of diagnoses. When organic material (e.g., food) is inhaled, it may go undetected for a time, but it eventually expands and an inflammatory reaction occurs in the bronchi. Organic material in the tracheobronchial tree can do one of three things: (1) it may be so small as to cause little if any obstruction; (2) it may cause complete obstruction during all phases of respiration, resulting in absorption atelectasis; or (3) it may cause obstructive emphysema secondary to air-trapping during expiration. (Obstruction is mainly expiratory because the increased intrathoracic pressure during expiration narrows the lower airway.)

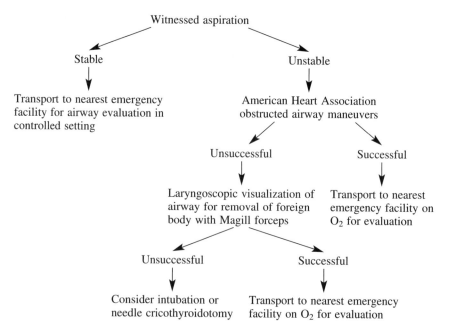

FIGURE 11.13. Algorithm outlining the management of airway foreign bodies. (From Bank,[17] with permission.)

When a child presents with symptoms of incomplete airway obstruction, the following X-ray views should be obtained:

Anterior–posterior (AP) and lateral neck
Inspiratory and expiratory chest
Barium swallow
Airway fluoroscopy

If the obstruction is caused by a radiolucent object at the level of the bronchi, the classical picture will be one of obstructive emphysema on the side where the foreign body is located. Although a chest X ray taken during inspiration may appear relatively normal, one during expiration will reveal hyperinflation on the affected side with a mediastinal shift toward the opposite side. It is therefore crucial to take chest X rays during both inspiration and expiration (Fig. 11.14).

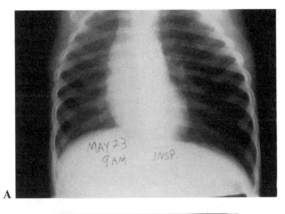

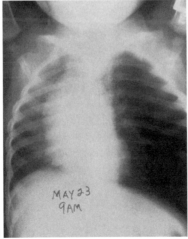

FIGURE 11.14. A radiolucent foreign body in the left bronchus. **A.** Inspiratory and, **B.** Expiratory films.

If a radiopaque object is lodged in the larynx, trachea, or a bronchus, radiological findings may be normal or may reveal ipsilateral obstructive emphysema or absorption atelectasis because the object is readily seen. If the object is inhaled, the diagnosis is much easier. (Incidentally, even a narrow foreign body accidentally swallowed may be large enough to encroach upon the airway and cause symptoms. For example, ingestion of a jack caused symptoms in the child shown in Figure 11.15). Any child with suspected foreign-body aspiration should be brought to a hospital immediately for further investigation.

The procedure for incomplete airway obstruction is as follows:

1. Immediate bronchoscopy for respiratory distress
2. Urgent bronchoscopy if no distress (wait for stomach to empty)

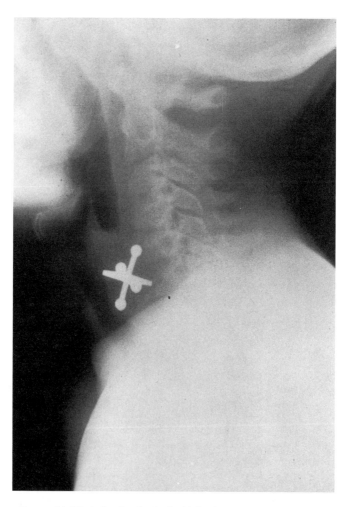

FIGURE 11.15. A foreign body (jack) in the esophagus of a child.

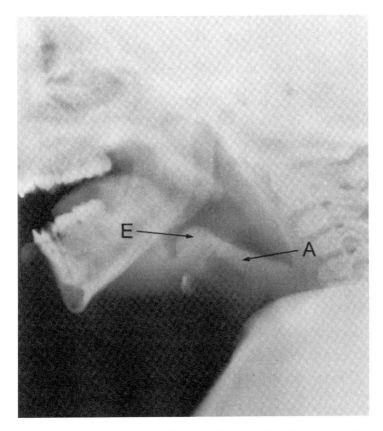

FIGURE 11.16. Epiglottitis in a 3-year-old boy produced marked thickening of the epiglottis (E) and aryepiglottic folds (A) seen on this lateral radiograph of the neck. Also note the overdistention of the pharynx. (From Gay BB. Radiographic anatomy and pathology of the child's airway. In: Murphy CH, Murphy MR, eds. *Radiology for Anesthesia and Critical Care.* New York: Churchill Livingstone; 1987:205, with permission.)

3. Semielective bronchoscopy after workup for suspected aspiration (within 24 to 48 hours)
4. Mist tent for 24 hours with oxygen enrichment after bronchoscopy
5. Chest physiotherapy after bronchoscopy

Figure 11.16 provides information about the anesthetic management of a child with incomplete airway obstruction.

Acute Epiglottitis

Acute epiglottitis is still one of the most feared forms of upper airway obstruction in children. Fortunately, the incidence of hemophilus influenza type B acute epiglottitis has decreased dramatically with the introduction of the conjugate vaccine. However, other organisms cause epiglottitis viz. *Staphylococcus aureus*,

Streptococcus pneumonia, and beta-hemolytic streptococci. *H. influenzae* type B disease still occurs in unvaccinated children. The disease usually occurs in children between ages 2 and 6 and occurs most frequently in the winter and spring months. The pathological features of acute epiglottitis include inflammation and swelling of mucous membranes covering the epiglottis, aryepiglottic folds, and other connective tissue structures and spaces in the supra- and paraglottic regions. The clinical features of acute epiglottis include: "a rapid onset of sore throat and pyrexia; airway obstruction may develop in less than 24 hours. Classically, the child appears toxic, adopts a sitting position, has a muffled cough, and experiences difficulty swallowing. As the condition progresses the child appears toxic, develops dysphagia, dysphonia and drooling." The classic posture of a child in advanced clinical stages of acute epiglottitis is as follows: the child is typically sitting bolt upright, leaning forward with the mouth wide-open, the jaw subluxed, and the head extended.

The white cell count is usually elevated ($> 10,000$) with marked neutrophilia, but the diagnosis is made on clinical grounds. In less acute cases, lateral neck X ray may be helpful (Fig. 11.16). A lateral X ray of the neck reveals the following classic radiologic features of acute epiglottitis: a thickened epiglottis (the "thumb sign") and swollen aryepiglottic folds; and the subglottic region appears normal.

When the diagnosis of acute epiglottitis is suspected, the opinions of the pediatrician, ENT surgeon, radiologist, and anesthesiologist should be sought. If the airway is severely obstructed, radiological studies should be deferred and arrangements made to transport the child to the operating room. An anesthesiologist should remain with the patient at all times.

Premature examination of the airway may precipitate acute obstruction from laryngospasm. In the past it was considered a major violation of protocol to examine the airway of a child with suspected acute epiglottitis while the child was awake. Common sense tells us the diagnostic yield from such an aggressive approach would be low, so therefore we recommend examination under anesthesia in most circumstances. However, if for some reason the examination is to be carried out in a conscious child, it should be carried out in an operating room and in the presence of airway experts who are prepared to intubate or intervene surgically at any time. Of course, awake intervention may be required without warning if complete airway obstruction occurs at any time or place. Most experts recommend airway examination under general anesthesia. The most experienced anesthesiologist available should be assigned to the task. Optimally, the child should remain sitting while oxygen and halothane or sevoflurane are administered by mask. Induction should be done slowly, with intravenous access established after the child has been anesthetized. It may take as long as 20 minutes to attain an adequate level of anesthesia to allow airway examination.

The vital signs need to be checked frequently throughout the induction, since these patients may be hypovolemic secondary to dehydration; thus, even a low concentration of halothane can cause hypotension. It is a good idea to administer about 10 ml/kg of a salt-rich solution once the intravenous line is established.

After adequate anesthesia has been achieved, the airway is exposed and an endotracheal tube is inserted under direct vision. It is important to have a wide selection of tubes available. On the initial intubation attempt, a tube at least one full size less than that predicted for the patient's age group should be used. Once the child has been stabilized, it is preferable to replace the oral tube with a correct-fitting nasal tube, which must be secured with great care. If intubation cannot be achieved, a tracheostomy must be performed.

Once the airway is established, antibiotic therapy should be instituted and must be effective against *H. influenzae* type B strains and other organisms capable of causing acute epiglottitis; blood cultures should be taken before commencing antibiotic therapy. The algorithm shown in Figure 11.17[17] may be helpful when confronted with a case of acute epiglottitis.

Croup

Croup is a crowing or barking sound caused by a narrowing of the upper airway in children. It is frequently associated with a viral laryngotracheobronchitis in small children. Parainfluenza virus types 1 and 2 are the most frequent offending agents and have an incidence of 1.5 per 100 children under 6 years of age per annum. Croup may also be caused by respiratory syncytial virus and influenza A and B. It may also occur secondary to trauma from upper airway manipulation. Croup is characterized by mucosal and submucosal edema of the mucous membranes of the airway in the subglottic region, which are typically loosely at-

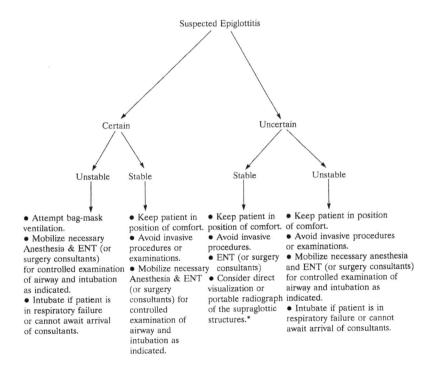

FIGURE 11.17. Algorithm outlining the management of epiglottis. *This should only be done in a controlled setting in which preparation for immediate intubation has been arranged. (From Bank and Krug,[17] with permission.)

tached to the larynx in this region and prone to edema. A 1-mm narrowing of the diameter of the airway in a 2-year-old causes a marked reduction in the cross-sectional area of the trachea (Fig 1.23). Viral diseases of the airway are also associated with an increased production of secretions, which are often viscous. These factors combine to reduce the cross-sectional area of an already small airway. Children with croup usually present with a brief history of an upper respiratory tract infection, with nasal discharge and a "croupy" cough and stridor. The stridor is most marked during inspiration. Fever is not a usual feature of the disease and the children do not usually appear to be sick, in contrast to acute epiglottitis. Children with croup do not usually complain of a sore throat. A–P and lateral neck X rays helps to rule out acute epiglottitis (Fig. 11.18).

One major problem in dealing with croup is deciding whom to admit to the hospital. Some 5% to 10% of children will require admission, but the remainder can usually be managed in the emergency room or at home. The vast majority are treated merely with a humidifier in the home. Any child who is hypoxic or has symptoms and signs of respiratory failure, tachypnea, dyspnea, cyanosis, lethargy, or retractions should be admitted to hospital.

The first line of treatment in the emergency room is humidification, and some patients respond solely to that treatment, even though humidification does nothing to reduce subglottic edema. Aerosolized racemic epinephrine is the treatment of choice for children with moderate to severe stridor. The recommended dose of epinephrine is 0.25 ml of a 1:1000 solution in children under 6 months; children older than 6 months should receive 0.5 ml. It is now considered safe to discharge a child

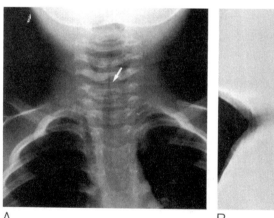
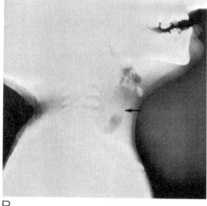

A   B

FIGURE 11.18. **A.** Croup in a $1^{1}/_{2}$-year-old boy caused the pharynx to be distended on inspiration. The laryngeal vestibule and subglottic area are narrowed (arrow). **B.** The lateral radiography of another patient with croup shows the subglottic area (arrow) to be narrow, and the trachea is distended during expiration. (From Gay BB. Radiographic anatomy and pathology of the child's airway. In: Murphy CH, Murphy MR, eds. *Radiology for Anesthesia and Critical Care.* New York: Churchill Livingstone; 1987:209, with permission.)

TABLE 11.9. Downes scoring system for upper airway obstruction

Physical finding	SCORE		
	0	1	2
Stridor	None	Inspiratory	Inspiratory and expiratory
Cough	None	Hoarse cry	Bark
Retractions and nasal flaring	None	Flaring with suprasternal retractions	Flaring with suprasternal, subcostal, and intercostal retractions
Cyanosis	None	In air	In 40% oxygen
Inspiratory breath sounds	Normal	Harsh with wheezing or rhonchi	Delayed

The maximum score is 10, normal 0. A score of 4 or more requires therapy. Any patient with a score of 7 or more who does not respond to medical management may require immediate insertion of an artificial tracheal airway.
Source: From Downes,[20] with permission.

from the emergency room after a suitable interval, following an aerosolized epinephrine treatment.[18] What role do steroids play in the treatment of croup? A recent metaanalysis involving several studies has shown that the need for endotracheal intubation is significantly reduced in hospitalized children who receive steroid treatment.[19] Dexamethasone is the steroid most frequently used and the recommended dose is 0.6 to 1 mg/kg IM, IV, or orally. Any child who receives an aerosolized racemic epinephrine treatment should also receive steroids.[17]

Airway intervention should be avoided if possible. However, if it becomes necessary, the preferred route is oral—at least initially. Tracheostomy is rarely necessary. To help answer the question of when an artificial airway should be placed, Downes[20] has devised a scoring system that should be used as a guide (Table 11.9).

Airway intervention is required when oxygenation and ventilation become compromised. This decision should be made in the operating room with an ENT surgeon and an anesthesiologist present. During laryngoscopy it is preferable to avoid narcotics, to allow these patients the full benefit of the respiratory drive. To reduce the amount of secretions, anticholinergic drugs should be administered. Many ENT surgeons prefer laryngoscopy under general anesthesia to determine the amount of swelling that remains. A final decision regarding intubation is then based upon these findings.

TABLE 11.10. Historical findings: croup and epiglottitis

	Croup	Epiglottitis
Onset	Gradual	Abrupt
Constitutional symptoms	Mild	Severe
Cough	Barking	Weak to none
Sore throat	Present	Severe
Dysphagia	May be present	Severe
Voice changes	Hoarseness	Muffled dysphonia progressing to aphonia
Drooling	Absent	May be present

Source: Diaz[21], with permission.

TABLE 11.11. Physical findings: croup and epiglottitis

	Croup	Epiglottitis
Protective posture	Absent	Present
Fever	Low	High
Cyanosis	Usually absent	Usually present
Stridor	Present	Mild to none
Nasal flaring	May develop	Usually present
Retractions	Initially mild when occur	Initially marked
Diaphragmatic and abdominal excursions	Not usually apparent	Marked
Heart rate	Sinus tachycardia	Sinus tachycardia, bradycardia with severe hypoxia and preceding cardiac arrest
Respiratory rate	Tachypnea	Tachypnea

Source: Diaz,[21] with permission.

The textbook descriptions of acute epiglottitis and croup are not always seen in clinical practice. Quite often there is considerable overlap between the two conditions.[21] If you are having difficulty distinguishing between acute epiglottitis and croup, Tables 11.10, 11.11, and 11.12 may be useful. Furthermore, always include foreign-body airway in the differential diagnosis. Complete details about the controversies surrounding these acute conditions are beyond the scope of this book. For further information, refer to articles by Barker[22] and Fried.[23] An algorithm outlining the management of croup is seen in Figure 11.19.

Acute Bacterial Laryngotracheobronchitis

This form of croup is clinically indistinguishable from the viral form, especially in the early stages, but with progression the secretions become copious and appear infected. It is much more incapacitating than viral croup. To determine the underlying etiology, you need cultures from the respiratory tract. The most common organisms cultured are *Streptococcus agalactiae, Streptococcus pneumoniae, Staphylococcus aureus,* and occasionally *Haemophilus influenzae.* The management is similar in many respects to that of the viral form. Humidification is instituted as soon as possible. Oxygen is administered if necessary. The ap-

TABLE 11.12. Management: croup and epiglottitis

	Croup	Epiglottitis
Oxygen	Essential	Essential
Airway	No intervention if possible, tracheostomy or short-duration nasotracheal intubation	Nasotracheal tube or tracheostomy
Humidification	Essential	Essential
Aerosolized vasoconstrictors	Beneficial	Ineffective
Steroids	Unproven	Unproven
Antibiotics	Ineffective	Essential

Source: Diaz,[21] with permission.

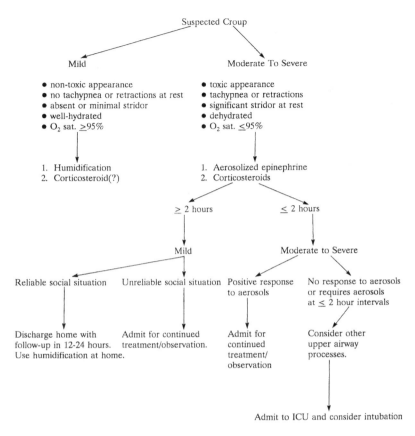

FIGURE 11.19. Algorithm outlining the management of croup. (From Bank and Krug,[17] with permission.)

propriate antibiotic therapy is commenced. Tracheostomy may be necessary to suction the secretions.

Spasmodic Croup

This condition is characterized by sudden laryngospasm of unknown etiology. Classically, it occurs at night and the child wakes up with a croupy cough. Fever, if present, is usually mild. Occasionally, the parent(s) will bring the child to the hospital and note a marked improvement on arrival. The condition also responds to humidification and racemic epinephrine. Steroids may be necessary, because in the early stages, the condition is indistinguishable from viral croup. Airway intervention is rarely needed.

Retropharyngeal Abscess

Retropharyngeal abscess is an infection in the space that lies between the buccopharyngeal fascia and the prevertebral fascia, which extends from the base of the skull down to T1 (see Fig. 1.9). Infection in this area may occur from direct trauma, or it may spread from a nasopharyngeal or middle ear infection, or from hematologic or lymphatic spread. Bacteria responsible for this infection include gram-negative rods, anaerobes, *Staphylococcus aureus*, and group A hemolytic streptococcus.

Retropharyngeal abscess usually occurs in children under 3 years of age. They usually complain of a sore throat and a stiff neck and they are quite often febrile. The diagnosis can be easily confused with acute epiglottitis. The symptoms and sighs are usually unilateral. A stiff neck and torticollis help distinguish this condition from acute epiglottitis.

If the clinical signs are confusing, a lateral X ray of the neck taken in extension is recommended. If the width of the retropharyngeal space at the level of C2 is twice that of the diameter of vertebral body, the likelihood of it being a retropharyngeal abscess is very high (sensitivity of approximately 90%).[24]

Airway compromise may occur in these cases, but generally once the diagnosis is made and the appropriate antibiotic prescribed, these children improve quickly. Surgical drainage may be required in some cases.

"Kissing Tonsils" and Sleep Apnea Syndrome

Occasionally, a patient will suffer from the peculiar syndrome of hypertrophied lymphoid tissue associated with sleep apnea. Anesthesiologists and other individuals taking care of these patients should be fully aware of the danger of administering narcotics, which can cause respiratory depression, during the preoperative and postoperative periods.

Laryngeal Edema (Allergic)

Occasionally, a patient will develop an acute allergic reaction following a bee sting or other insect bite that leads to life-threatening laryngeal edema. These children must be treated aggressively with epinephrine, corticosteroids, and antihistamines. And if airway compromise occurs, prompt intubation or tracheostomy may be necessary.

For a more complete summary of upper airway obstruction in children, refer to Maze and Block.[25]

Management of the Child with Impending Airway Obstruction

In no area of medicine is closer cooperation required between the anesthesiologist, surgeon, and nursing personnel than when treating a child with upper airway obstruction. Traditionally, in many large centers, children presenting with acute epiglottitis are treated by protocol, and it would be logical if we instituted the same protocol when dealing with any child with upper airway obstruction. In most instances, the anesthesiologist has time to prepare for the emergency. However, if a child presents *in extremis*, there may be no other option but to secure the airway immediately. The first line of approach should always be bag/mask ventilation with 100% oxygen. In many instances, immediate improvement follows. If bag/mask ventilation does not work, you should insert an LMA. If, and when, oxygenation improves, the next step would be to attempt oral endotracheal intubation. Failing that, your only option is a surgical airway. Cricothyrotomy is not recommended in children age 12 and under because of the risk of serious permanent disruption of the airway. Needle cricothyrotomy only should be used as a "last ditch" procedure in children.

The moment the anesthesiologist is alerted that a child has upper airway obstruction, he or she must remain with the patient at all times. Children presenting with upper airway obstruction are often extremely apprehensive, and every effort must be made to calm them. It is often helpful to have one parent remain with the child, at least until the procedure is about to begin. Children suffering from upper airway obstruction usually find the supine position intolerable. Therefore, they should be allowed to remain in the sitting position for as long as possible.

In many situations, proper handling of acute upper airway obstruction in the child requires general anesthesia. With the child in the sitting position, the anesthesiologist should gradually induce anesthesia by delivering a mixture of oxygen and an inhalation agent. Firm application of the mask to the patient's face will only frighten the patient and lead to further agitation. The anesthesia circuit, without mask, should be gradually brought closer to the patient's face. Individuals in the operating room should be encouraged to go about their business without making too much noise. When unconsciousness occurs, an IV should be established. (A tracheostomy set should already be opened.) Some patients suffering from airway obstruction may be volume-depleted because of fever and the inability to eat or drink; therefore, you should be very careful about administering potent inhalation agents, which can cause hypotension. The blood pressure should be carefully monitored. If a significant airway problem is suspected, an arterial line should be inserted to obtain subsequent blood samples.

Sometimes it is quite difficult to judge the depth of anesthesia in these patients. However, with an IV in place, it is reasonable to supplement the inhalation agent by administering thiopental, propofol, and lidocaine. There is considerable controversy about the use of neuromuscular blocking drugs in children with impending upper airway obstruction. Although succinylcholine is used routinely by clinicians in some centers, others shun the use of neuromuscular blockers altogether in this situation. Thus, there are no hard-and-fast rules; however, if you do paralyze a child in the process of securing the airway, the onus rests heavily upon you to maintain adequate oxygenation at all times.

An array of endotracheal tubes and laryngoscope blades should be ready for immediate use. Atropine in a dose of 0.01 mg/kg should be administered intravenously. When an adequate level of anesthesia is achieved, laryngoscopy is performed, and an endotracheal tube that is at least one size smaller than normal should be inserted. When the airway is secured, the ENT surgeon is likely to perform a laryngoscopy with the endotracheal tube in place. If the airway was easy to secure, it may be reasonable to switch to a nasotracheal tube at this time. The

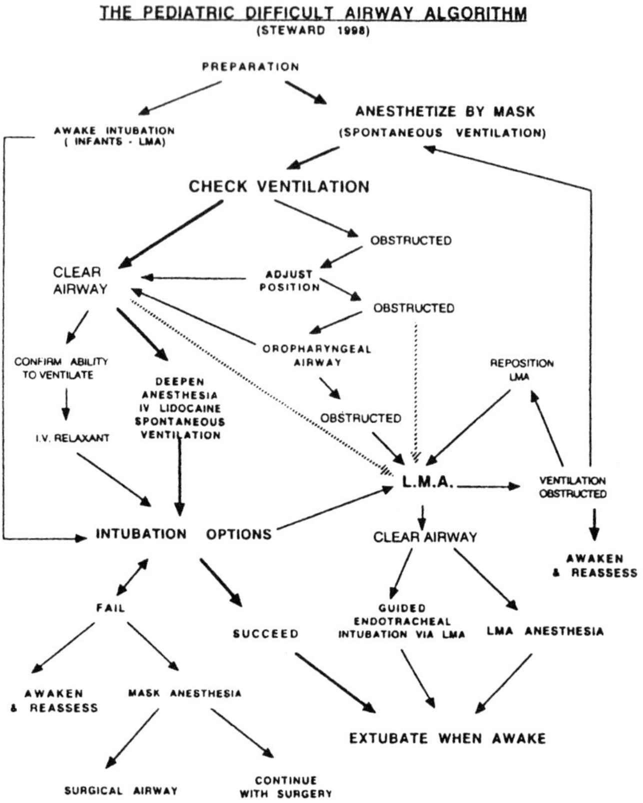

THE PEDIATRIC DIFFICULT AIRWAY ALGORITHM
(STEWARD 1998)

PREPARATION

AWAKE INTUBATION
(INFANTS - LMA)

ANESTHETIZE BY MASK
(SPONTANEOUS VENTILATION)

CHECK VENTILATION

OBSTRUCTED

CLEAR
AIRWAY

ADJUST
POSITION

OBSTRUCTED

CONFIRM ABILITY
TO VENTILATE

OROPHARYNGEAL
AIRWAY

REPOSITION
LMA

DEEPEN
ANESTHESIA
IV LIDOCAINE
SPONTANEOUS
VENTILATION

OBSTRUCTED

I.V. RELAXANT

L.M.A.

VENTILATION
OBSTRUCTED

INTUBATION OPTIONS

CLEAR AIRWAY

AWAKEN
& REASSESS

FAIL

GUIDED
ENDOTRACHEAL
INTUBATION VIA LMA

LMA ANESTHESIA

SUCCEED

AWAKEN
& REASSESS

MASK ANESTHESIA

EXTUBATE WHEN AWAKE

SURGICAL AIRWAY

CONTINUE
WITH SURGERY

FIGURE 11.20. (From Steward D,[26] with permission.)

endotracheal tube should be securely taped, and the child should be sedated and should have restraints placed on his arms before he awakens. Nursing personnel must be given instructions as to how to handle this child postoperatively. In addition to ensuring that the endotracheal tube remains in place, the nurse must suction it on a regular basis to prevent it from becoming obstructed. The inspired gases should be humidified and a minimum amount of continuous positive air pressure (CPAP) should be applied. A physician capable of reintubating the tracheal should be immediately at hand at all times.

Steward has recommended the following algorithm for the child presenting with airway obstruction (Fig. 11.20).[26]

Tracheostomy in the Child

Tracheostomy may occasionally be a lifesaving procedure in children, but many have died as a result of immediate or late complications of tracheostomy. In fact, the mortality rate is quoted as 10% for each year that the tracheostomy remains in place.

Emergency tracheostomy in the child is dangerous at all stages. Not only is the anatomy smaller and more difficult to expose, but general anesthesia is almost always essential to perform this operation satisfactorily.

Preparation

The following recommendations should be adhered to if possible: 100% oxygen should be administered, if at all possible; nitrous oxide should not be used. Ideally, tracheostomy is performed after first securing the airway with an endotracheal tube. Unfortunately, this is not always possible, and you may have to "make do" with bag/mask ventilation with or without an anesthetic. Children with severe airway obstruction often can be adequately oxygenated but inadequately ventilated. Carbon dioxide narcosis then makes them insensible to the pain of surgery. The worst situation is having to perform a tracheostomy in some remote part of the hospital with inadequate lighting. The operating room is the ideal place for this operation.

Technique

Tracheostomy in children is quite a difficult procedure simply because the structures are so much smaller than in adults. If at all possible, this procedure should be performed by ENT or other surgeons trained to do so. Refer to an ENT textbook for technical details about this procedure.

Complications

Tension pneumothorax is a danger before, during, and after tracheostomy. The anesthesiologist is well advised to use the educated hand to detect subtle changes in compliance of the lungs during bag ventilation rather than commit these patients to the mechanical ventilation. The surgeon should always insert durable sutures on either side of the tracheal incision to facilitate rapid replacement of the tracheostomy tube, should it come out. Excessive torque exerted by the breathing circuit may force the tube from the stoma. Occasionally, tracheostomy tubes may be incorrectly replaced and false passages created, leading to subcutaneous emphysema and tension pneumothorax. Nursing care, including tracheobronchial toilet, is also vitally important in preventing complications. Mucous plugs are a constant danger. These children should be closely watched at all times, especially within the first week of surgery. Given the mortality rate associated with this procedure, they should never be alone for any length of time.

One of the major problems when dealing with airway problems in children is the lack of uniformity when it comes to selecting endotracheal tubes, bronchoscopes, and tracheostomy tubes. It is a constant source of confusion to anesthesiologists, ENT surgeons, and others who deal with these problems on a day-today basis. Ideally, the nomenclature needs to be standardized for all airway equipment.

Summary

This chapter familiarized you with some of the special airway problems encountered in pediatric practice. The pediatric airway is different from that of the adult, not just in caliber but also in structure and function. In order to clarify some of these points, the anatomy of the airways of the adult and infant were compared. The differences in basic airway management and CPR in infants and children also were highlighted. Resuscitation of the newborn is a demanding task that should only be delegated to clinicians well versed in neonatology and airway management. The salient points of resuscitation of the newborn and the technical aspects of airway management including endotracheal intubation in infants and children were covered. Finally, information on the more common airway problems occurring in this age group was presented. With this information you should be in a much better position to deal competently with airway problems in children.

References

1. Godinez RI. Special problems in pediatric anesthesia. *Int Anesthesol Clin.* 1985;23:88.
2. Pueschel SM. Atlanto-axial subluxation in Downs syndrome [letter]. *Lancet.* 1960:1983.
3. Introduction to the international guidelines 2000 for CPR and ECG [part 1]. *Circulation.* 2000;102(suppl 1):1–3421.
4. Standard Guideline CPR JAMA 1992;268;21:2172–83.
5. Ayre P. Anaesthesia for intracranial operation: new technique. *Lancet.* 1937;1:561.
6. Rees GJ. Neonatal anesthesia. *Br Med Bull.* 1958;14:38.
7. Roy RN, Betheras FR. The Melbourne Chart—a logical guide to neonatal resuscitation. *Anaesth Intensive Care.* 1990;18:348–357.
8. Apgar V. Proposal for a new method of evaluation of the newborn infant. *Curr Res Anesth Analg.* 1953;32:260.
9. Elliott RD. Neonatal Resuscitation: the NRP Guidelines. *Can J Anaesth.* 1994;41: 742–752.
10. Paterson SJ, Byrne PJ, Molesky MG, Seal RF, Finucane BT. Neonatal resuscitation using the laryngeal mask airway. *Anesthesiology.* 1994;80:1248–1253.
11. *Injury Chart Book, Health in the US 1996–1997.* Washington, D.C.: National Center for Health Statistics; 1997:25–26.
12. Donnelly KJ, et al. Three-dimensional magnetic resonance imaging evaluation of pediatric tracheobronchial tree. *Laryngoscope.* 104:1425–1429.
13. National Safety Council. *Accident Facts.* 1984.
14. Harris CS, et al. Children asphyxiation by food: a national analysis and overview. *JAMA.* 1984;251:2231.
15. Lima J. Laryngeal foreign bodies in children: a persistent, life-threatening problem. *Laryngoscope.* 1989;99:415–420.

16. Esclamado R, Richardson M. Laryngeal foreign bodies in children: a comparison with bronchial foreign bodies. *Am J Dis Child.* 1987;141:259–262.
17. Bank DE, Krug SE. New approaches to upper airway disease. *Emerg Med Clin North Am.* 1995;13(2):473–487.
18. Kelley P, Simon J. Racemic epinephrine use in croup and disposition. *Am J Emerg Med.* 1992;10:181–183.
19. Cressman W, Myer C. Diagnosis and management of croup and epiglottitis. *Ped Clin North Am.* 1994;41:265–276.
20. Downes JJ. Pediatric intensive care: Annual refresher course lectures. ASA, 1974.
21. Diaz JH: Croup and epiglottitis in children. *Anes Analg.* 1985;64:621–633.
22. Barker GA. Current management of croup and epiglottitis. *Ped Clin North Am.* 1979;26:565.
23. Fried MP. Controversies in the management of supraglottitis and croup. *Ped Clin North Am.* 1979;26:931.
24. Coulthard M. Retropharyngeal abscess. *Arch Dis Child.* 1991;66:1227–1230.
25. Maze A, Block E. Stridor in patients. *Anesthesiology.* 1979;50:132.
26. Steward D. *IARS Review Course Lectures.* 1999.

12
Mechanical Ventilation and Respiratory Support

In the last decade, new strategies involving the management of mechanical ventilation and intensive respiratory support have been introduced. Much work has been directed toward understanding the causes, pathology, and the treatment of patients with acute lung injury/acute respiratory distress syndrome (ALI/ARDS).

Ventilator design and technology has advanced, offering more options to the clinician. New weaning techniques have been proposed. Ethical considerations are being debated with respect to patients' wishes about the need for intubation. Importantly, research is being designed to evaluate many of the aspects of mechanical ventilation and respiratory support that were previously taken for granted, dropped from practice, or introduced with little or no scientific justification.

Since airway management does not stop with intubation, the first part of this chapter will cover the **basic aspects of ventilatory and respiratory support** in detail. The reader should understand the indications for mechanical ventilation, how to manage a ventilator, how to wean a patient from mechanical support, when and how to extubate, and how to troubleshoot basic problems.

The second part of the chapter will present many of the recent (and sometimes controversial) practices and therapies now under scrutiny.

Basic Aspects of Ventilatory and Respiratory Support

The basic goals of respiratory support are **oxygenation** and **ventilation** of the patient. A third goal of **airway protection** is implied. This section of the chapter will be presented sequentially from selection of a ventilator, initial ventilatory orders, weaning, and extubation. Finally, complications and troubleshooting will be discussed.

Selection of a Ventilator

Practically speaking, the ventilators used in a typical intensive care unit are positive-pressure units delivering ventilation to an intubated patient. Other types of ventilation (negative pressure and mask ventilation) will be mentioned in the last section of the chapter.

The respiratory therapy department of a hospital, with input from clinicians, selects, operates, and maintains the ventilatory equipment. Modern ventilators are computer-controlled units that can deliver all of the popular modes of ventilatory support. These modes include the following:

Commonly Utilized Modes of Ventilation[1]

CMV: Controlled mechanical ventilation
IMV: Intermittent mandatory ventilation
SIMV: Synchronous intermittent mandatory ventilation
PSV: Pressure support ventilation
PCV: Pressure-controlled ventilation
PACV: Pressure-assisted controlled ventilation
IRV: Inverse-ratio ventilation
VCV: Volume-controlled ventilation
VAV: Volume-assisted ventilation
VACV: Volume-assisted controlled ventilation

TABLE 12.1. Application of breath function (phase variables)

Function	Mode	Primary parameter	Comment
Initiation	Control	Predetermined time interval	Machine triggered
	Assist	Threshold negative airway pressure	Patient triggered
Limit	Volume	Delivery at preset tidal volume	Airway pressure variable
	Pressure	Attainment of preset airway pressure	Tidal volume variable
Cycle-off	Volume	Preset volume achieved	
	Pressure	Preset pressure achieved	
	Time	Predetermined time interval passed	Inspiratory pause (zero flow)
	Flow	Decline to preset minimum flow rate	Patient inspiratory flow pattern

Source: Sladen,[1] with permission.

The mode of ventilation selected is dictated by the condition of the patient and the preference of the clinician.

In addition, the ventilator delivers gas flow to patients breathing spontaneously as well as supports various end-expiratory maneuvers such as **CPAP** (continuous positive airway pressure) and **PEEP** (positive end-expiratory pressure).

The ventilator also monitors various patient ventilatory parameters, preset mechanical parameters, and ventilator function. Alarms alert the clinician or the therapist if preset limits are not maintained.

The ventilatory cycle is defined by three functions (phase variables): **initiation, limit,** and **cycle-off.** Table 12.1 summarizes these functions that change with the **mode** of ventilation selected.

The type of breath delivered is defined both by the machine and the patient as tabulated in Table 12.2.

Many companies manufacture ventilators that are in current use. Following is a description of one ventilator that is used in many institutions. It is offered as an example of a machine that incorporates the latest technology with practical design applications.

Siemens Servo Ventilator 300/300A
(Siemens-Elema AB, SE-171 95 Solna, Sweden)

The Siemens Servo Ventilator 300/300A (Fig. 12.1) will be described to exemplify a popular ventilator in widespread clinical use. The versatile design of this ventilator features current technological advancements in mechanical respiratory

TABLE 12.2. Breath types defined by the machine vs. patient control phase variable

Breath type	Initiation (trigger)	Limit (target)	Cycle-off
Mandatory	Machine	Machine	Machine
Assisted	Patient	Machine	Machine
Supported	Patient	Machine	Patient
Spontaneous	Patient	Patient	Patient

Source: Sladen,[1] with permission.

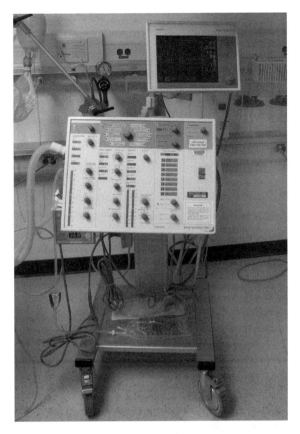

FIGURE 12.1. Siemens Servo Ventilator. (From Siemens,[3] with permission.)

support. The graphic monitor display allows the practitioner to access many physiologic parameters. Following is a summary of the ventilator's salient features.

General Description

The Siemens Servo Ventilator is a lung ventilator intended for neonatal, pediatric, and adult use. The ventilator has two main units, the control unit and the patient unit. A third unit, the Servo Screen 390 V2.0/3.X, with or without a carbon dioxide (CO_2) analyzer, provides a display of waveform and parameter information.[2] The Servo 300 is essentially the same as the 300A without the "Automode" function.[3]

The control unit contains the circuitry necessary to control ventilation. The patient unit is the ventilator.

Control Unit

The control unit has **knobs** that are used to set ventilator parameters, and **touch-pads** used to read alarm messages in memory, for use when setting the "Set Parameter Guide," for alternative information on the respiratory pattern displays, and during calibration procedures. The control unit also has many digital displays that are easy to read. Flow measurements and indicated volumes are referenced to standard pressure (760 mm Hg.)

Patient Unit

Ventilator gas flow is regulated by two gas modules, one for air and one for oxygen. Both modules contain bacterial filters. Flow and pressure are continuously measured by transducers, the information from which is compared with the control unit settings. Differences are corrected by flow valves. Pressures and flows are monitored in the inspiratory and expiratory limbs of the circuit. Oxygen concentration is also monitored. The expiratory limb contains a moisture trap. The distending airway pressure (PEEP) is regulated by the expiratory valve. Finally, patient breathing efforts used to trigger various modalities of ventilation are sensed in the expiratory limb of the circuit.

Technical Specifications of the Servo 300/300A

Following are some of the technical specifications of the Siemens Servo Ventilator 300/300A.[3]

General
Patient range: neonatal, pediatric, adult

Gas and Power Supply
Inlet gas pressure: (air and oxygen) 29 to 94 psi
Gas delivery system: microprocessor-controlled valves
Power supply: wall and battery backup (30 min.)

Alarms
Airway pressure
High continuous pressure
Oxygen concentration
Expired minute volume (upper and lower settings)
Apnea
Gas supply
Battery
Technical

Monitoring
Frequency (breath cycle time)
Pressures
Airway pressure
Tidal volumes (inspiratory and expiratory)
Flow rate
Oxygen concentration
Supply pressure
Battery voltage

Knob Settings
CMV frequency
SIMV frequency
Inspiration time
Pause time
Pressure control
Pressure support
PEEP
Trigger sensitivity
Trigger bias flow
Inspiration rise time
Preset tidal volume
Oxygen breaths
Start breath
Pause hold
Alarm silence (2-minute or reset)
Oxygen concentration
Automode (300A)

In summary, the Siemens Servo Ventilator 300/300A (Table 12.3) is one example of a popular, versatile, and clinically respected ventilator for use with all ages of patients. All clinically useful modalities of ventilation can be delivered with this ventilator. The company publishes many manuals describing the ventilator and provides company-sponsored seminars designed to promote safe and efficient use of the machine.[4]

TABLE 12.3. Modes of ventilation for the Siemens 300 and 300A

Controlled ventilation	
PC	Pressure-controlled ventilation
VC	Volume-controlled ventilation
PRVC	Pressure-regulated volume-controlled ventilation
Supported ventilation	
VS	Volume-supported ventilation
PS	Pressure-supported ventilation
CPAP	Continuous positive airway pressure
Combined ventilation	
SIMV (VC) + PS	Synchronized intermittent mandatory ventilation based on volume-controlled ventilation with pressure support
SIMV (PC) + PS	Synchronized intermittent mandatory ventilation based on pressure-controlled ventilation with pressure support
Combined ventilation SV 300A (automode)	
Pressure control/support (PC/S)	After two consecutive patient triggers, the ventilator
Volume control/support (VC/S)	shifts from controlled to supported ventilation and
Pressure reg. volume	remains in the support mode as long as the patient
Control/support	keeps triggering. If the patient stops breathing, the ventilator shifts back to the control mode.

Initial Ventilator Settings

After the patient is intubated, the tube position verified, the tube secured, and the ventilator tested, the initial ventilator orders can be written. Ventilator orders vary depending on the patient's age, pathology, weaning expectations, and operator preferences. Serial blood gas analyses verify oxygenation and ventilation. The initial blood gas can be taken 15 minutes after beginning support. The therapist and/or clinician should observe the patient and ventilator to ensure that the patient is well oxygenated and that the machine is functioning properly.

Five parameters are set when ventilatory support is initiated. The parameters are specified, along with limits, by orders from a physician. For example, the following orders could be written for an adult patient who does not have very severe or unusual pulmonary dysfunction:

Ventilatory Orders (Adult)

1. **FiO_2**
   100% until first blood gas result has been obtained. (FiO_2 may be decreased as the disease state permits, but oxyhemoglobin saturation should remain at or above 90%).
2. **Tidal Volume**
   8 to 12 cc/kg body weight (see discussion of acute respiratory distress syndrome (ARDS) later in the chapter
3. **Frequency**
   8 to 10 breaths per minute (IMV = 8 to 10/min)
4. **Distending Airway Pressure**
   The amount of CPAP or PEEP to be applied depends on the degree of shunt (venous admixture), the patient's lung compliance, and functional residual capacity (FRC). (Five cm H_2O is considered "physiologic PEEP" and should be applied if ventilatory support is extended beyond a few minutes.)
5. **Modality of Ventilation**
   The modality of ventilation depends on patient variables such as strength, depth of sedation, mental and nutritional status, and type and magnitude of pathology or injury. Weaning expectations and clinical preference also play roles in the modality of ventilation selected. Currently PSV, IMV, and PRVC (pressure-regulated volume-controlled ventilation) with appropriate levels of PEEP and CPAP are popular modalities of ventilation.

Comments on the Modality of Ventilation

No single modality of ventilation has proven to be superior to all others. Some modalities decrease the work of breathing, others allegedly increase patient comfort, and some are more likely to produce barotrauma, at least theoretically, while others demand patient participation. Clinical bias and experience often dictate the modality of ventilation selected. One should consider the expected duration

TABLE 12.4. Modalities of ventilation

Target	Mode	Breath trigger	Comments
Volume	CMV (VCV)	Mechanical	1. No spontaneous patient breath 2. Eliminates work of breathing 3. Pressure limit set at 60 cm H_2O 4. Patients often heavily sedated, anesthetized, paralyzed
Volume	VAV	Patient	1. Assisted breaths delivered at full volume 2. May induce respiratory alkalosis, hypokalemia, arrhythmias
Volume	VACV	Mechanical and patient	1. Machine delivers backup 2. May induce respiratory alkalosis
Volume	IMV	Mechanical and patient	1. Useful weaning modality 2. Preset IMV rate 3. No assisted breaths; therefore, hemodynamics may be improved with less likelihood of developing respiratory alkalosis 4. Higher work of breathing than with PSV
Pressure	PSV	Patient	1. High degree of patient-ventilator interaction 2. ? Improved patient comfort 3. Decreased work of breathing 4. Lower peak airway pressures 5. If PS level high, may induce respiratory alkalosis
Pressure	PCV and IRV	Mechanical	1. I:E ratio greater than 1:2 for IRV 2. May evoke patient discomfort 3. May adversely affect hemodynamics 4. May produce intrinsic PEEP
Pressure	PACV	Mechanical and patient	1. May be weaned to PSV as patient's condition improves and mean airway pressure decreases to 15 cm H_2O and inspiratory time < 0.8 s

of ventilatory support, the type and degree of pathology, as well as the weaning strategy when selecting the modality of ventilation. Table 12.4 presents a few salient comments on various modalities of ventilation summarized from an excellent review article on the subject.[1]

Pediatric and Neonatal Ventilation

Historically, neonates and premature infants were ventilated with IPPV (intermittent positive-pressure ventilation) and CPAP.[5] Over the past two decades, a better understanding of the pathogenesis of hyaline membrane disease (HMD), bronchopulmonary dysplasia (BPD), and retrolental fibroplasia have led clinicians to introduce many new therapeutic agents and techniques (surfactant, steroids, lower FiO_2) and to utilize newer monitors such as transcutaneous oxygen, carbon dioxide analyzers, and oxyhemoglobin saturation monitors. Many of the current modalities of ventilation have been used to support neonatal and pediatric patients, such as PSV,[6] proportional-assist ventilation,[7] and various assisted modalities.[5] Ventilators such as the Siemens 300 are designed for neonatal and pediatric use. It is beyond the scope of this book to discuss, in detail, the merits of each of these modalities. However, if the patient does not have severe lung disease, the following ventilator orders can be written for the typical patient under 10 kg:

Ventilator Orders for the Infant under 10 kg

1. FiO$_2$	Start with 100%, but wean to keep oxyhemoglobin saturation greater than 90%
2. Frequency	18 to 20 breaths per minute
3. Airway pressures	Inspiratory: limit to 18 to 20 cm H$_2$O
	Expiratory: 2 cm H$_2$O
4. PEEP or CPAP	As clinically indicated
5. Arterial blood gases	As indicated

Larger children may be ventilated with the same targets and goals as an adult. If a neonatal or premature patient presents with **severe** pulmonary dysfunction, a neonatalogist or pediatrician must be consulted to manage ventilatory support.

Weaning the Patient from Mechanical Ventilation

As the patient's condition improves, the pathology resolves, his alertness approaches his normal level, and paralytic agents are discontinued, mechanical support can be weaned toward eventual discontinuation and extubation. The rapidity of weaning depends primarily on resolution of the disease or condition that necessitated the initiation of ventilatory support. The five parameters delineated in the initial orders may be weaned in the following fashion:

1. FiO$_2$

   The FiO$_2$ should be weaned as quickly as possible to below 40%. The oxyhemoglobin saturation should remain at 90% or greater and the PaO$_2$ at or above 60 mm Hg.

2. Tidal Volume

   The volume delivered by the ventilator remains constant.

3. Frequency

   The preset ventilator rate can be weaned when the patient starts breathing spontaneously. Wean the rate to keep the arterial pH in the normal range (7.35 to 7.45).

4. PEEP or CPAP Level

   The level of distending airway pressure may be weaned by titrating it against the patient's PaO$_2$, the FiO$_2$ needed to maintain oxygenation goals, and clinical signs of the patient's work of breathing such as spontaneous respiratory rate and tidal volume. If high levels of PEEP or CPAP are required, above 15 cm H$_2$O, a pulmonary catheter can be inserted and pulmonary artery blood gas obtained to calculate the shunt fraction. Distending airway pressure should be applied to maintain a shunt fraction at or below 18%.

5. Modality of Ventilation

IMV:	Wean by decreasing the IMV rate
PSV:	Wean the "plateau pressure" in 1 to 2 cm H_2O increments to 10 to 15 cm H_2O. Do not wean below 8 cm H_2O.
CMV:	Allow the paralytic agents and sedatives to wear off, then convert to IMV.
Assisted modalities:	Incrementally decrease the frequency.

Finally, the clinician should consider a final **T-tube trial** for a relatively short interval before final discontinuation of ventilatory support. With a T-tube the patient receives supplemental oxygen without ventilatory support.

Extubation Criteria

Extubation can be considered when **all** of the following criteria are met:

• Adequate oxygenation and ventilation can be maintained by the patient. The oxyhemoglobin saturation is at or above 90% with an FiO_2 of 40% or less, and CPAP is less than or equal to 5 cm H_2O. The pH should be above 7.35 while the patient receives 2 or fewer mechanical breaths per minute. The level of pressure support should be in the range of 8 to 10 cm H_2O.
• The measured vital capacity is at least 15 ml/kg and the negative inspiratory force is less than -20 cm H_2O.
• The patient is alert, cooperative, and oriented. He has an active cough and gag and swallow reflexes. (The competence of the cough reflex can be tested when the trachea is stimulated during suctioning. The gag reflex can be tested by stimulating the pharynx with a tongue blade.)
• No airway obstruction after extubation is anticipated.

If all of these criteria are met, a safe extubation should be accomplished. If a patient displays permanent loss of reflexes, such as after a stroke, tracheostomy should be considered.

Troubleshooting Ventilator Problems

Modern ventilators are equipped with many monitors and alarms to assure proper mechanical function and patient safety. However, ventilators can fail or become disconnected. Furthermore, the patient may develop a new condition that hinders ventilation, often quickly and dramatically. Emergency equipment that must be immediately available to assist in these circumstances include an oxygen wall outlet with proper connectors, a self-inflating ventilation bag, intubation, mask ventilation, and suctioning equipment. If a ventilator appears to be malfunctioning or the patient develops distress or obvious hypoxemia, **hand ventilate the patient with a self-inflating bag and 100% oxygen and call for the respiratory therapist to assist with the machine.**

Table 12.5 lists some common problems and complications that might make ventilation difficult.

Figure 12.2 may help guide your approach to evaluating ventilatory difficulty.

TABLE 12.5. Difficulty with ventilation

Patient problems	Equipment problems
Chest wall	Misplacement of tube
Obesity	Endobronchial
Stiff chest syndrome	Esophageal
Pleura	Submucosal
Hemothorax	Laryngeal (cuff between vocal cords)
Hydrothorax	Extubation
Pneumothorax	Obstruction
Tumor	Kinking
Lung parenchyma	Biting
Adult respiratory distress syndrome	Foreign body
Aspiration	Blood/secretions
Atelectasis	Cuff
Chronic obstructive pulmonary disease	Overinflated
Pulmonary edema	Herniation
Tumor	Leaks
Bronchi	Circuit
Obstruction	Valves
Reactive airway disease	Leaks
Larynx and trachea	Soda lime exhaustion
Stenosis	Increased resistance
Tumor	Ventilator
Mouth	Disconnects
Oral hygiene	Loss of power
Loose teeth	O_2 delivery
Nose	Failure
Sinusitis	Crossed gas lines/contamination
Bleeding	Disconnects

Recent Developments in Mechanical Ventilation and Respiratory Care

Over the past decade, many new practices, strategies, and therapies have been introduced. Some of these developments have been adopted and are now in clinical use. The efficacy of others is still being investigated. Some of the new practices involve old treatment modalities that have been updated. The remainder of the chapter will discuss some of the recent developments that have received much consideration in the literature.

ALI/ARDS (Acute Lung Injury/Acute Respiratory Distress Syndrome)

The term *adult respiratory distress* was first used by Ashbaugh et al in 1967 to describe a pulmonary syndrome in adults that resembled respiratory distress in infants.[8] For years, the condition was referred to as **ARDS (adult respiratory distress syndrome).** The syndrome was characterized by acute onset, tachypnea,

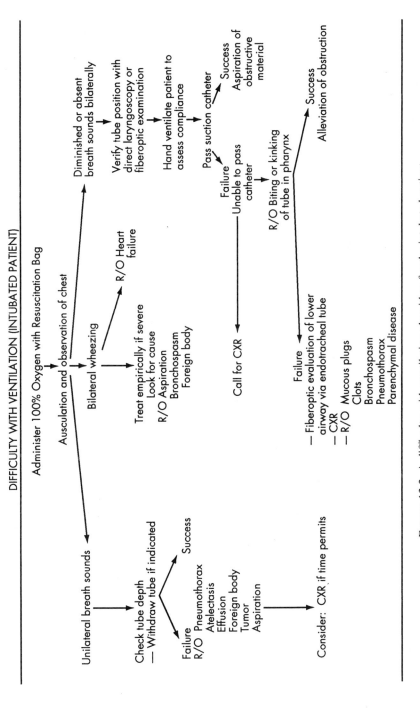

DIFFICULTY WITH VENTILATION (INTUBATED PATIENT)

Administer 100% Oxygen with Resuscitation Bag

Auscultation and observation of chest

Diminished or absent breath sounds bilaterally

Verify tube position with direct laryngoscopy or fiberoptic examination

Hand ventilate patient to assess compliance

Pass suction catheter

Success
Aspiration of obstructive material

Failure
Unable to pass catheter

R/O Biting or kinking of tube in pharynx

Success
Alleviation of obstruction

Failure
— Fiberoptic evaluation of lower airway via endotracheal tube
— CXR
— R/O Mucous plugs
   Clots
   Bronchospasm
   Pneumothorax
   Parenchymal disease

Bilateral wheezing

R/O Heart failure

Treat empirically if severe
Look for cause
R/O Aspiration
   Bronchospasm
   Foreign body

Call for CXR

Unilateral breath sounds

Check tube depth
— Withdraw tube if indicated

Success

Failure
R/O Pneumothorax
   Atelectasis
   Effusion
   Foreign body
   Tumor
   Aspiration

Consider: CXR if time permits

FIGURE 12.2. A difficulty-with-ventilation algorithm for the intubated patient.

429

hypoxemia, poor lung compliance, and bilateral pulmonary infiltrates. The hypoxemia could be treated with PEEP. The mortality rate was reported to be as high as 90%. It was recognized that ARDS was not necessarily a primary disease but rather the pulmonary manifestation of many different pathologic and traumatic processes. ARDS was often associated with multiple organ dysfunction and failure. In 1994, the European-American Consensus Committee on ARDS agreed on the following definitive features of the syndrome:

European-American Consensus Committee on ARDS:
1994[8–10] Definitive Features of ALI/ARDS

1. Acute onset
2. Bilateral infiltrates on chest X ray
3. Hypoxemia:
   ALI: PaO_2/FiO_2 ratio less than 300 mm Hg
   ARDS: PaO_2/FiO_2 ratio less than 200 mm Hg
4. No evidence of left atrial hypertension:
   (Pulmonary artery occlusion pressure [wedge] less than 18 mm Hg)

The committee also recommended that the syndrome be called **acute respiratory distress syndrome** rather than **adult respiratory distress syndrome.**

Investigators studied many therapeutic and supportive interventions to improve the outcome of patients with ARDS. With the recognition that the syndrome represented the pulmonary component of many different processes and the introduction of PEEP to improve oxygenation so the patient would not die of simple hypoxemia, the mortality rate has dropped to the 25% to 50% range. More recently, a better understanding of the pulmonary effects of PPV and PEEP, the hormonal and humeral components of the syndrome, and the early discovery of loss of surfactant with ARDS have led to a multitude of proposals to "treat" ARDS.

Fortunately, McIntyre et al[8] have reviewed the literature in a comprehensive paper published in 2000. They considered the findings of 285 papers dealing with various aspects of ARDS-related clinical trials. They evaluated the "quality of evidence" supporting various conclusions and practices. Furthermore, they rated the conclusions and practices in terms of the level of recommendation. Table 12.6 summarizes their evaluation of the literature.

Following is a summary of the rating systems used by McIntyre et al in their paper.

Rating Systems for Scientific Evidence and Recommendations[8]

Rating System for Quality of Evidence

Level 1: Large, randomized, prospective, controlled investigations
Level 2: Small, randomized, prospective, controlled trials with uncertain results
Level 3: Nonrandomized, concurrent, or historical cohort investigations
Level 4: Peer-reviewed state-of-the-art articles, review articles, editorials, or substantial case series

TABLE 12.6. An evaluation of ARDS-related clinical trials

Clinical modality	Quality of evidence (levels)	Recommendation rating
Noninvasive positive pressure ventilation	2 and 4	C
Lung protective ventilation	1	B
Inverse ratio ventilation	3 and 4	D
Extracorporeal life support		Recommend new prospective clinical trials
Prone ventilation	3	D
Liquid ventilation	4	E
Fluid management (restriction and/or diuretics)	2	C
Surfactant	3	C
Nitric oxide	1	Nitric oxide not recommended
Almitrine	3	C
Prostacyclin	3	C
Immune modulation Strategies		
• Prostaglandin E1	1	Not recommended
• Ketoconazole	1 and 2	Not recommended
• Antioxidants	2	Not recommended
• Corticosteroids	2	C

Source: McIntyre,[8] with permission.

Level 5: Non-peer-reviewed published opinions, such as textbook statements or official organizational publications

Rating System for Recommendations

A. Convincingly justifiable on scientific evidence alone (2 Level 1 investigations)
B. Justifiable by available scientific evidence (1 Level 1 investigation)
C. Reasonably justifiable by available scientific evidence and strongly supported By expert critical care opinion (Level 2 investigations only)
D. Adequate scientific evidence is lacking but widely supported by available data and expert critical care opinion (Level 3 data)
E. No scientific data exists to justify support (Level 4 and 5 publications)

Of all of the therapeutic interventions reviewed, only one, the **lung protective ventilator strategy,** is strongly recommended. Lower tidal volumes and airway pressures should be used when ventilating patients with ALI/ARDS. Utilizing this strategy, tidal volumes are delivered in the range of 6 ml/kg with driving pressures (PSV plateau and peak inspiratory pressure delivered with IMV or CMV) in the range of 20 to 25 cm H_2O above PEEP levels. One may have to tolerate "permissive hypercapnia" with this ventilatory strategy.

Conclusions from the McIntyre, et al Paper

Only 5% of patients with ARDS die from respiratory failure. Most deaths result from sepsis and multiple organ failure. McIntyre et al propose that the changes in outcome over the years "are likely attributable to several factors, including improved ventilator management, sophisticated monitoring devices, fluid management, nutritional support, and antibiotic therapy."[8] Finally, they suggest that previous researchers have not accounted for the "heterogeneity of patients with ARDS." Future studies should identify specific subgroups and define more specific endpoints. With **"mortality"** as the only endpoint, many physiologic and pathologic subtleties will be overlooked.

The Future of ARDS Research

In the future, clinical trials will have to be more carefully designed and controlled, and they will have to enroll larger numbers of patients if valid scientific conclusions are to be justified. More specific endpoints will have to be defined. Current publications have shown favorable results in many areas. These results will lead to future research with extracorporeal life support,[9] hormonal and humeral regulation, high frequency and other modalities of ventilation, liquid ventilation, carbon dioxide washout techniques, and positioning (prone vs. supine). The role of nitric oxide with respect to ARDS deserves further research. The effects of alveolar recruitment will be investigated. Hopefully, the **best combination of supportive and therapeutic modalities** will be defined.

Alternative Modalities of Ventilation

Many alternative modalities of ventilation are reported in the literature. Table 12.7 lists a few of the more commonly mentioned modes and the reported benefits and utility of each.

A more detailed discussion of some of these modalities is offered in comprehensive textbooks on the subject of mechanical ventilation.[24,25]

TABLE 12.7. Alternative modalities of ventilation

Modality	Comments
High-frequency ventilation[11,12]	Surgical field avoidance procedures
	Lower airway pressures
Noninvasive mask ventilation[13]	Patient refusal to be intubated
	? Adjunct to weaning from ventilation
Negative-pressure ventilation[14]	Surgical field avoidance
Airway pressure release ventilation[15,16]	Lower airway pressures
	Hemodynamic stability
Differential lung ventilation[17]	Lung isolation
	Lung-specific therapeutic intervention
Apneic ventilation/oxygenation[18–20]	Difficult airway management
	Carbon dioxide washout techniques
Zero deadspace endotracheal tube[21]	Requires special tube
Proportional-assist ventilation[22]	Improved pulmonary mechanics
Intermittent CPAP[23]	Ventilatory efficacy demonstrated in anesthetized patients

TABLE 12.8. Causes of difficult weaning

Inadequate Respiratory Center Output
• Residual effect of sedative drugs
• CNS damage
• Severe metabolic alkalosis
Increase in Respiratory Workload
• Increased minute ventilation
  ○ Hyperventilation from pain, anxiety, restlessness
  ○ Increased metabolic rate from excessive feeding or sepsis
  ○ Increased physiologic dead space
• Increased elastic workload
  ○ Low thoracic or lung compliance
  ○ Intrinsic PEEP
• Increased restrictive workload
  ○ Lower airway obstruction
  ○ Thick or copious airway secretions
  ○ Artificial airway (endotracheal tube)
  ○ Ventilator circuitry and demand valve
  ○ Postextubation upper airway obstruction
Respiratory Pump Failure
• Thoracic wall abnormality or disease
• Peripheral neurologic disorder
  ○ Phrenic nerve injury
  ○ Cervical spine damage
  ○ Critical care neuropathy
  ○ Guillain-Barre syndrome
• Muscular Dysfunction
  ○ Malnutrition, muscular catabolism
  ○ Pulmonary hyperinflation
  ○ Severe electrolyte and metabolic disorders
  ○ Prolonged postneuromuscular blockade effect
Left Ventricular Failure
• Left ventricular dysfunction
• Coronary artery disease

Source: Lessard and Brochard,[26] with permission.

New Weaning Strategies

Weaning from mechanical ventilation is usually straightforward. However, many factors can lead to trouble. Table 12.8 shows causes that may make weaning difficult.

Many indexes of spontaneous ventilatory effort have been proposed in an attempt to predict the success of weaning. The most useful is the **f/Vt ratio.**[26] If the **f/Vt ratio** is greater than or equal to 100 breaths/min/L, weaning is likely to fail (f = frequency [breaths/min]; V_t = tidal volume [liters]).

To facilitate difficult weaning, consider the points listed in Table 12.9.[26]

Complications of Mechanical Ventilation

Many of the complications associated with mechanical ventilation such as equipment failure, upper airway trauma and injury, and barotrauma have already been mentioned. More recent investigators are looking into many new and intriguing

TABLE 12.9. Things to consider to facilitate difficult weaning

1. Recognize and correct the causes of weaning failure.
2. Define a patient-specific weaning program.
3. Consider psychological factors (gain patient cooperation, mobilization, sleep at night, oral feeding, TV, radio, newspapers, hypnosis).[27]
4. Provide adequate nutritional support.
5. Correct metabolic abnormalities.
6. Optimize cardiac function.
7. Reduce the imposed work of breathing (aspirate airway, consider bronchodilators and corticosteroids, replace a partially obstructed endotracheal tube, consider tracheotomy, optimize ventilator settings [inspiratory flow], optimize sensitivity of ventilator triggers, carefully add external PEEP [in patients with intrinsic PEEP and expiratory flow limitation—e.g., COPD], allow permissive hypercarbia).
8. Improve the patient's respiratory capacity (consider theophylline), consider respiratory muscle training program.
9. Consider deflating the endotracheal tube cuff[28] to improve the patient's ability to handle secretions and to decrease airway flow resistance.[29]
10. Consider alternative ventilatory modalities such as mask ventilation.[28,30]
11. Manage the case with a specialized team.

areas of research associated with mechanical ventilation. For example, investigators have begun to define specific lung injury caused by mechanical ventilation itself. Suter[31] summarized biochemical components of lung injury in ventilated subjects. He states:

"It has become evident that MV (mechanical ventilation) using large tidal volumes without PEEP and/or causing overdistension of lung units produces significant inflammatory changes in the lung. In experimental and human studies, a marked increase in leukocytes and proinflammatory cytokines was noted in bronchoalveolar lavage fluid during the application of more "aggressive" ventilatory strategies as compared with more "protective" modes, i.e., lower Vt applied on the steeper part of the pressure-volume curve, thereby avoiding repeated opening and closing, and also overdistension, of the lung. It has also been shown that regular stretching of alveolar cells in culture produces release of cytokines when small amounts of lipopolysaccharides are present. These data provide a cellular explanation of the inflammatory changes observed."

Many other investigators are studying the humoral and cellular effects of mechanical ventilation. As a result of this research, as has been noted, clinicians are more prone to use lower tidal volumes and to utilize modalities of ventilation that create lower overall airway pressures.

With respect to the issue of infection, one paper found that **ventilator-associated pneumonia** did not appear to be an independent risk factor for death in their study population.[32] This finding has been challenged.[33] More research will deal with the causes and treatment of pneumonia in ventilated patients. Safer techniques and protocols will be proposed.

Finally, swallowing dysfunction in patients receiving ventilatory support is being investigated.[34] This area of research may lead to new weaning strategies and ways to make the immediate postextubation period safer for the patient.

Portable Ventilators

For the sake of completeness, mention should be made of a class of ventilators designed to be of utility when transporting and resuscitating patients. One such ventilator, the Pneupac Ventipac portable gas-powered ventilator, is described by McCluskey and Gwinnutt.[35] Before using any medical device, such as a ventilator, you must receive expert training in its operation.

Hyperbaric Oxygenation

Hyperbaric oxygenation has been reported to reverse both the clinical symptoms and EKG changes of cardiac ischemia in two case reports of patients with profound anemia.[36] The technique requires a hyperbaric chamber and expert operation to avoid complications. Other uses for hyperbaric oxygenation may be introduced to critical care practitioners.

Ethical Considerations of Mechanical Ventilation

Recently, investigators have begun to examine and report on various ethical considerations associated with mechanical ventilation. One such paper deals with the development of a questionnaire to elicit patient preferences with respect to intubation.[37] Decisions made when treating ventilated patients are often profound, if not life-ending. Patients, families, and physicians need to develop better means to communicate.

Summary

This chapter has offered the reader a practical review of the basic concepts of mechanical ventilatory support. Current equipment and practices have been described. In addition, recent innovations and research have also been presented to introduce the reader to ongoing developments in this area of patient care. Effectively applying the techniques of modern ventilatory support takes years of training and experience. The goal of therapy is to maintain oxygenation and ventilation in patients who are often critically ill. When managing patients, set specific and realistic goals and utilize the newest monitors. Finally, remember that **ventilators sometimes fail** or the **patient's condition may deteriorate quickly.** In these situations, **revert to the basics. Check the endotracheal tube, administer 100% oxygen with a self-inflating resuscitation bag, auscultate the chest for breath sounds, keep a finger on the pulse, and reassess the monitored information. Do not hesitate to call for help!**

References

1. Sladen, RN. Current concepts of mechanical ventilation. *IARS Review Course Lectures.* 1999;86–92.
2. Siemens Servo Screen 390 V2.0/3.X operating manual.

3. Siemens Servo Ventilator 300/300A operating manual 8.1/9.1.

4. Ouellet P. Seimens Waveform and Loop Analysis in Mechanical Ventilation (Siemens-Elema AB, SE-171 95 Solna, Sweden).

5. Kossel H, Versmold H. 25 Years of respiratory support of newborn infants. *J Perinat Med.* 1997;25:421–432.

6. Tokioka H, et al. Pressure support ventilation augments spontaneous breathing with improved thoracoabdominal synchrony in neonates with congenital heart disease. *Anesth. Analg.* 1997;85:789–793.

7. Schulze A, et al. Proportional assist ventilation in low birth weight infants with acute respiratory disease: a comparison to assist/control and conventional mechanical ventilation. *J Pediatrics.* 1999;135(3):339–344.

8. McIntyre RC, et al. Thirty years of clinical trials in acute respiratory distress syndrome. *Crit Care Med.* 2000;28:3314–3331.

9. Shapiro MB, et al. Respiratory failure: conventional and high-tech support. *Surg Clin North Am.* 2000;80(3):871–883.

10. Bernard GR, et al. The American-European Consensus Conference on ARDS: definitions, mechanisms, relevant outcomes, and clinical trial coordination. *Am J Respir Crit Care Med.* 1994;149:818–824.

11. MacIntyre NR. High-frequency ventilation. In: Tobin MJ. *Principles and Practice of Mechanical Ventilation.* New York: McGraw-Hill, Inc.; 1994.

12. Sakuragi T, et al. High-frequency jet ventilation during fiberoptic laser resection of tracheal granuloma in a small child. *Anesth Analg.* 1996;82:889.

13. Meduri GU, et al. Noninvasive mechanical ventilation via face mask in patients with acute respiratory failure who refused endotracheal intubation. *Crit Care Med.* 1994; 22(10):1584–1590.

14. Natalini G, et al. Negative pressure ventilation vs external high-frequency oscillation during rigid bronchoscopy. *Chest.* 2000;118(1):18–23.

15. Neumann P, Hedenstierna G. Ventilatory support by continuous positive airway pressure breathing improves gas exchange as compared with partial ventilatory support with airway pressure release ventilation. *Anesth Analg.* 2001;92:950–958.

16. Smith RPR, Fletcher R. Airway pressure release ventilation in cardiac surgery patients. *Br J Anaesth.* 2000;84(2):272.

17. Branson RD, Hurst JM. Differential lung ventilation. In: Peral A, Stock MC. *Handbook of Mechanical Ventilatory Support.* Baltimore: Williams and Wilkins; 1992:185–193.

18. Smith RB. Continuous flow apneic ventilation. In: Perol A, Stock MC. *Handbook of Mechanical Ventilatory Support.* Baltimore: Williams and Wilkins; 1992:175–184.

19. Okazaki J, et al. Usefulness of continuous oxygen insufflation into trachea for management of upper airway obstruction during anesthesia. *Anesthesiology.* 2000;93(1): 62–68.

20. Wolf AR. Blood gas changes during apnoeic oxygenation in infants and children. *Br J Anaesth.* 1997;78(4):473.

21. Liebenberg CS, et al. Small tidal volume ventilation using a zero deadspace tracheal tube. *Br J Anaesth.* 1999;82(2):213–216.

22. Ranieri VM, et al. Effects of proportional assist ventilation on inspiratory muscle effort in patients with chronic obstructive pulmonary disease and acute respiratory failure. *Anesthesiology.* 1997;86:79–91.

23. Bratzke E, et al. Intermittent CPAP. *Anesthesiology.* 1998;89:334–340.

24. Perel A, Stock MC. *Handbook of Mechanical Ventilatory Support.* Baltimore: Williams and Wilkins; 1992.

25. Tobin MJ. *Principles and Practice of Mechanical Ventilation*. New York: McGraw-Hill, Inc.; 1994.

26. Lessard MR, Brochard LJ. Weaning from ventilatory support. *Clin Chest Medicine*. 1996;17(3):475–489.

27. Treggiari-Venzi MM, et al. Successful use of hypnosis as an adjunctive therapy for weaning from mechanical ventilation. *Anesthesiology*. 2000;92:890–892.

28. Shneerson JM. Are there new solutions to old problems with weaning? [editorial] *Br J Anaesth*. 1997;78(3):238–240.

29. Bapat P, et al. Cuff deflation for easier weaning from ventilation. *Br J Anaesth*. 1997;79(1):145.

30. Girault C, et al. Noninvasive ventilation as a systemic extubation and weaning technique in acute-on-chronic respiratory failure. *Am J Respir Crit Care Med*. 1999;160:86–92.

31. Suter PM. Does mechanical ventilation cause lung injury? *IARS Review Course Lectures*. 2001:104–105.

32. Bregeon F, et al. Is ventilator-associated pneumonia an independent risk factor for death? *Anesthesiology*. 2001;94:554–560.

33. Kollef MH. What's new about ventilator-associated pneumonia [editorial]. *Anesthesiology*. 2001;94:551–553.

34. Tolep K, et al. Swallowing dysfunction in patients receiving prolonged mechanical ventilation. *Chest*. 1996;109(1):167–172.

35. McLuskey A, Gwinnutt CL. Evaluation of the pneupac ventipac portable ventilator: comparison of performance in a mechanical lung and anaesthetized patients. *Br J Anaesth*. 1995;75(5):645–650.

36. Greensmith JE. Hyperbaric oxygen reverses organ dysfunction in severe anemia. *Anesthesiology*. 2000;93:1149–1152.

37. Dales RE, et al. Intubation and mechanical ventilation for COPD: development of an instrument to elicit patient preferences. *Chest*. 1999;116(3):792–800.

13
The Laryngeal Mask Airway (LMA)

LMA and LMA model names are registered trademarks of the Laryngeal Mask Company
Ltd: LMA North America, Inc., San Diego, CA.

The LMA was invented by Dr. Archie Brain in 1981.[1] Commercial products were introduced in 1988. Since then, various models of the LMA have been developed and marketed worldwide.

Dr. Brain stated: "The aim [of developing the LMA] was to form a direct connection with the patient's airway which might afford greater security and convenience than the face-mask."[1] When the LMA is inserted correctly, the tip rests against the upper esophageal sphincter, the sides face into the pyriform fossae, and the upper border faces the base of the tongue. Proper positioning of the LMA brings the glottic and airway aperatures into alignment. The LMA "forms a seal around the laryngeal, not the pharyngeal, perimeter."[1] Two practical features of the LMA are that it provides a "much more reliable airway than the face-mask,"[1] and when secured, the practitioner can use both hands to perform other tasks. The LMA was designed for use with patients breathing spontaneously or for those whose ventilation is controlled. Dr. Brain has consistently warned that the LMA is *not* a substitute for an endotracheal tube when the latter device is *clearly indicated*. The LMA does not necessarily protect the patient from aspiration of regurgitated gastric contents, and the glottic sphincter may still close with the LMA in place, especially if the patient is inadequately anesthetized or the airway is used by "less experienced"[1] clinicians.

Over the past 13 years the LMA and its various modifications have revolutionized airway management. The device has been accepted enthusiastically by anesthesiologists and other practitioners who deal with the airway. It has become a fundamental component in the armamentarium of airway equipment.

It is beyond the scope of this book to analyze and summarize the voluminous world literature on the LMA. The reader is directed to the book entitled *The Laryngeal Mask Airway: A Review and Practical Guide.*[2] The book comprehensively covers the subject up to 1997, though much has been written concerning the LMA since then.[3] A comprehensive bibliography concerning the LMA is provided by LMA North America, Inc., at their website: www. LMANA.com.

The primary objective of this chapter is to describe the LMA, the various LMA modifications, and the common uses of the LMA. In addition, subsequent sections will be devoted to the following considerations:

1. Comments concerning LMA size, modified insertion techniques, etc.
2. Cuff and mucosal pressures and the LMA
3. Esophageal reflux and the risk of aspiration
4. Positive-pressure ventilation (PPV) and the LMA
5. Use of the LMA with pediatric patients
6. Innovative uses of the LMA
7. Using the LMA with adjunctive airway equipment
8. Adverse effects and problems associated with the LMA
9. The LMA and the "difficult airway"

Indications for LMA Use

The LMA manual[4] lists the indications for LMA use to be the following:

1. As an alternative to the face mask in routine and emergency procedures
2. For use in known or unknown difficult airway situations
3. For use during resuscitation in the "profoundly unconscious patient with absent"[4] airway reflexes

Note: The LMA is not indicated as a replacement for endotracheal intubation.

Contraindications Against LMA Use

The LMA manual[4(p5)] lists the contraindications against LMA use to be the following:

1. Electively, the LMA should not be used with patients who have not fasted or who might likely have retained gastric contents, such as those who are obese, pregnant, injured, or in pain, or who have any condition associated with delayed gastric emptying such as opiate use.
2. Patients with hiatal hernia, "unless effective measures have been taken to empty their stomach contents beforehand."[4(p5)]
3. Patients with decreased pulmonary or chest wall compliance, as the mask forms a "low-pressure seal around the larynx"[4(p5)] and high positive pressure could inflate the stomach.
4. In the emergency setting of resuscitation, the LMA should not be used if the patient is not "profoundly unresponsive."[4(p5)] If the patient is not "profoundly unresponsive" or if oropharyngeal trauma is present, you must weigh the risks and benefits of the LMA as compared to other airway devices and interventions.

Cautions and Warnings

Consult the LMA manuals concerning various cautions and warnings. Steam autoclaving is the "only recommended method for sterilization of the LMA."[4(p6)] The Manual also stresses careful examination of each LMA to make sure that the device has not been damaged by cleaning or usage. Make sure that the mask inflates to the "test volume" (see following text) without leaking and that no wires protrude from the walls of the LMA-Flexible airway tube.

LMA Design Description

The LMA is an airway device made of latex-free medical-grade silicone rubber. The device is reusable after proper sterilization (see LMA manuals for cleaning instructions). The three main components of the LMA are the airway tube, the mask, and the mask inflation line (Fig. 13.1).

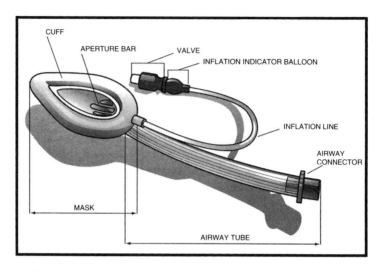

FIGURE 13.1. The components of the LMA-Classic. *LMA Manual*. 2000: figure 1, p. 1. (Reproduced with permission of LMA North America, Inc.)

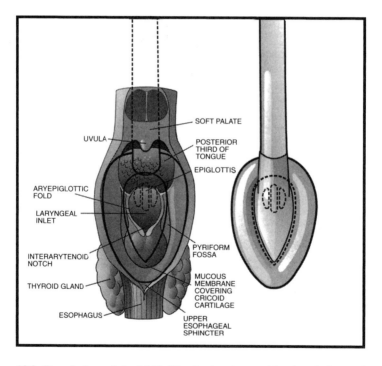

FIGURE 13.2. Dorsal view of the LMA-Classic showing position in relation to the pharyngeal anatomy. Note that the aperature of the airway and the glottic opening are aligned when the LMA is properly positioned. (Reproduced with permission of LMA North America, Inc.) (*LMA Manual*. 2000: figure 2, p. 2.)

TABLE 13.1. LMA-Classic size selection guidelines

LMA size	Patient size
1	Neonates/Infants up to 5 kg
$1^{1}/_{2}$	Infants 5 to 10 kg
2	Infants/children 10 to 20 kg
$2^{1}/_{2}$	Children 20 to 30 kg
3	Children (small adults) 30 to 50 kg
4	Adults 50 to 70 kg
5	Adults 70 to 100 kg
6	Large adults over 100 kg

When the LMA is placed in correct position, the airway aperture and the glottic opening are aligned as shown in Figure 13.2.

LMA Models

There are five models of LMA currently marketed. These include the LMA-Classic, the LMA-Flexible, the LMA-Unique, the LMA-ProSeal, and the LMA-Fastrach (known as the Intubating LMA outside of the United States).

LMA-Classic

The Classic is the standard LMA in use. This airway is shown in Figures 13.1 and 13.2. The Classic is designed for use with pediatric and adult patients and comes in the recommended sizes[4(p21)] shown in Table 13.1.

Once inserted into the patient, the cuff inflation volumes recommended for each LMA are listed in Table 13.2.[4(p28)]

The volumes to be used to "test" the mask shape and airway integrity for leakage before insertion are listed in Table 13.3.[4(p17)]

LMA-Flexible

The LMA-Flexible has a wire-reinforced flexible airway tube. This LMA is useful when the airway tube has to be positioned so that it will not interfere with

TABLE 13.2. Maximum cuff inflation volumes

LMA size	Cuff volume (air)
1	Up to 4 ml
$1^{1}/_{2}$	Up to 7 ml
2	Up to 10 ml
$2^{1}/_{2}$	Up to 14 ml
3	Up to 20 ml
4	Up to 30 ml
5	Up to 40 ml
6	Up to 50 ml

TABLE 13.3. Test cuff inflation volume

LMA size	Air volume
1	6 ml
$1^1/_2$	10 ml
2	15 ml
$2^1/_2$	21 ml
3	30 ml
4	45 ml
5	60 ml
6	75 ml

the surgical field. The LMA-Flexible comes in the following sizes: 2, $2^1/_2$, 3, 4, 5, 6. The patient sizes and maximum cuff volumes are the same as for the LMA-Classic.

LMA-Unique

The LMA-Unique is designed to be a disposable airway for one-time use. It can be used in the operating room or elsewhere for emergency airway management. The Unique comes in sizes 3 through 6 with the same patient size and maximum cuff volume recommendations as the Classic (Fig. 13.3).

LMA-ProSeal

The LMA-ProSeal is an airway made with dual tube design. The airway tube is wire-reinforced and the aperture is of modified size and shape (Fig. 13.4). A second tube allows for esophageal-gastric suctioning and venting when the LMA is positioned properly. According to the manufacturer, the ProSeal provides an "improved laryngeal seal for higher airway seal pressure during PPV (positive pressure ventilation)"[5] The ProSeal comes with an introducer, which allows insertion without placement of fingers in the patient's mouth. The tube also has a built-in "bite block."

The LMA-ProSeal comes in sizes 3 through 5 and the patient sizes and cuff volumes are the same as for the LMA-Classic. It is recommended that the cuff pressure be inflated to 60 cm H_2O.

A size 16 French orogastric tube or a 14 French Salem Sump can be passed through the drainage channel of the size 3 or 4 airway. An 18 French orogastric tube or a 16 French Salem Sump can be passed through the size 5 airway. A suction tube should be passed through the ProSeal as part of the positioning test to confirm patency and proper placement.

LMA-Fastrach[6]

The LMA-Fastrach (or the Intubating LMA, in countries outside of the United States) is designed for one-handed insertion and is designed to facilitate "blind"

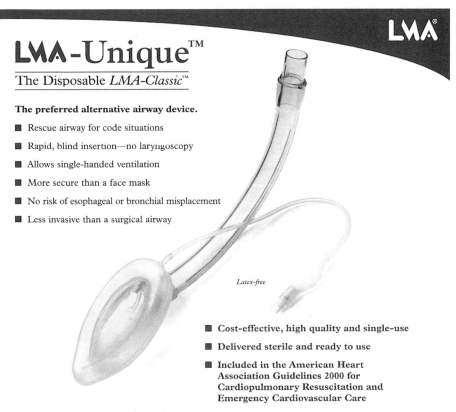

LMA-Unique™
The Disposable LMA-Classic™

The preferred alternative airway device.

■ Rescue airway for code situations

■ Rapid, blind insertion—no laryngoscopy

■ Allows single-handed ventilation

■ More secure than a face mask

■ No risk of esophageal or bronchial misplacement

■ Less invasive than a surgical airway

Latex-free

■ **Cost-effective, high quality and single-use**

■ **Delivered sterile and ready to use**

■ **Included in the American Heart Association Guidelines 2000 for Cardiopulmonary Resuscitation and Emergency Cardiovascular Care**

The Only Disposable LMA™ Airway for Resuscitation.

FIGURE 13.3. The LMA-Unique Disposable Airway. (Reproduced with permission of LMA North America, Inc.) (From LMA-Unique advertisement.)

intubation of the trachea. It comes in sizes 3 through 5 and the patient sizes and cuff volumes are the same as for the Classic. The Fastrach should be used with reusable LMA-Fastrach endotracheal tubes, which come in sizes 7.0, 7.5, and 8.0-mm I.D (Euromedical ILM Endotracheal Tube Euromedical, Malaysia). The Fastrach has proven to be a useful adjunct to fiberoptic intubation. The technique of "blind" intubation and use of the Fastrach for fiberoptic intubation will be described later in the chapter (Fig. 13.5).

LMA-Classic Insertion Techniques[4(pp21–37)]

The LMA instruction manual describes two techniques for the device's insertion: the standard technique and the thumb technique.[7] Both of these techniques may be used for adult as well as pediatric patients. These techniques are applicable to all of the models of LMA except the Fastrach.

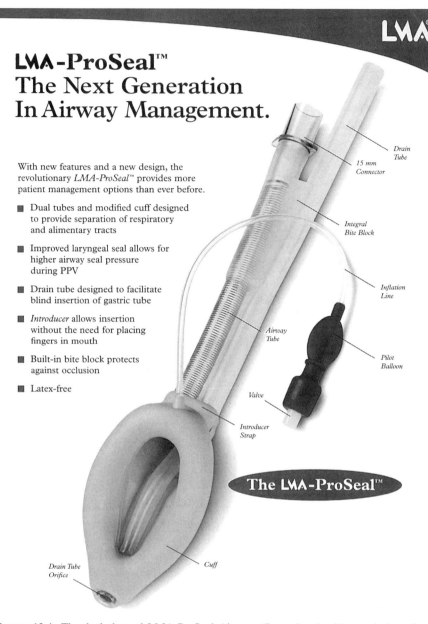

LMA®

LMA-ProSeal™
The Next Generation
In Airway Management.

With new features and a new design, the
revolutionary *LMA-ProSeal™* provides more
patient management options than ever before.

■ Dual tubes and modified cuff designed
to provide separation of respiratory
and alimentary tracts

■ Improved laryngeal seal allows for
higher airway seal pressure
during PPV

■ Drain tube designed to facilitate
blind insertion of gastric tube

■ *Introducer* allows insertion
without the need for placing
fingers in mouth

■ Built-in bite block protects
against occlusion

■ Latex-free

Drain
Tube

15 mm
Connector

Integral
Bite Block

Inflation
Line

Airway
Tube

Pilot
Balloon

Valve

Introducer
Strap

The LMA-ProSeal™

Drain Tube
Orifice

Cuff

FIGURE 13.4. The dual-channel LMA-ProSeal Airway. (Reproduced with permission of
LMA North America, Inc.) (From LMA-ProSeal advertisement.)

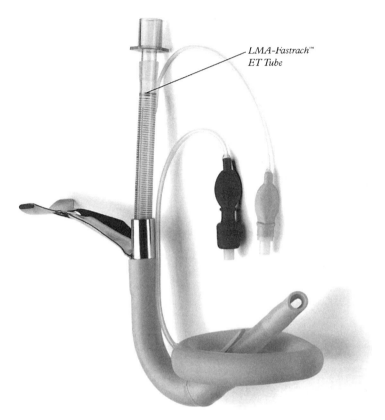

LMA-Fastrach™
ET Tube

FIGURE 13.5. The LMA-Fastrach. (Reproduced with permission of LMA North America, Inc.) (From LMA-Fastrach advertisement.)

Standard Insertion Technique

"To position the LMA correctly, the cuff tip must avoid entering the valleculae or the glottic opening, and must not become caught up against the epiglottis or the arytenoids. Therefore, keep the cuff tip pressing against the posterior pharyngeal wall during insertion."[4(p23)] To get the tip of the LMA to pass into the proper position, you must exert cranially directed pressure on the tube with the index finger during insertion.

1. After the equipment has been checked and the patient prepared, place the patient's head in the normal intubating position ("sniff position": neck flexion and head extension).
2. Prepare the LMA by completely deflating the cuff and lubricating its posterior surface.

The next steps are illustrated in Figures 13.6 through 13.12, which are taken from the LMA instruction manual.

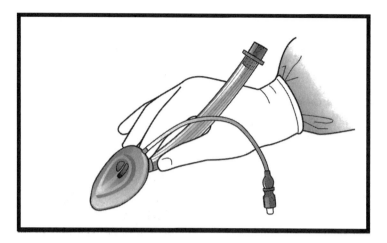

FIGURE 13.6. Method for holding the LMA for insertion. The index finger is placed at the junction of the cuff and the tube. (Reproduced with permission from LMA North America, Inc.) (*LMA Manual*. 2000: figure 7, p. 23.)

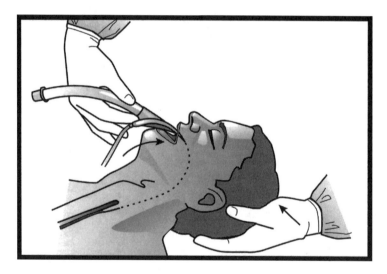

FIGURE 13.7. With the head extended and the neck flexed, carefully flatten the LMA tip against the hard palate. (Reproduced with permission from LMA North America, Inc.) (*LMA Manual*. 2000: figure 8, p. 24.)

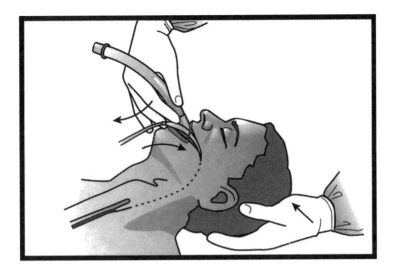

FIGURE 13.8. To facilitate LMA introduction into the oral cavity, gently press the middle finger down on the jaw. (Reproduced with permission from LMA North America, Inc.) (*LMA Manual*. 2000: figure 9, p. 25.)

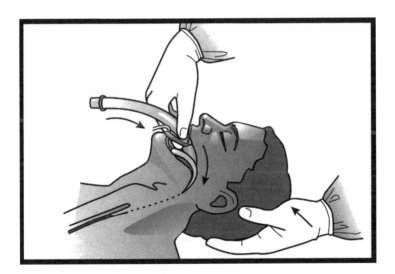

FIGURE 13.9. The index finger pushes the LMA in a cranial direction following the contours of the hard and soft palates. (Reproduced with permission from LMA North America, Inc.) (*LMA Manual*. 2000: figure 10, p. 25.)

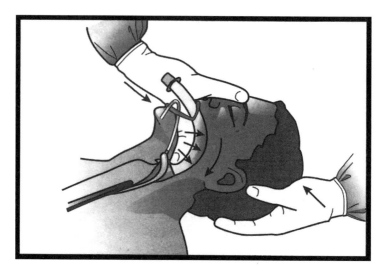

FIGURE 13.10. Maintaining pressure with the finger on the tube in the cranial direction, advance the mask until definite resistance is felt at the base of the hypopharynx. Note the flexion of the wrist. (Reproduced with permission from LMA North America, Inc.) (*LMA Manual*. 2000: figure 11, p. 26.)

Inflate the cuff with enough air to obtain an airway seal at 18–20 cm H_2O. Do not exceed the maximum volume recommended for the cuff (see Table 13.2).

Finally, secure the tube, insert a bite block, and attach the tube to the ventilation equipment.

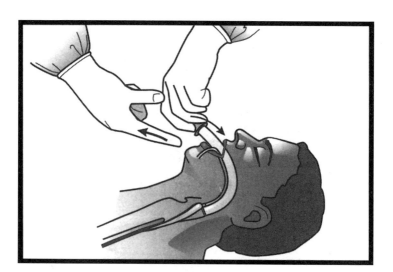

FIGURE 13.11. Gently maintain cranial pressure with the non-dominant hand while removing the index finger. (Reproduced with permission from LMA North America, Inc.) (*LMA Manual*. 2000: figure 12, p. 26.)

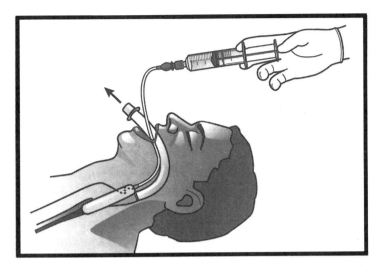

FIGURE 13.12. Inflation without holding the tube allows the mask to seat itself optimally. (Reproduced with permission from LMA North America, Inc.) (*LMA Manual*. 2000: figure 13, p. 27.)

Thumb Insertion Technique

The thumb insertion technique may be useful if the LMA is inserted with the operator facing the patient from below or from the side. With this technique, the thumb takes the place of the index finger to guide the LMA into place and to maintain cranially directed pressure on the mask during insertion. Figures 13.13 through 13.17 are taken from the LMA instruction manual and illustrate the thumb insertion technique.

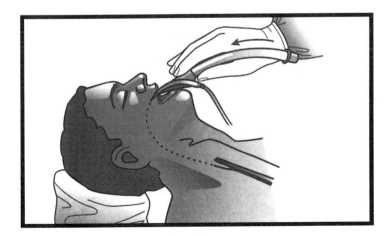

FIGURE 13.13. Method for holding the LMA for thumb insertion. (Reproduced with permission from LMA North America, Inc.) (*LMA Manual*. 2000: figure 14, p. 29.)

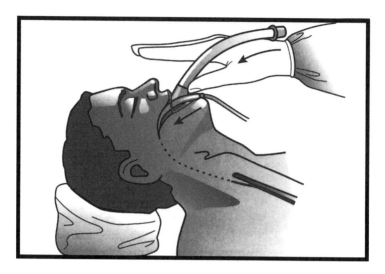

FIGURE 13.14. With the fingers extended, press the thumb along the posterior pharynx. (Reproduced with permission from LMA North America, Inc.) (*LMA Manual*. 2000: figure 15, p. 29.)

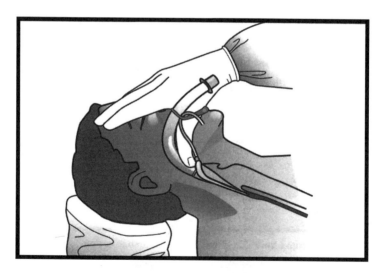

FIGURE 13.15. Advance the thumb to its fullest extent. (Reproduced with permission from LMA North America, Inc.) (*LMA Manual*. 2000: figure 16, p. 30.)

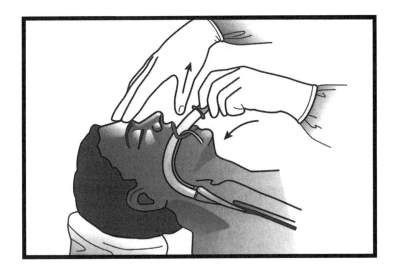

FIGURE 13.16. Press gently into place with the non-dominant hand while removing the thumb. (Reproduced with permission from LMA North America, Inc.) (*LMA Manual*. 2000: figure 17, p. 30.)

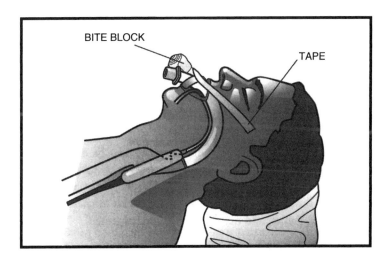

FIGURE 13.17. Tape the bite block and airway tube together with the tube taped downward against the chin. (Reproduced with permission from LMA North America, Inc.) (*LMA Manual*. 2000: figure 18, p. 31.)

LMA-ProSeal Insertion Using the Introducer

The LMA-ProSeal can be inserted with the techniques described above or with an introducer as described in the LMA-ProSeal instruction manual.[7]

During insertion, keep the introducer blade close to the patient's chin and rotate the airway smoothly following the curve of the introducer.

Figures 13.18 through 13.25 illustrate insertion of the ProSeal with the introducer.

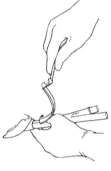

FIGURE 13.18. Place the tip of the introducer into the strap of the LMA-ProSeal. (Reproduced with permission from LMA North America, Inc.) (*LMA-ProSeal Manual*. 2000: figure 5a, p. 21.)

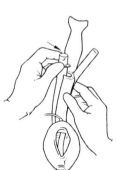

FIGURE 13.19. Fold the tubes around the introducer and fit the proximal end of the airway tube in the matching slot. (Reproduced with permission from LMA North America, Inc.) (*LMA-ProSeal Manual*. 2000: figure 5b, p. 21.)

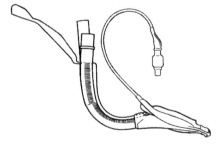

FIGURE 13.20. LMA-ProSeal with the introducer in place. (Reproduced with permission from LMA North America, Inc.) (*LMA-ProSeal Manual*. 2000: figure 6, p. 23.)

FIGURE 13.21. Press the tip of the cuff against the hard palate. (Reproduced with permission from LMA North America, Inc.) (*LMA-ProSeal Manual.* 2000: figure 7, p. 23.)

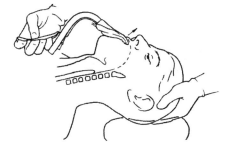

FIGURE 13.22. Press the cuff further into the mouth, maintaining pressure against the palate. (Reproduced with permission from LMA North America, Inc.) (*LMA-ProSeal Manual.* 2000: figure 8, p. 23.)

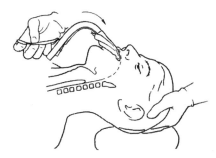

FIGURE 13.23. Swing the device inward with a circular motion, pressing against the contours of the hard and soft palate. (Reproduced with permission from LMA North America, Inc.) (*LMA-ProSeal Manual.* 2000: figure 9, p. 24.)

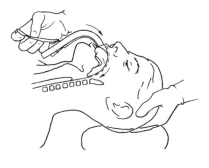

FIGURE 13.24. Advance the LMA-ProSeal into the hypopharynx until resistance is felt. (Reproduced with permission from LMA North America, Inc.) (*LMA-ProSeal Manual.* 2000: figure 10, p. 24.)

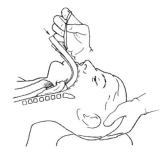

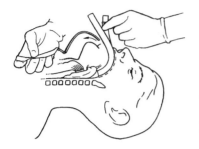

FIGURE 13.25. Hold the ProSeal tube in place while removing the introducer. (Reproduced with permission from LMA North America, Inc.) (*LMA-ProSeal Manual*. 2000: figure 11, p. 24.)

Testing the ProSeal for Proper Positioning: "Malpositioning Test"

All of the recommendations suggested by the manufacturer should be followed to assure that the airway is properly inserted. Pass a tube through the drainage channel of the airway to make sure it is not occluded. Perform a "malpositioning test" by placing a small bolus of lubricant gel at the proximal end of the drainage tube, then deliver a positive pressure breath through the airway. If the gel is ejected, the mask is not positioned properly.

LMA-Fastrach Insertion Technique

Once properly positioned, the LMA-Fastrach can be used as the primary airway or it can serve as a guide for fiberoptic or blind endotracheal intubation. The manufacturers of the Fastrach recommend using specially designed LMA-Fastrach silicone rubber endotracheal tubes for intubation. These tubes come in three sizes: 7.0-, 7.5-, and 8.0-mm ID (Euromedical ILM Endotracheal Tube Euromedical, Malaysia).

The Fastrach has the following noteworthy design features[8]:

1. The airway has a rigid anatomically curved airway tube with a handle designed to facilitate single-handed insertion.
2. The handle also makes positioning and removal of the airway easier.
3. The airway can be used on patients who have limited mouth opening (as little as 20 mm).
4. The epiglottic elevating bar of the airway displaces the epiglottis when an endotracheal tube is passed into the trachea.

The patient and equipment are prepared in the same manner as for LMA-Classic insertion. Lubricate the posterior surface of the Fastrach and be sure that the cuff is completely deflated.

Standard Insertion Technique

Figures 13.26 through 13.30 illustrate the LMA-Fastrach and the standard insertion technique.

Cautionary Note: The LMA-Fastrach has been shown to exert significant pressure on surrounding mucosal surfaces. Some investigators recommend that the

FIGURE 13.26. Features of the LMA-Fastrach. (Reproduced with permission from LMA North America, Inc.) (*Fastrach Manual*. 1998: figure 1, p. 4.)

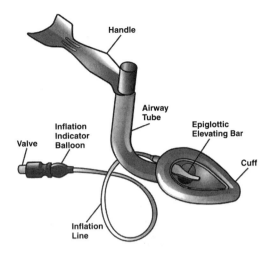

FIGURE 13.27. Rub the lubricant over the anterior hard palate with the device in position as shown. (Reproduced with permission from LMA North America, Inc.) (*Fastrach Manual*. 1998: figure 4, p. 18.)

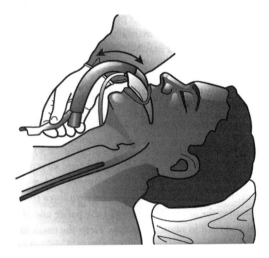

FIGURE 13.28. Swing the mask into place in a circular movement, maintaining pressure against the palate and posterior pharynx. (Reproduced with permission from LMA North America, Inc.) (*Fastrach Manual*. 1998: figure 5, p. 19.)

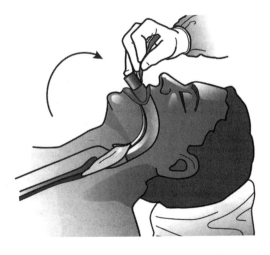

457

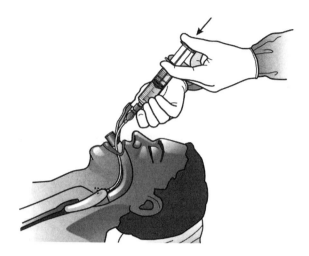

FIGURE 13.29. Inflate the mask, without holding the tube or handle, to a pressure of approximately 60 cm H_2O. (Reproduced with permission from LMA North America, Inc.) (*Fastrach Manual*. 1998: figure 6, p. 19.)

Fastrach not be left in place for long periods of time. (See section on measured mucosal pressures later in this chapter.)

Intubation through the LMA-Fastrach

Before intubating the patient, assure adequate oxygenation. Lubricate the special endotracheal tube with a small amount of water-soluble lubricant and gently insert the endotracheal tube into the airway after stabilizing its position with the handle.

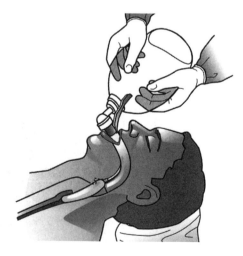

FIGURE 13.30. LMA-Fastrach can be used to ventilate the patient on its own. (Reproduced with permission from LMA North America, Inc.) (*Fastrach Manual*. 1998: figure 7, p. 20.)

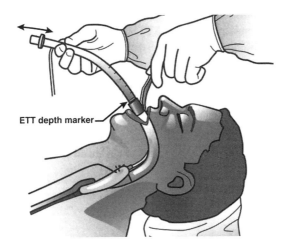

FIGURE 13.31. Hold the LMA-Fastrach handle steady while gently inserting the endotracheal tube into the metal shaft up to the 15-cm transverse depth marker. (Reproduced with permission from LMA North America, Inc.) (*Fastrach Manual*. 1998: figure 9, p. 22.)

Rotate the endotracheal tube and pull it in and out of the airway to lubricate the channel. Proceed with intubation as illustrated in Figures 13.31 and 13.32.

Insert the 15-mm adapter into the endotracheal tube, inflate the cuff, and ventilate the patient.

If you want to remove the Fastrach but leave the endotracheal tube in place, first remove the 15-mm adapter and proceed as illustrated in Figures 13.33 to 13.37.

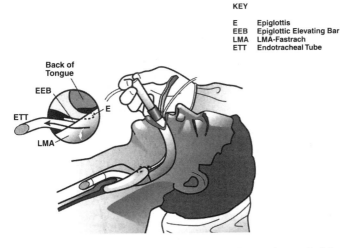

FIGURE 13.32. Advance the endotracheal tube 1.5 cm. If no resistance is felt, continue to advance the tube, while holding the LMA-Frastrach steady until intubation has been accomplished. (Reproduced with permission from LMA North America, Inc.) (*Fastrach Manual*. 1998: figure 10, p. 23.)

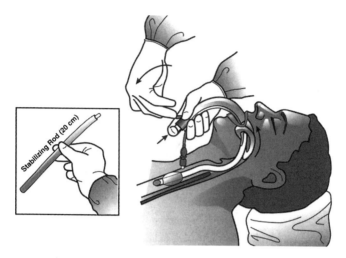

FIGURE 13.33. After fully deflating the cuff, swing the mask out of the pharynx into the oral cavity while applying counterpressure to the tracheal tube with the finger as shown. This maneuver is performed before the Fastrach Stability Rod is inserted into the tube. (Reproduced with permission from LMA North America, Inc.) (*Fastrach Manual.* 1998: figure 13, p. 25.)

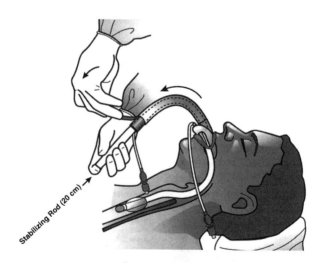

FIGURE 13.34. Insert the Stabilizing Rod into the end of the airway until it comes into contact with the end of the endotracheal tube. Slide the LMA-Fastrach over the endotracheal tube and Stabilizing Rod until it is clear of the mouth. (Reproduced with permission from LMA North America, Inc.) (*Fastrach Manual.* 1998: figure 14, p. 26.)

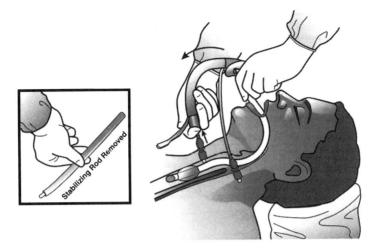

FIGURE 13.35. Remove the Stabilizing Rod and steady the endotracheal tube at the level of the incisors. (Reproduced with permission from LMA North America, Inc.) (*Fastrach Manual*. 1998: figure 15, p. 26.)

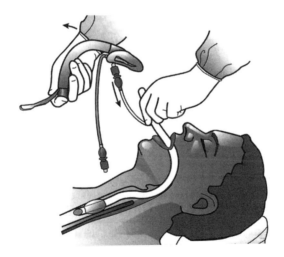

FIGURE 13.36. Remove the LMA-Fastrach completely, gently unthreading the inflation line and pilot balloon of the endotracheal tube. (Reproduced with permission from LMA North America, Inc.) (*Fastrach Manual*. 1998: figure 16, p. 27.)

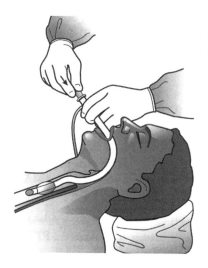

FIGURE 13.37. Replace the 15-mm adapter to the endotracheal tube and ventilate the patient. (Reproduced with permission from LMA North America, Inc.) (*Fastrach Manual*. 1998: figure 17, p. 27.)

Intubating through the LMA-Fastrach Using a Fiberoptic Endoscope

The Fastrach is inserted with the standard technique.

Place an endotracheal tube onto the lubricated fiberoptic bundle of the endoscope. Next, pass the endotracheal tube into the Fastrach to the 15-mm depth marker. Insert the fiberoptic scope to the end of the tube. You should see the Epiglottic Elevating Bar lying across the epiglottis. Next, insert the endotracheal tube 1.5 cm. Pass the endoscope to the end of the endotracheal tube. The view should be of the glottic opening with the Epiglottic Elevating Bar pushed anteriorily. If this is the view, pass the endotracheal tube into the trachea, remove the scope, confirm position of the endotracheal tube, reconnect the 15-mm adapter and ventilate the patient. The fiberoptic endoscope should not be pushed beyond the Epiglottic Elevating Bar. Figure 13.38 illustrates use of a fiberoptic endoscope with the LMA-Fastrach.

Evaluating LMA Position after Insertion

After inserting the LMA, one must evaluate the airway's positon in the hypopharynx. The manufacture of the LMA suggests that the signs of correct placement include the following:

1. Slight outward movement of the LMA upon cuff inflation
2. The presence of a smooth oval swelling in the neck around the thyroid and cricoid area.
3. No cuff visible in the oral cavity.[4(p28)]

Many other tests are used by the clinician to evaluate the position of the LMA. These include:

1. Movement of the anesthesia circuit bag when the patient breathes spontaneously

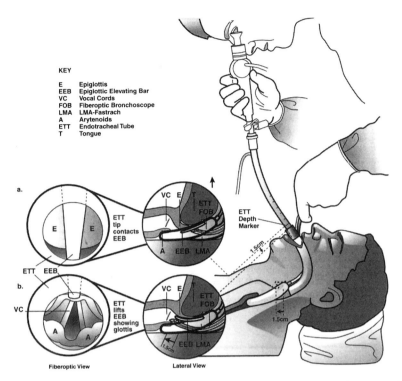

KEY

E	Epiglottis
EEB	Epiglottic Elevating Bar
VC	Vocal Cords
FOB	Fiberoptic Bronchoscope
LMA	LMA-Fastrach
A	Arytenoids
ETT	Endotracheal Tube
T	Tongue

FIGURE 13.38. Intubation with fiberoptic bronchoscope. **A.** Illustrates the view seen when the endotracheal tube is inserted to the 15-cm mark. **B.** Illustrates the view when the endotracheal tube is passed 1.5 cm further and the tip of the tube elevates the Epiglottic Elevating Bar. (Reproduced with permission from LMA North America, Inc.) (*Fastrach Manual.* 1998: figure 12, p. 24.)

2. Midline position of the LMA "black marker"
3. Anterior displacement of the larynx
4. Ability to ventilate the patient manually
5. Capnographic detection of carbon dioxide upon exhalation
6. Adequate sealing of the airway within the manufacturer's recommended cuff volume and pressure ranges.

With experience, proper seating can be achieved easily in nearly every application of the airway.

In an evaluation of positioning tests, Joshi et al[9] found that the ability to manually ventilate the patient and to generate an airway pressure of 20 cm H_2O were the best correlates of proper LMA positioning as verified by fiberoptic examination. Each clinician should develop his own set of tests and observations to check proper LMA placement. When in doubt, fiberoptic endoscopy can verify airway positioning.

Removing the LMA

The LMA is well tolerated by patients as they emerge from general anesthesia if the cuff pressure is kept around 60 cm H_2O.[4(p36)] Keep the monitors on the patient to assure that vital signs are stable and oxygenation is adequate. Leave the cuff inflated, avoid pharyngeal or tracheal suctioning, do not disturb the patient by movement or other bodily manipulations or interventions, and allow the patient to emerge from anesthesia. Observe for the return of airway reflexes (swallowing). Allow the patient to wake up and follow commands. Deflate the cuff and remove the LMA and the oral airway simultaneously when the patient opens his mouth on command. Verify ventilation and suction the pharynx if necessary. Nunez et al[10] verified that removal of the LMA in accordance with the manufacturer's recommendations resulted in fewer complications than when the LMA was removed with the patient still anesthetized. Many clinical considerations are taken into account when deciding when to remove the LMA. Whether you remove the LMA in the operating room or the recovery area, and whether you strictly adhere to the manufacturer's recommendations concerning removal, you should be ready to intervene immediately if the patient experiences any post-removal airway problems.

Educational Materials

Manuals and videotapes are available from LMA North America, Inc., that describe all of the applications of each model of LMA. The literature and videotapes also contain much more information concerning the LMA, including warnings, cleaning instructions, and complications and problems associated with the LMA. Read the manuals and review the videotapes before using the LMA.

Additional Considerations Concerning the LMA

Studies, case reports, and comments concerning the LMA and its applications have received widespread exposure in the literature. As early as 1996, Brimacombe and Berry[11] estimated that LMA usage in the United Kingdom ranged between 30% and 60% of all general anesthetic cases. One of the reasons the LMA was accepted so quickly was because investigators documented the device's safety and efficacy shortly after it was introduced. In 1996, Verghese and Brimacombe[12] published the results of LMA use in nearly 12,000 patients. They concluded that the device was successfully inserted in 99.8% of patients and that use of the LMA was safe and effective for patients ventilated with positive pressure as well as for those breathing spontaneously. They reported that the LMA had been used to gain airway control in patients whose airways could not be managed with conventional techniques. Investigators have continued to study many facets of LMA use and to document complications and problems associated with the device.

Subsequent sections of this chapter will examine several topics of interest concerning the LMA.

LMA Size

The manufacturer of the LMA suggests guidelines for mask size based on the weight of the patient. Kagawa and Obara[13] have suggested a formula to estimate LMA size based on the patient's weight:

$$LMA\ Size = Square\ Root\ of\ (Patient\ Weight\ (kg)/5)$$

Much debate regarding the appropriateness of weight-based sizing has appeared in the literature. Many clinicians select a size used for adult patients based on the sex of the patient. Whether you use a gender-based size (for the average adult) of size 3 for females and size 4 for males[14] or a size 4 for females and size 5 for males,[15,16] you should adjust the cuff volume to achieve a minimum effective sealing pressure at which an airway leak is noted (18 to 20 cm H_2O) when positive pressure is delivered to the patient. If the cuff's volume cannot be adjusted to secure a seal below the manufacturer's recommended maximum volume, replace the LMA and try a different size. When comparing different studies, carefully examine the methods (patient demographics, anesthetic techniques) and endpoints (postoperative sore throat vs. airway leak) before reaching conclusions concerning LMA size.

Modified Insertion Techniques

Clinicians insert the LMA utilizing techniques that differ from those suggested by the device's manufacturer. One technique is to partially fill the cuff with air before insertion. Wakeling et al[17] reported that this modification facilitated insertion and decreased both the incidence of postoperative sore throat as well as blood observed on the LMA after removal. Brimacombe[18] commented that this technique could facilitate insertion "to compensate for suboptimal insertion skills," a hypothesis with which Wakeling[19] did not agree. Another modification of the insertion technique is for the operator to initiate insertion with a partially inflated LMA introduced into the mouth with the breathing grille pointing toward the hard palate. The LMA is advanced into the hypopharynx, then twisted 180 degrees[20] (the "Charlottetown twist"). Dugois et al reported that a distinct "pop" is felt when the LMA seats itself. Brimacombe[21] has questioned the safety of this maneuver. Dugois[22] reported that the maneuver had not caused "arytenoid dislocation," in response to Brimacombe's comments.

Other airway maneuvers have been studied as to their effect on LMA positioning and function. Aoyama et al reported that the triple airway maneuver, a combination of head extension, mouth opening, and jaw thrust used on anesthetized/paralyzed patients, resulted in less epiglottic downfolding by the LMA.[23] The same group reported that the application of cricoid pressure to anesthetized/paralyzed patients impeded the positioning of and ventilation through the LMA.[24]

Learn the recommended insertion techniques before experimenting with modifications. Future studies will document the efficacy and safety of modified techniques that are in widespread clinical use.

LMA Insertion and Mallampati Grading

McCrory and Moriarty[25] compared the ease of insertion of the LMA in patients with various Mallampati grades of airway anatomy. They concluded "that the Mallampati classification indicates difficulty not only in tracheal intubation but also in achieving an adequate airway with the LMA." Brimacombe and Berry[26] cited many methodological problems with the study and reported their findings with larger patient populations. They concluded that LMA insertion by skilled clinicians was not affected by Mallampati grades I through III airway anatomy. They had "insufficient data to be certain about Mallampati grade IV patients" at the time they published their comments.

Comparing Anesthetic Techniques and LMA Insertion

It is beyond the scope of this book to compare the myriad of anesthetic techniques and drugs used to facilitate LMA insertion. You may consult recent anesthesiology textbooks with regard to this subject. Let it suffice to say that the LMA can best be inserted with the patient anesthetized appropriately. Airway reflexes should be absent and the patient relaxed (though not necessarily paralyzed).

Cuff and Mucosal Pressures and the LMA

It has been postulated that complications such as sore throat and nerve damage may be related to pressure exerted by the LMA on airway structures. Recent and ongoing research is testing of this hypothesis. Defining the precise mechanisms of airway injury associated with LMA use is an area of active investigation.

It is important to keep in mind that the traditionally accepted magnitude of capillary perfusion pressure to tracheal and pharyngeal tissues ranges between 20 and 40 mm Hg (27 and 54 cm H_2O). Should external pressures exceed these levels, ischemic injury may result.

The following sections deal with various pressure-related topics associated with LMA use.

Calculated Versus Measured Mucosal Pressures

Marjot[27] warned that the calculated transmitted pharyngeal pressure exerted by size 2 to size 4 LMA's on hypopharyngeal tissue ranged from 103 to 251 mm Hg (139 to 339 cm H_2O). He postulated that these pressures could cause tissue ischemia by exceeding the capillary perfusion pressure of the airway tissue. However, in 1999, Keller et al[28] challenged this conclusion. With microsensors attached to a size 5 LMA, they documented that actual measured pharyngeal mucosal pressures ranged between 2 and 14 cm H_2O (mean pressure) at various cuff sensor locations. These pressures are below the accepted capillary perfusion pressure of pharyngeal tissue. They concluded that the calculated pressures were a poor indicator of the actual pressure exerted against the pharyngeal tissues in their model.

In a series of papers, Keller and Brimacombe reported that the measured pharyngeal mucosal pressures, as documented by an array of microsensors affixed to an LMA, were consistently less than assumed capillary perfusion pressure for the LMA-Classic,[29–32] LMA-Flexible,[30] LMA-Unique,[31] and the LMA-ProSeal.[32] The measured pharyngeal pressures for all of these airways ranged generally between 2 and 20 cm H_2O at all of the 6 or 7 sensor locations directed toward different pharyngeal surfaces. With respect to the LMA-Fastrach (Intubating LMA), these same investigators found that the measured pharyngeal mucosal pressures exerted by the Fastrach were higher when compared to the LMA-Classic and that the pressures exerted by the Fastrach "always exceeded capillary perfusion pressure."[33] They recommended that the Fastrach should be removed after intubation and that the Fastrach should not be used as a routine airway.

Pharyngeal Mucosal Pressure Versus Airway Sealing Pressure

Brimacombe and Keller[34] demonstrated that the pharyngeal mucosal pressure and airway sealing pressure showed no correlation at any location measured by an array of microsensors affixed to a size 5 LMA in anesthetized patients. They noted that the mucosal pressures were highest in the oropharynx. When the cuff was inflated with more than 20 ml of air and the cuff pressure exceeded 69 cm H_2O, the mean mucosal pressure was reported to be 41 cm H_2O, a level higher than the capillary perfusion pressure. One can conclude that the cuff should be sealed with the lowest volume required to achieve an effective seal.

Head and Neck Position, Oropharyngeal Leak Pressure, and Cuff Position

Keller and Brimacombe[35] compared the leak pressure and the cuff position (fiberoptically verified) with different head and neck positions in 20 anesthetized patients. They found that head position (extension, flexion, and rotation compared to neutral) caused little change in oropharyngeal leak pressure and no change with respect to cuff position. The small change noted for the leak pressure led to the suggestion that a more efficient seal might be obtained with flexion and by avoiding extension of the head.

Neuromuscular Blockade, Mode of Ventilation and Respiratory Cycle, and Pharyngeal Mucosal Pressures

Keller and Brimacombe[36] compared measured pharyngeal mucosal pressures with their microsensor model under the following conditions in anesthetized patients (1) apneic, nonparalyzed patients, (2) spontaneously breathing, nonparalyzed patients, (3) ventilated, paralyzed patients, (4) nonventilated, paralyzed patients. They found that the conditions did not affect the measured **pharyngeal mucosal pressures** at any sensed location in the airway.

Cuff Volume, Oropharyngeal Leak Pressure, and Fiberoptic View

Keller et al[37] and Brimacombe[38] reported that the most efficient cuff seal and the best fiberoptic view through the LMA are achieved with cuff volumes below the maximum volumes suggested by the manufacturer. They recommend using about 15 ml of air for a size 4 LMA and between 20 and 30 ml of air for a size 5 LMA to achieve these endpoints.

Comparison of Methods to Assess LMA Airway Sealing Pressures

Many clinical tests are used to assess the efficiency of the airway seal when an LMA is positioned. You should use an appropriately sized airway and inject the smallest volume of air necessary to achieve a seal at around 20 cm H_2O. Keller et al[39] compared four tests to assess the airway seal as follows: (1) detection of audible noise by listening over the mouth; (2) capnography: detection of carbon dioxide by a sampling tube placed 5 cm inside the mouth alongside of the LMA; (3) manometric stability: observing "an aneroid manometer dial as the pressure from the breathing system increased and noting the airway pressure at which the dial reached stability"; (4) auscultation: "detection of an audible noise using a stethoscope placed just lateral to the thyroid cartilage." In their subjects, the mean airway sealing pressure ranged between 19.5 and 21.3 cm H_2O. All of the tests were deemed to be excellent for clinical purposes. The manometric stability test was determined to have the best interobserver reliability. These tests, and others, should be used to verify that the LMA is in proper position and inflated to a safe and effective volume.

Esophageal Reflux and the Risk of Aspiration with the LMA

In the previously cited study of Verghese and Brimacombe,[12] the LMA was used to manage the airways of 11,910 patients who underwent general anesthesia and surgery. These authors reported that "regurgitation occurred in four patients (0.03%), vomiting in two patients (0.017%), and aspiraton occurred once (0.009%)."

However, the possibility that the LMA could reflexly trigger or at least facilitate gastroesophageal reflux remained a concern to many clinicians. Roux et al[40] compared esophageal pH values in anesthetized, spontaneously ventilating patients. They reported that the incidence of reflux into the lower but not the midesophagus was higher for patients managed with an LMA as compared to those managed with an oral airway. McCrory and McShane[41] reported a high frequency of reflux when the LMA was used in patients placed in the lithotomy position, though methodological details in their abstract are lacking. Brain et al[42] and Brimacombe et al[43] have raised many methodological concerns with respect to LMA related reflux studies.

Recent studies evaluate the interactions between the LMA and esophagus. Keller et al[44,45] demonstrated in controlled cadaver studies that the Classic, the ProSeal, and the Flexible LMA all attenuated the flow of liquid between the esophagus and pharynx. Keller and Brimacombe[46] demonstrated that in awake subjects with topically anesthetized airways, the LMA did not change the resting gastroesophageal barrier pressure or the upper esophageal sphincter pressure.

Positive-Pressure Ventilation (PPV) and the LMA

The LMA was designed to be used for cases and situations in which the clinician would traditionally use a face mask.[4(p4)] The LMA was not designed to replace an endotracheal tube or to be used to manage patients where the face mask was not indicated. Brimacombe et al[47] noted that "the LMA was designed for use at peak airway pressures (PAP) less than 20 cm H_2O and tidal volumes 8–10 mL/Kg."

To this formula, one could add the recommendation that the cuff of the LMA should be inflated with just enough air to achieve a seal at about 18 to 20 cm H_2O.

LMA Versus the Face Mask Used with PPV

Ho-Tai et al[48] compared the ventilatory mechanics and incidence of gastric insufflation in patients managed with an LMA or a standard face mask. Both groups of patients received PPV. They reported that both devices established efficient airways. The incidence of gastric insufflation with the LMA ranged between 1.6% and 5%, depending on the peak airway pressure (20 to 30 cm H_2O). The incidence of gastric insufflation with the face mask ranged between 5% and 26.6% over the same pressure range. A study by Weiler et al[49] demonstrated that "gastric insufflation occurred in 27% of the patients [managed with an LMA] at inspiratory pressures between 19 and 33 cm H_2O." The median maximum inspiratory pressure used in study subjects was reported to be 30.7 cm H_2O. Weiler et al cited a previous face mask study they had conducted[50] and compared results with their LMA study. They concluded that the LMA was not better than the standard face mask "in preventing airway pressure transmission to the esophagus" when the patient was ventilated with positive pressure. Brimacombe et al[47] noted that the peak airway pressures quoted in the Wieler study exceeded recommended pressures to be used with the LMA. It is fair to say that at some airway pressure, about 30 cm H_2O, esophageal insufflation could occur with either device in place.

Modes of Ventilation

In most LMA studies, patients are managed with spontaneous or controlled PPV. Recently, the modality of pressure support ventilation (PSV) has been studied. Brimacombe et al[51] reported that PSV at a plateau of 5 cm H_2O above a CPAP level of 5 cm H_2O provided better carbon dioxide exchange, higher tidal volume, and higher oxyhemoglobin levels than those achieved with CPAP alone. Cochran et al[52] reported that patients showed improved ventilatory mechanics when PSV was added to a "maximum" level at which respiratory rate dropped below 8/min or a leak around the LMA was detected. Pressure support ventilation levels were titrated up to 14 cm H_2O, with adjustments made if breathing became irregular.

Select the most appropriate modality of ventilation and apply it to the LMA as you would with a face mask or an endotracheal tube *as long as the recommended peak airway pressures, airway leak pressures, cuff pressures, and cuff volumes are not exceeded.*

The LMA, Gastric Distention, Reflux, and PPV: Clinical Studies

In 1996, Verghese and Brimacombe[12] reported their findings after studying 11,910 patients managed with an LMA. Of these patients, 5,240 (44%) received PPV, 2,222 for intraabdominal surgical procedures. The incidence of experiencing a critical event was 0.21% for patients receiving PPV, vs. 0.11% for those breathing spontaneously (not statistically different). As previously noted, only one case of aspiration was reported.

Many clinical studies support using the LMA with PPV, assuming that the manufacturer's volume and pressure recommendations are observed. Wainwright[53] reported a series of 1,958 ophthalmic surgery patients, 1,424 of whom were ventilated with PPV. No signs of aspiration were noted for any patient. Other investigators have published prospective clinical studies examining use of the LMA with PPV for a variety of surgical procedures. The reports of Bapat and Verghese[54] and Skinner et al[55] support use of the LMA with patients undergoing gynecological laparoscopic surgery by showing that the risk of significant clinical gastric regurgitation is extremely low in their study populations. (Esophageal pH probe evidence documented the incidence of reflux to be 15% of patients ventilated with positive pressure, vs. 5% for those breathing spontaneously.)[55] Agro et al[56] reported no evidence of reflux in patients receiving PPV for orthopedic surgery. They did *not* reverse neuromuscular blocking drugs with antagonists because antagonists might increase the risk of passive or active gastric regurgitation. Finally, Maltby et al[57] reported that patients undergoing laparoscopic cholecystectomy who were ventilated with positive pressure experienced the same amount of "gastric distension" whether they were managed with an LMA or an endotracheal tube.

Pediatric Use of the LMA and PPV

Positive-pressure ventilation via an LMA has been used with pediatric patients for many years. Many investigators cautioned against the routine use of the LMA because they observed a high incidence of gastric distention in their patients. Two prospective studies by Ruiz et al[58] and Gursoy et al[59] documented that the use of PPV and the LMA with pediatric patients undergoing a variety of surgical procedures did not lead to "major gastric insufflation."[58] The authors cautioned that close "monitoring of airway integrity, gas leak, and abdominal distension"[59] be maintained, as well as low peak positive ventilating pressures (10 to 18 cm H_2O).

LMA-ProSeal: Cautionary Notes

Brimacombe[60] reported a case in which a ProSeal was inserted and the initial malposition test indicated proper positioning. Gastric distention was noted 20 minutes after the start of surgery. Upon fiberoptic examination, the authors noted that the distal mask was folded under the proximal mask, thus occluding the distal drainage channel of the airway. The upper esophageal sphincter was observed to open with each positive-pressure breath. The tube was repositioned and the airway functioned properly for the rest of the case. The authors recommended that after initial positioning, a tube be passed through the drainage channel to make sure that it is not occluded by malpositioning.

Stix et al[61] reported two cases of air entrainment into the esophagus during spontaneous ventilation. In one case, the ProSeal was positioned correctly. In the other, the cuff of the airway caused partial airway obstruction. When these patients took a spontaneous breath, negative pleural pressures (that were lower because of partial airway obstruction) were transmitted to the esophagus and air was entrained down the drainage tube into the stomach.

Both of these cases stress the importance of proper airway positioning, testing the drainage tube for patency and proper seating, and observing for gastric distention and changes in airway positioning during management of the patient.

External Airway Maneuvers and the LMA

As already noted, flexion, though not extension, of the head can improve the airway seal of the LMA. Brimacomabe and Berry[62] report that gentle, gradual pressure applied with the palms "to the front and/or sides of the neck" can improve the LMA seal; but take care not to dislodge the airway. They also report that an alternative to using manual pressure is "to place two sandbags on either side of the neck to obliterate [a] leak."

Asai et al[63] report that the application of cricoid pressure can decrease the gastric insufflation of gas during PPV; however, the maneuver may also decrease the tidal volume delivered to the patient.

Conclusions Regarding the Use of PPV and the LMA

Current literature supports the contention that the LMA can be used safely with PPV provided that the manufacturer's pressure and volume recommendations are observed. An important corollary is that the clinician placing the LMA is experienced and can assure that the LMA is properly positioned.

The LMA can be used when it would be appropriate to use a face mask. The LMA is not a substitute for the endotracheal tube.

Use of the LMA with Pediatric Patients

Insertion Techniques

In commenting on LMA insertion in children, Brain[64] reconfirmed that the standard technique described for adults is applicable to children. He stressed the need to maintain "firm flexion of the neck with head extension by the nondominant hand," a maneuver that opens the space behind the larynx. Brain also wrote that "the inserting finger must imitate the action of the tongue, which requires the person doing the insertion to point his or her finger toward his or her own umbilicus during the whole insertion maneuver. This means the direction of applied pressure is different from the direction in which the mask moves, a point rarely appreciated."

Clinicians, however, have devised modified insertion techniques. One such technique is described by Elwood and Cox.[65] They reported that a Mac #2 laryngoscope could be used to help insert an LMA in a series of patients ranging in age from 8 months to 10 years. The laryngoscope was inserted in the standard manner and the LMA was inserted under direct vision. They concluded that the LMA was inserted easily either with or without laryngoscopic assistance. However, they documented fiberoptically that the epiglottis was in the proper position (out of view) in 10 of 25 patients who received laryngoscopic assistance but in only 1 of 22 patients in whom the LMA was inserted blindly. Cox[76] stated that he routinely used the standard (blind) method to insert an LMA in children. He used "the rotary method and the laryngoscopic method, should the blind method fail." Yih[67] found that a straight laryngoscope blade could also be used to assist insertion of an LMA in children.

Removal of the LMA in Pediatric Patients

Controversy exists as to whether the LMA should be removed with the patient "deep" (still anesthetized) or "awake," having regained all airway reflexes and being responsive to command or stimuli, as recommended by the manufacturer.[68]

Kitching et al[69] compared removal of the LMA from anesthetized vs. "awake" patients who ranged in age from 12 months to 8 years. They reported that the patients who had the LMA removed when they were "awake" experienced more coughing and desaturation during the coughing spells. As a result of their study and others, the authors state, "For older infants and young children we now advocate removal of the LMA at a deep plane of anaesthesia to remove the stimulating effect on the airway."

Parry et al[70] challenged the conclusions of Kitching, citing that the LMA had not been removed in accordance with the recommendations of the manufacturer and inventor of the device. Parry et al reported their group's experience with LMA removal and quoted other papers supporting the opinion that the LMA should be left in place until spontaneously ejected by the patient.

Finally, Samarkandi[68] published a study of 165 pediatric patients who ranged in age from 2 months to 13 years and concluded that "there was no difference in the incidence of airway complications whether the LMA was removed in the anaesthetized or the awake child."

More study regarding LMA removal in pediatric patients needs to be undertaken. The main problem when comparing current studies is the lack of control for important variables such as anesthetic and analgesic techniques, site of surgery, LMA removal criteria, and the level of experience and training of recovery room personnel. At the present time, opinions vary as to the most appropriate time to remove the LMA from a pediatric patient emerging from general anesthesia.

Use of the LMA to Manage Patients with Congenital Airway Anomalies

Many congenital syndromes are associated with abnormal airway anatomy. When devising a plan to care for these patients, consider using the LMA. Specify the device's place in the airway management algorithm. While no technique or device is guaranteed to be effective, the LMA has been used to manage the airways of children with many different types of congenital anomalies. These include the following: Freeman-Sheldon syndrome,[71] Pierre-Robin syndrome,[72,73] Schwartz-Jampel syndrome,[74] Beckwith-Wiedemann syndrome,[75] and laryngo-tracheo-esophageal clefts.[76] Many more congenital anomalies affecting airway anatomy are referenced in the bibliography at www.LMANA.com.

The LMA and Neonatal Resuscitation

As early as 1995, Brimacombe and Berry[77] suggested that the LMA should receive serious consideration for inclusion in neonatal resuscitation protocols. Paterson et al[78] evaluated the use of the LMA to manage the airways of 21 neonates in a prospective resuscitation study. The LMA was inserted successfully in every patient and PPV was quickly established. A size 1 airway was used for all patients. All of the LMAs were successfully inserted on the first attempt in an average of 8.6 seconds. The investigators recommended that further studies were needed to more clearly define the role of the LMA in neonatal resuscitation. Arkoosh[79] has made the same recommendation.

Use of the LMA in Pediatric Surgical Patients with Upper Respiratory Tract Infections (URIs) and Mild Bronchopulmonary Dysplasia (BPD)

Tait et al[80] compared the LMA to the endotracheal tube as the method of airway management in 82 patients ranging in age from 3 months to 16 years. All of the patients had an active URI at the time of surgery. None of the surgical procedures were performed on the airway. No statistically significant difference between groups was noted for the incidence of perioperative coughing, laryngospasm, breath-holding, arrhythmias, excitement, or excessive secretions. The severity of coughing was assessed to be higher in the endotracheal tube group of patients, as was the incidence of mild bronchospasm. The total number of episodes of breath-holding, laryngospasm, bronchospasm, and oxygen desaturation was significantly greater in the endotracheal tube group. At least one case of laryngospasm was noted in each group. All airway complications were easily managed. The authors concluded that if surgery had to be performed on patients with a URI, the LMA should be considered an airway management option.

Ferrari and Goudsouzain[81] compared the use of the LMA with that of the endotracheal tube in 27 former premature patients undergoing eye surgery. All of the patients were diagnosed with mild BPD. They found no statistically significant differences with respect to airway complications in the intraoperative period. Patients in the LMA group opened their eyes and were discharged from the recovery room sooner than those in the endotracheal tube group. Three children in the endotracheal tube group had transient postoperative respiratory complications. They concluded that children with mild BPD could be managed with an LMA during minor surgical procedures. Mayhew and Dalmeida[82] disagreed with Ferrari and Goudsouzain concerning the safety of the LMA to manage surgical pediatric patients with mild BPD. In response, Ferrari[83] maintained that the purpose of their study was to "present to anesthesiologists our unique experience of safety utilizing the laryngeal mask airway (LMA) in children with chronic lung disease with bronchopulmonary dysplasia as the model." Ferrari and Goudsouzain did not claim to have published conclusive evidence that the LMA was superior to the endotracheal tube to manage patients with BPD. Future studies with larger numbers of subjects will define the role of the LMA in managing this challenging group of patients.

Diagnostic Fiberoptic Bronchoscopy with LMA Assistance

Diagnostic fiberoptic bronchoscopic examination to evaluate conditions such as stridor or pulmonary infiltrate is common in pediatric tertiary care hospitals. Traditionally, airway management included: (1) fiberoptic examination with no supportive airway intervention, (2) examination through a modified face mask that allowed passage of the endoscope, or (3) examination through an endotracheal tube. Many clinicians now use the LMA to facilitate diagnostic fiberoptic examinations in pediatric patients.[84,85]

The Learning Curve for Pediatric LMA Use

Lopez-Gil et al[86] studied 8 third-year anesthesiology residents with no prior experience using the LMA. Each resident was observed performing 75 LMA insertions on pediatric patients using the standard insertion technique. The overall rate of experiencing problems with insertion declined from 62% to 2%, comparing the first 15-case epoch to the last. The residents with the highest insertion problem rates after 60 insertions all recorded rates less than 10%. The authors concluded: "Pediatric anesthesiologists with problem rates greater than 10% should determine if they are using the device suboptimally."

Innovative Uses of the LMA

It is beyond the scope of this book to describe all of the special and innovative applications of the LMA. Table 13.4 presents a sample from the literature describing use of the LMA in ways that might have seemed improbable when the device was introduced. Uses that were first deemed impractical, such as tonsillectomy performed with LMA airway management, are now accepted by many clinicians. *Not all of the applications on the list are accepted by all clinicians.* Many represent one-time case reports. However, Table 13.4 is presented to document the variety of ways the LMA has been used to help manage patients with rather complicated airway problems.

Many other applications have been reported. To reference a particular application, consult the bibliography at the website of LMA North America, Inc. (www.LMANA.com).

TABLE 13.4. Innovative and special uses of the LMA

1. Oral and maxillofacial surgery[87]
2. Neurosurgery[88–90]
3. Tonsillectomy
4. Ventilation through a tracheostomy stoma[91]
5. A route for tracheal drug administration[92]
6. Dental surgery[93]
7. To manage a patient with laryngeal polyposis[94]
8. To facilitate gastroscopy[95,96]
9. To facilitate transesophageal echocardiography[97]

Using the LMA with Adjunctive Airway Equipment

Learning to use the LMA to facilitate fiberoptic intubation is one of the skills the advanced airway manager must master. Any type of LMA can be used. Consider the type of opening that sits above the glottis when selecting an LMA. The standard grill will probably have to be modified (cut out a few of the gill slits to allow for passage of the endoscope and endotracheal tube). The Fastrach has an Epiglottic Elevator Bar that will push the epiglottis out of the way when the tube is inserted. When using the Fastrach remember to pass the endoscope to the end of the tube and advance the two pieces of equipment together until the Epiglottic Elevator Bar pushes the epiglottis out of view.

Another important use of the LMA is to facilitate insertion of the percutaneous tracheostomy tube as described in Chapter 10.

Another technique to learn is the insertion of the LMA under fiberoptic videoscopic guidance.[98] Hamaguchi et al describe this technique that would be very useful as an educational tool. They "suggest that after a fiberscope, which is connected to a closed-circuit television, is inserted into the laryngeal mask, the mask is inserted while the fiberoptic view is being shown on the television. This method enables one to see the anatomical course of the mask, in relation to the tongue, epiglottis or glottis during insertion."

Endotracheal intubation through the LMA-Classic has been described many times. The fiberoptic endoscope is usually used to facilitate this technique. The most perplexing step in the technique involves deciding what to do with the LMA after the intubation is completed. Various techniques have been described to remove the LMA. Some involve using various forceps techniques[99] to hold the endotracheal tube in place while the LMA is withdrawn over the forceps. Other techniques involve devising "tube extenders" such as smaller endotracheal tubes wedged into each other, end-to-end, and inserted into the tube used for intubation. (Remove the 15-mm adapters from all tubes.) The LMA can be withdrawn over the series of tubes, the tubes disconnected, and the adapter replaced into the endotracheal tube that has been left in place. Two authors suggest using long microlaryngeal tubes (30 to 33 cm in length) to intubate through the LMA.[100,101] These tubes are long enough to extend out of the LMA and serve as stabilizers when the LMA is removed. The tubes can then be cut off to the standard length. The tubes are manufactured by Mallinckrodt (St. Louis, MO) and Rusch, Inc. (Duluth, GA). The tubes are called microlaryngeal tubes (MLTs) and they come in different sizes. Most intubations through an LMA, whether blindly or fiberoptically guided, are facilitated by use of the LMA-Fastrach, which is specially designed for intubation. The Extender or Stabilizer Rod is used to hold the endotracheal tube in place as the LMA is removed, as described earlier in the chapter.

Finally, many authors report using a portable flexible lighted catheter or stylet inserted through an LMA as a guide to intubation.[102,103] The Fastrach may prove to be the best LMA to use with the lighted stylet, as problems with the standard LMA have been reported.[104,105] With the LMA in place, the lighted stylet is inserted through the airway into the trachea and the glow from the tip of the stylet is observed in the trachea below the thyroid cartilage at the level of the cricothyroid membrane. When the glow is seen, the tube is slipped off the lighted stylet into the trachea. Remember that the lighted stylet is rather rigid and should never be forced into the trachea. The LMA may need subtle manipulation to position its opening before passing the lighted stylet into the trachea. One type of stylet is the Trachlight Wand (Laerdal Medical Corp, NY).

Adverse Effects and Complications Associated with the LMA

A list of adverse effects associated with the LMA is presented in the LMA instruction manual.[4(pp10,11)] The authors of the manual state the following:

1. The incidence of aspiration associated with LMA use is estimated to be 2:10,000 applications.
2. The incidence of sore throat is estimated to be 10% (0-70% reported in various studies).
3. There have been *no reports of death* directly attributable to the LMA.

The manual lists the adverse effects related to LMA use (Table 13.5).

Other problems associated with LMA use have appeared in recent literature. One of these includes a case of acute transient submandibular sialadenopathy.[106] Brimacombe and Keller[107] comment that increased anterior pressure exerted by a malpositioned LMA could possibly cause sialadenopathy. Ogata et al[108] reported ul-

TABLE 13.5. Adverse events reported with LMA use

Aspiration	Regurgitation	Vomiting	
Pharyngolaryngeal reflexes			
Bronchospasm	Hiccup	Coughing	Laryngeal spasm
Gagging	Transient glottic closure	Retching	Breathholding
Trauma			
Arytenoid dislocation	Larynx	Minor abrasions	Tonsils
Epiglottis	Posterior pharyngeal wall	Uvula	
Neurovascular			
Tongue cyanosis	Vocal cord paralysis	Hypoglossal nerve paralysis	Parotid gland swelling
Lingual nerve paralysis	Tongue macroglossia		
Postoperative			
Dry mouth	Sore throat	Dysphonia	Pharyngeal ulcer
Dysphagia	Mouth ulcer	Hoarseness	
Feeling of fullness	Dysarthria	Stridor	
Coincidental			
Pulmonary edema	Stridor	Laryngeal hematoma	Head and neck edema
Nonairway			
Myocardial ischemia	Dysrhythmias		

Source: Brain, Denman, and Goudsouzian, 2000.[4(pp10–11)]

trasonic evidence that the submandibular gland could be deformed by insertion of the LMA, especially if excessively large volumes of air were injected into the cuff.

Two cases of negative-pressure pulmonary edema have been reported, one by Sullivan[109] in a patient who experienced airway obstruction once he was placed in the lateral position, and one by Devys et al,[110] in which the patient caused airway obstruction by biting the LMA. Both patients were breathing spontaneously when the obstruction occurred.

Maltby et al[111] reported a case of acute *unilateral* macroglossia following use of the LMA. The swelling resolved spontaneously and uneventfully. The authors speculated that the cause of the tongue swelling was related to "pressure-induced venous thrombosis," although the swelling could have been related to an "allergic reaction or angioneurotic oedema, damage to the right hypoglossal nerve, or obstruction of venous return." They reported that the LMA had been inserted easily and properly.

Branthwaite[112] reported a case of esophageal rupture related to LMA use. He reported that an intubating LMA had been inserted with difficulty: "The mask was replaced at least once and intubation was only achieved successfully on the fifth attempt." Signs of airway trauma were documented as blood was suctioned from the pharynx. Postoperatively, esophageal perforation was documented radiographically. The patient subsequently died as a result of other complications. "At the inquest into the patient's death, the Coroner returned a verdict of 'misadventure,' defined at law as the unintentional adverse outcome of a deliberate, lawful, human act." The author of the paper attributed the perforation to the LMA or to the endotracheal tube, although the exact mechanism of the injury could not be defined. The patient's airway had also been instrumented with a suction catheter and a nasogastric tube, devices that could have caused the perforation. Reports like this stress the absolute necessity to follow standard instructions that warn against forceful insertion.

Equipment problems have also been reported that include a fractured LMA mask,[113] a damaged LMA-Fastrach endotracheal tube,[114] and an LMA with a hole in the pilot tube.[115] As recommended by the manufacturer, always visually inspect the LMA-related equipment and test for leaks before use.

Finally, remember that LMA insertion can be made difficult or impossible if the patient has grossly abnormal airway anatomy or pathology.[116–118]

In conclusion, use of the LMA is not without risk. However, the device has a long and spectacular safety record. As with the selection of any piece of equipment, consider the risks and benefits of the LMA and weigh these against the risks and benefits of alternative devices used to manage the airway. Learn to use the LMA properly and *exercise clinical judgment!*

The LMA and the "Difficult Airway"

Many reports have verified the utility of the LMA in managing patients with known or unknown difficult airways. The LMA has a high rate of success (establishing and maintaining an oxyhemoglobin saturation greater than 90%) even when used in rescue situations after a difficult ventilation/difficult intubation crisis had developed. Parmet et al[119] reported that an airway emergency team, responding to urgent calls within the hospital, established a satisfactory rescue airway in 16 of 17 cases in which the LMA was the first device used to establish the airway. The failed case involved a patient who had a tracheal clot resulting from a previous cricothyroid puncture. Other reports support use of the LMA in the emergency setting. Recent studies in the anesthesiology literature have evaluated the LMA-Fastrach used to manage the airways of surgical patients presenting with known or suspected difficult airway anatomy.[120–123] These studies demonstrated that the LMA-Fastrach had a very high success rate when used to direct "blind" intubation (93%–100%). The LMA-Fastrach performed as well or better than the fiberoptic endoscope when used to facilitate endotracheal intubation. Langeron et al[123] advised that "blind" Fastrach-directed intubation was not recommended for use in patients with "previous radiotherapy" to the neck and pharynx. Ferson et al,[124] studying 254 patients with "difficult-to-manage airways," reported that the "overall success rates for blind and fiberoptically guided intubations through the LMA-Fastrach were 96.5 and 100.0%, respectively." Most of these intubations were carried out in the operating room, though 11 were performed in the ICU, emergency room, or the radiology suite. The patients had a variety of airway abnormalities including cervical spine pathology (see the section on use of the LMA to manage these patients).

The LMA and the American Society of Anesthesiologists (ASA) Difficult Airway Algorithm

The ASA published its first Difficult Airway Algorithm in 1991. Soon after, the LMA was approved for use in the United States and was recognized to be a useful tool to manage patients with difficult airways. The current ASA Difficult Airway Algorithm[125] includes the LMA as an option that should be considered on its "Emergency Pathway Limb" as an "Emergency-Nonsurgical Ventilation Device." Benumof[126] suggested that the LMA could fit into the **algorithm** at five different places to be used as a ventilation device or a conduit for fiberoptic intubation (Fig. 13.39).

Use of the LMA to Manage the Difficult Airway in Obstetric Patients

Management of the difficult airway in obstetric patients has received much consideration. Godley et al[127] reported a case in which the LMA was used to facilitate awake intubation prior to cesarean section. Gataure and Hughes[128] reported that of 209 anesthesiologists who responded to a survey sent to 250 obstetric centers, 72% "were in favor of using the LMA to maintain oxygenation when tracheal intubation had failed and ventilation using a face mask was inadequate." After inserting the LMA, the clinician must decide whether to proceed with sur-

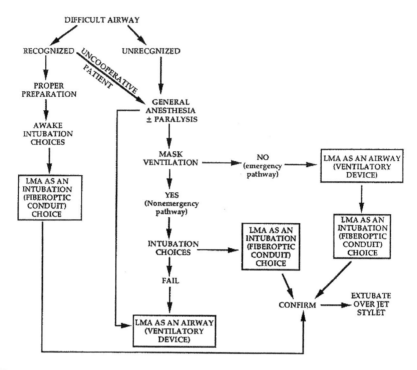

FIGURE 13.39. LMA and the ASA Difficult Airway Algorithm: *Five Points of Entry into the algorithm.* (From Benumof, 1996.[126])

gery, allow the patient to wake up, or to intubate the trachea through the LMA before proceeding with surgery. This is often a difficult decision to make and is based on the condition of the mother and the baby. Remember that the application of cricoid pressure might alter the LMA cuff seal or make passage of an endotracheal tube more difficult. The LMA should be stocked with the standard equipment in the obstetric suite. Define its place in the Difficult Obstetric Airway Algorithm before an airway emergency arises!

Difficult Pediatric Airway

The LMA has been used to establish an airway in pediatric patients who have morphologic and pathologic congenital airway anomalies. Two recent papers described strategies on how to intubate these patients through an LMA. Osses et al[129] reported on 6 patients (3 newborns and 3 infants). Under anesthesia, they examined the airway with a laryngoscope and could not see the epiglottis in any patient. After removing the laryngoscope, they inserted an LMA and verified correct position with capnography. They then blindly passed an oral RAE tube (Mallinckrodt Medical) through the unmodified LMA into the trachea and confirmed its position. They removed the 15-mm adapter from the tube, attached an adult intubating stylet onto the endotracheal tube, and used the stylet to hold the tube in place as the LMA was withdrawn over the stylet. The 15-mm adapter was reinserted and the patient ventilated. They achieved success in all 6 patients.

Walker[130] reported using the LMA to facilitate fiberoptic intubation in 21 children on 31 occasions. The patients ranged in age from 5 months to 18 years and had a variety of airway abnormalities. Under general anesthesia, an LMA was inserted. A fiberoptic endoscope was passed through the LMA into the trachea. A guide wire was passed through the scope into the trachea down to the right mainstem bronchus. The scope was removed and a "stiffening" catheter was passed over the guide wire. The wire was removed and the stiffening catheter was left in the trachea. An attempt was made to monitor carbon dioxide through the catheter to verify position. The LMA was removed and an endotracheal tube was passed over the catheter into the trachea. The catheter was then removed and the tube's position verified. The author reported successful intubation in all cases.

These and other reports support LMA use in the Difficult Pediatric Airway Algorithm.

The LMA and the Morbidly Obese Patient

Traditionally, the LMA has not been recommended for use with morbidly obese patients. However, these patients often present the anesthesiologist with difficult airway challenges, including difficulty maintaining mask ventilation and establishing endotracheal intubation. Recognizing that these challenges exist, Keller et al[131] reported a study that included 60 morbidily obese patients who were managed with an LMA-ProSeal airway. The patients were preoxygenated and anesthetized with an intravenous anesthetic. A ProSeal was inserted when there was "no response to jaw thrust." A size 5 ProSeal was used. All tubes were inserted with the manufacturer's "introducer tool." The cuff was inflated until a square wave capnograph was established and no audible leak was detected with peak airway pressures greater than 12 cm H_2O during manual ventiation. Once the tube was properly positioned, the patients were paralyzed and mechanical ventilation started. The intracuff pressure was set to 60 cm H_2O. All patients were ventilated with 8 ml/kg tidal volume at a rate of 12/min and an I:E ratio of 1:1.5. The patients were ventilated for 3 minutes, observations were taken, and then the ProSeal was replaced with an endotracheal tube for surgery. The authors reported that the LMA was inserted easily, 90% on the first attempt, 10% on the second. The average time to establish an airway was 15 seconds. Oropharyngeal leak pressure averaged 32 cm H_2O. No gastric or drainage tube air leaks were detected. Ventilation with a tidal volume of 8 ml/kg was possible in 95% to 98% of the patients. The authors listed the limitations of the study, notably the short duration of PPV and lack of controls. However, they concluded that the LMA was an effective *temporary ventilatory device* in grossly obese anesthetized patients.

The ASA Difficult Airway Algorithm does not specify which airway devices should be used to manage patients based on weight. Clinical judgment must be exercised. The study cited in this section established ventilatory parameters for the study population. Extrapolation to other patient populations is not justified.

However, the authors demonstrated that under the conditions of the study, an LMA can be used to deliver PPV to morbidly obese patients. Each clinician must decide the conditions under which an LMA will be used when faced with a "cannot ventilate/cannot intubate" scenerio.

Role of the LMA Outside of the Operating Room

The LMA was introduced for use by anesthesiology personnel in the operating room. Most of the studies evaluating the LMA's utility and operational parameters have been conducted in the operating room under the supervision of an anesthesiologist. However, it has become evident that the LMA could be very useful outside of the operating room. For example, the LMA could be used to establish an airway during resuscitation before definitive intubation of the trachea, especially if mask ventilation proved difficult with a standard oral airway. In 1994, Brimacombe[132] presented reasonable evidence that the LMA had a role in emergency airway management outside of the operating suite. He wrote that two national authorities, one in Japan and the other in the United Kingdom, had approved of programs to train "paramedical staff" in the use of the LMA. He cited reports of the successful use of the LMA to manage the airway in a variety of emergency settings. One example was use of the LMA to establish an airway in a crash victim who could not be intubated due to his position. He suggested that controlled trials were needed to define the role of the device outside of the operating room. A recent review by Pollack,[133] written for emergency physicians, stated that it was appropriate to use the LMA in the emergency setting. He wrote that a pilot study conducted in his emergency department to train emergency medicine residents had proven successful.

Future studies will more thoroughly define how the LMA should be used in emergency settings outside of the operating room. If the LMA is to be used *safely,* training and testing protocols will need to be established to insure *appropriate and proficient* use of the device.

Use of the LMA in Patients with Cervical Spine Pathology

The LMA has been used to establish an airway and to serve as an aid to facilitate fiberoptic intubation in patients with many types of cervical spine pathology, including neck trauma, extensive neck contracture,[134] previous cervical radiotherapy,[135] and patients with stiff necks such as those in fixed flexion.[136]

The recommended position of the head and neck for insertion of the LMA is the standard intubating position (slight flexion of the neck with head extension: the sniff position). This position differs from the neutral position, with in-line traction used to stabilize patients with many types of cervical spine pathology.

The application of neck stabilization devices and maneuvers such as neutral in-line cervical support may affect LMA use.

Ferson et al[124] reported using the Fastrach to ventilate and intubate 12 of 12 patients whose necks were immobilized with stereotactic frames. They concluded their paper with the comment that the Fastrach proved to be a "particularly valuable" tool and that its use should be considered "in the treatment of patients with immobilized cervical spines."

Asai et al[137] compared the time and ease of insertion of a standard LMA in anesthetized, paralyzed patients who were placed either in the sniff position or in a neutral position with manual in-line stabilization. They reported that it was significantly easier and faster to insert the LMA when the patients were placed in the recommended sniff position. The difference in insertion times was 11.7 vs. 20.1 seconds. They were able to insert the airway on the first attempt in 20 of 20 patients in the "sniff" position and 19 of 20 patients fixed in the neutral position. The clinical significance of the differences was not commented upon.

Another study by Asai et al[138] compared the Fastrach to the standard LMA with respect to the time and ease of insertion in anesthetized, paralyzed patients whose heads were held in the neutral position with manual in-line stabilization. They reported that the Fastrach was faster and easier to insert. They did not try to intubate through the LMA airways.

Nakazawa et al[139] reported that 36 of 40 patients with cervical spine disease (24 of whom had limited or prohibited neck extension and 10 of whom presented in stabilization devices) were blindly intubated through an LMA-Fastrach. The other 4 patients were intubated with fiberoptic assistance through the Fastrach. They attributed failure to intubate to the use of an inappropriately sized LMA.

Wakeling and Nightingale[140] studied use of the LMA-Fastrach to intubate simulated cervical spine–injured patients in a cervical collar with cricoid pressure applied. The patients were anesthetized and paralyzed for the study. They reported that presence of the collar (Stifneck Select; Laerdal Medical Corp., Wappinger's Falls, NY) made insertion of the Fastrach difficult because of limited mouth opening. They also reported that blind passage of the endotracheal tube was also difficult, if not impossible, in the majority of their patients. They concluded that the Fastrach was not "recommended as an adjunct for intubation in patients wearing semi-rigid neck collars."

By comparison, Moller et al[141] reported that the stiff neck collar "produced no serious obstacle to insertion, ventilation and blind intubation through the ILMA" in their case series. Obviously, more controlled studies need to be undertaken to assess the degree of impediment produced by various neck stabilization devices.

Cervical Pressures and Movement During Use of the LMA

Brimacombe et al[142] studied the pressure exerted on the second and third cervical vertebrae during standard LMA insertion. In a series of 20 fresh cadavers, they reported that pressure exerted on the vertebrae during insertion rose transiently to 224 cm H_2O and decreased rapidly to less than 20 cm H_2O after seating of the LMA. The pressure was caused by the index finger used to exert posterior pressure on the mask to hold it against the palate and posterior pharynx during insertion. They suggested that further research was needed to determine the clinical implications of their findings. They recommended "that clinicians be careful to avoid excessive posterior force when using the LMA in [patients with an] unstable cervical spine." They also did not recommend using an LMA-Fastrach (Intubating LMA) as an alternative to the standard LMA because a recent study had shown that the Fastrach had "been shown to exert substantial static pressures (approximately 160 cm H_2O) against the mucosa overlying the cervical vertebrae, and the implications of this have not been evaluated."

Kihara et al[143] studied segmental cervical spine movement related to the LMA-Fastrach insertion in 20 anesthetized patients with cervical spine pathology. All patients were stabilized with neutral manual in-line traction maintained by a neurosurgeon during LMA insertion. They recorded cervical movement with single-frame lateral radiographic imaging. Transillumination with a lightwand was used to direct intubation. They took care not to exert posterior pressure on the handle of the Fastrach. They reported that the LMA was easily inserted on the first attempt in all patients. To facilitate intubation, 10 patients required between 2 and 4 adjusting maneuvers. During LMA insertion, intubation, and LMA removal, various cervical segments were flexed between 1 and 4 degrees. Posterior movement ranged between 0.5 and 1.0 mm on insertion and intubation. No movement was observed with removal of the LMA. The neurological symptoms of all patients improved after surgery. The authors concluded that Fastrach insertion, lightwand-directed intubation, and LMA removal produced segmental movement of the cervical spine in spite of the application of in-line cervical traction. They noted that the movement caused was flexion, the opposite of that observed with laryngoscopic intubation.

Before initiating airway management in patients with cervical spine problems, a thorough airway examination must be undertaken and the surgeon responsible for the patient's care should be consulted. The safety of head and neck movement, the extent and direction of allowable movement, and stabilization precautions and measures should be discussed. In many cases, the sniff position is safe for the patient and the LMA should be inserted as recommended. In some cases, the patient should remain in the neutral position.

To summarize this section, consider the following. Insertion of the LMA may be more difficult if the patient is maintained in the neutral position with in-line stabilization. The application of cricoid pressure may impede LMA placement and intubation through the airway. In-line traction does not necessarily immobilize the neck during LMA insertion, intubation, or removal. Excessive posterior pressure should not be applied with the index finger in the posterior direction. Finally, if an LMA-Fastrach is used, it should not be left in place after intubation because of the posterior mucosal pressures it exerts. Clinical judgment and experience are required to manage the airways of patients with cervical spine pathology, whether or not an LMA is used.

Summary

The LMA is a revolutionary airway device. Its use in anesthesiology has become routine. The LMA is more than an alternative to the oral airway. It is used to assist in the management of complex airway problems and its place in the ASA

Difficult Airway Algorithm is firmly established. Future research will define new roles and establish extended safety parameters for the LMA in all fields of airway management.

References

1. Brain AIJ. *The Intavent Laryngeal Mask: Instruction Manual.* Tidmarsh, Berkshire; UK: Brain Medical Ltd.; 1992:1.
2. Brimacombe JR, Brain AIJ, Berry AM. *The Laryngeal Mask Airway: A Review and Practical Guide.* [CITY]: WB Saunders Company Ltd; 1997.
3. Joo H. Book review. *Can J Anaesth.* 1998;45(8):825.
4. Brain AIJ, Denman WT, Goudsouzian NG. *LMA-Classic and LMA-Flexible Instruction Manual.* San Diego: LMA North America, Inc.; 2000.
5. LMA-ProSeal advertisement. San Diego: LMA North America, Inc. LMA-178 Rev C.
6. LMA-Fastrach advertisement. San Diego: LMA North America, Inc. LMA-210 Rev A.
7. *LMA-ProSeal Instruction Manual.* San Diego: LMA North America, Inc.: 21–33.
8. Brain AIJ, Verghese C. *LMA-Fastrach Instruction Manual.* San Diego: LMA North America, Inc.: 4.
9. Joshi S, et al. A prospective evaluation of clinical tests for placement of laryngeal mask airways. *Anesthesiology.* 1998;89:1141.
10. Nunez J, et al. Timing of removal of the laryngeal mask airway. *Anaesthesia.* 1998;53:126.
11. Brimacombe J, Berry A. The laryngeal mask airway—anatomical and physiological implications. *Acta Anaesth Scand.* 1996;40:201.
12. Verghese C, Brimacombe JR. Survey of laryngeal mask airway usage in 11,910 patients: safety and efficacy for conventional and nonconventional usage. *Anesth Analg.* 1996;82(1):129.
13. Kagawa T, Obara H. An easy formula to remember the laryngeal mask airway size-patient weight relationship. *Anesthesiology.* 2000;92(2):631.
14. Nott MR, Hill RP. Letter. *Br J Anaesth.* 1998;81(4):656–657.
15. Asai T, et al. Appropriate size and inflation of the laryngeal mask airway. *Br J Anaesth.* 1998;80(4):470.
16. Brimacombe J, Keller C. Laryngeal mask airway size selection in males and females: ease of insertion, oropharyngeal leak pressure, pharyngeal mucosal pressures and anatomical position. *Br J Anaesth.* 1999;82(5):703.
17. Wakeling HG, et al. The laryngeal mask airway: a comparison between two insertion techniques. *Anesth Analg.* 1997;85(3):687.
18. Brimacombe JR. Laryngeal mask insertion techniques [letter]. *Anesth Analg.* 1998; 86(6):1337.
19. Wakeling HG. Response to Brimacombe [letter]. *Anesth Analg.* 1998;86(6):1337.
20. Dubois JY, et al. The Charlottetown LMA twist. *Can J Anesthesia.* 1998;45(8):823.
21. Brimacombe J, Gardiner D. The Charlottetown click. *Can J Anesthesia.* 1999;46(5):512.
22. Dubois JY. Response to Brimacombe and Gardiner [letter]. *Can J Anesthesia.* 1999; 46(5):512.
23. Aoyama K, et al. The triple airway manoeuvre for insertion of the laryngeal mask airway in paralyzed patients. *Can J Anaesth.* 1995;42(11):1010.
24. Aoyama K, et al. Cricoid pressure impedes positioning and ventilation through the laryngeal mask airway. *Can J Anaesth.* 1996;43(10):1035.
25. McCrory CR, Moriarty DC. Laryngeal mask airway positioning is related to Mallampati grading in adults. *Anesth Analg.* 1995;81:1001.

26. Brimacombe JR, Berry AM. Mallampati grade and laryngeal mask placement [letter]. *Anesth Analg*. 1996;82(5):1112.

27. Marjot R. Pressure exerted by the laryngeal mask airway cuff upon the pharyngeal mucosa. *Br J Anaesth*. 1993;70:25.

28. Keller C, et al. Calculated vs measured pharyngeal mucosal pressures with the laryngeal mask airway during cuff inflation: assessment of four locations. *Br J Anaesth*. 1999;82(3):399.

29. Keller C, Brimacombe J. Mucosal pressures from the cuffed oropharyngeal airway vs the laryngeal mask airway. *Br J Anaesth*. 1999;82(6):922.

30. Brimacombe J, Keller C. Comparison of the flexible and standard laryngeal mask airways. *Can J Anesth*. 1999;46(6):558.

31. Keller C, Brimacombe J. Mucosal pressure, mechanism of seal, airway sealing pressure, and anatomic position for the disposable versus reusable laryngeal mask airways. *Anesth Analg*. 1999;88:1418.

32. Keller C, Brimacombe J. Mucosal pressure and oropharyngeal leak pressure with the ProSeal versus laryngeal mask airway in anaesthetized paralysed patients. *Br J Anaesth*. 2000;85(2):262.

33. Keller C, Brimacombe J. Pharyngeal mucosal pressures, airway sealing pressures, and fiberoptic position with the intubating versus the standard laryngeal mask airway. *Anesthesiology*. 1999;90(4):1001.

34. Brimacombe J, Keller C. A comparison of pharyngeal mucosal pressure and airway sealing pressure with the laryngeal mask airway in anesthetized adult patients. *Anesth Analg*. 1998;87(6):1379.

35. Keller C, Brimacombe J. The influence of head and neck position on oropharyngeal leak pressure and cuff position with the flexible and the standard laryngeal mask airway. *Anesth Analg*. 1999;88:913.

36. Keller C, Brimacombe J. Influence of neuromuscular block, mode of ventilation and respiratory cycle on pharyngeal mucosal pressures with the laryngeal mask airway. *Br J Anaesth*. 1999;83(3):480.

37. Keller, C, et al. Influence of cuff volume on oropharyngeal leak pressure and fibreoptic position with the laryngeal mask airway. *Br J Anaesth*. 1998;81(2):186.

38. Brimacombe J. Letter. *Br J Anaesth*. 1999;82(1):150.

39. Keller C, et al. Comparison of four methods for assessing airway sealing pressure with the laryngeal mask airway in adult patients. *Br J Anaesth*. 1999;82(2):286.

40. Roux M, et al. Effect of the laryngeal mask airway on oesophageal pH: influence of the volume and pressure inside the cuff. *Br J Anaesth*. 1999;82(4):566.

41. McCrory C, McShane AJ. Laryngeal mask airway is associated with reflux in the lithotomy position. *Br J Anaesth*. 1996;77(5):693.

42. Brain AIJ, et al. Letter. *Br J Anaesth*. 1995;74(4):489.

43. Brimacombe JR. Letter. *Anesth Analg*. 1996;82(1):215.

44. Keller C, et al. Do laryngeal mask airway devices attenuate liquid flow between the esophagus and pharynx? A randomized, controlled cadaver study. *Anesth Analg*. 1999;88:904.

45. Keller C, et al. Does the ProSeal laryngeal mask airway prevent aspiration of regurgitated fluid? *Anesth Analg*. 2000;91:1017.

46. Keller C, Brimacombe J. Resting esophageal sphincter pressures and deglutition frequency in awake subjects after oropharyngeal topical anesthesia and laryngeal mask device insertion. *Anesth Analg*. 2001;93:226.

47. Brimacombe JR, et al. Letter. *Anesth Analg*. 1998;86(4):914.

48. Ho-Tai, et al. Gas leak and gastric insufflation during controlled ventilation: face mask versus laryngeal mask airway. *Can J Anesth.* 1998;45(3):206.

49. Weiler N, et al. Respiratory mechanics, gastric insufflation pressure, and air leakage of the laryngeal mask airway. *Anesth Analg.* 1997;84:1025.

50. Weiler N, et al. Assessment of pulmonary mechanics and gastric inflation pressure during mask ventilation. *Prehospital Disaster Med.* 1995;10:101.

51. Brimacombe J, et al. Pressure support ventilation versus continuous positive airway pressure with the laryngeal mask airway: a randomized crossover study of anesthetized adult patients. *Anesthesiology.* 2000;92(6):1621.

52. Cochran D, et al. Pressure support ventilation in the anaesthetized patient using the laryngeal mask airway [abstract]. *Br J Anaesth.* 1999;83(3):530.

53. Wainwright AC. Positive pressure ventilation and the laryngeal mask airway in ophthalmic anaesthesia. *Br J Anaesth.* 1995;75(2):249.

54. Bapat PP, Verghese C. Laryngeal mask airway and the incidence of regurgitation during gynecological laparoscopies. *Anesth Analg.* 1997;85:139.

55. Skinner HJ, et al. Gastro-oesophageal reflux with the laryngeal mask during daycase gynaecological laparoscopy. *Br J Anaesth.* 1998;80(5):675.

56. Agro F, et al. Laryngeal mask airway and incidence of gastro-oesophageal reflux in paralysed patients undergoing ventilation for elective orthopaedic surgery. *Br J Anaesth.* 1998;81(4):537.

57. Maltby JR, et al. Gastric distension and ventilation during laparoscopic cholecystectory: LMA-Classic vs. tracheal intubation. *Can J Anesth.* 2000;47(7):622.

58. Ruiz J, et al. Mechanical ventilation with laryngeal mask airway and gastric insufflation in paediatric anaesthesia. *Br J Anaesth.* 1999;82(suppl 1):150.

59. Gursoy F, et al. Positive pressure ventilation with the laryngeal mask airway in children. *Anesth Analg.* 1996;82(1):33.

60. Brimacombe J, et al. Gastric insufflation with the ProSeal laryngeal mask. *Anesth Analg.* 2001;92:1614.

61. Stix MS, et al. Esophageal aspiration of air through the drain tube of the ProSeal laryngeal mask. *Anesth Analg.* 2001;93:1354.

62. Brimacombe J, Berry A. Letter. *Can J Anaesth.* 1996;43(5):537.

63. Asai T, et al. Cricoid pressure applied after placement of the laryngeal mask prevents gastric insufflation but inhibits ventilation. *Br J Anaesth.* 1996;76(6):772.

64. Brain, AIJ. Letter. *Anesth Analg.* 1995;81(1):212.

65. Elwood T, Cox RG: Laryngeal mask insertion with a laryngoscope in paediatric patients. *Can J Anaesth.* 1996;43(5):435.

66. Cox RG. Letter. *Can J Anesth.* 1999;46(12):1195.

67. Yih PSW. Letter. *Can J Anesth.* 1999;46(6):617.

68. Samarkandi A. Awake removal of the laryngeal mask airway is safe in paediatric patients. *Can J Anaesth.* 1998;45(2):150.

69. Kitching AJ, et al. Removal of the laryngeal mask airway in children: anaesthetized compared with awake. *Br J Anaesth.* 1996;76(6):874.

70. Parry M, et al. Removal of LMA in children. *Br J Anaesth.* 1997;78(3):337.

71. Cruickshanks GF, et al. Anesthesia for Freeman-Sheldon syndrome using a laryngeal mask airway. *Can J Anesth.* 1999;46(8):783.

72. Baraka A. Laryngeal mask airway for resuscitation of a newborn with Pierre-Robin syndrome. *Anesthesiology.* 1995;83(3):645.

73. Hansen TG, et al. Laryngeal mask airway guided tracheal intubation in a neonate with Pierre Robin syndrome. *Acta Anaesth Scand.* 1995;39:129.

74. Theroux MC, et al. Laryngeal mask airway and fiberoptic endoscopy in an infant with Schwartz-Jampel syndrome. *Anesthesiology.* 1995;82(2):605.
75. Goldman LJ, et al. Successful airway control with the laryngeal mask in an infant with Beckwith-Wiedemann syndrome and hepatoblastoma for central line catheterization. *Paed Anaesth.* 2000;10:445.
76. Fraser J, et al. The use of the laryngeal mask airway for inter-hospital transport of infants with type 3 laryngotracheo-oesophageal clefts. *Intensive Care Med.* 1999;25:714.
77. Brimacombe J, Berry A. The laryngeal mask airway—a consideration for the Neonatal Resuscitation Programme guidelines? *Can J Anaesth.* 1995;42(1):88.
78. Paterson SJ, et al. Neonatal resusitation using the laryngeal mask airway. *Anesthesiology.* 1994;80(6):1248.
79. Arkoosh VA. Neonatal resuscitation: what the anesthesiologist needs to know. *A.S.A. Refresher Course Lectures.* 2001:242.
80. Tait AR, et al. Use of the laryngeal mask airway in children with upper respiratory tract infections: a comparison with endotracheal intubation. *Anesth Analg.* 1998; 86(4):706.
81. Ferrari LR, Goudsouzian NG. The use of the laryngeal mask airway in children with bronchopulmonary dysplasia. *Anesth Analg.* 1995;81:310.
82. Mayhew JF, Dalmeida RE. Letter. *Anesth Analg.* 1996;82(4):886.
83. Ferrari LR, Goudsouzian N. Response to Mayhew, Dalmeida [letter]. *Anesth Analg.* 1996;82(4):886–887.
84. Badr A, et al. Bronchoscopic airway evaluation facilitated by the laryngeal mask airway in pediatric patients. *Ped Pulm.* 1996;21:57.
85. Bandla HPR, et al. Laryngeal mask airway facilitated fibreoptic bronchoscopy in infants. *Can J Anaesth.* 1997;44(12):1242.
86. Lopez-Gil, et al. Laryngeal mask airway in pediatric practice: a prospective study of skill acquisition by anesthesiology residents. *Anesthesiology.* 1996;84(4):807.
87. Bennett J, et al. Use of the laryngeal mask airway in oral and macillofacial surgery. *J Oral Macillofac Surg.* 1996;54:1346.
88. Agarwal A, Shobhana N. Letter. *Can J Anaesth.* 1995;42(8):750.
89. Agarwal A, Shobhana R. Letter. *Can J Anaesth.* 1995;42(12):1176.
90. Silva LC, Brimacombe JR. Letter. *Anesth Analg.* 1996;82(2):430.
91. Morita Y, Takenoshita M. Laryngeal mask airway fitted over a tracheostomy orifice: a mean to ventilate a tracheotomized patient during induction of anesthesia. *Anesthesiology.* 1998;89(5):1295.
92. Alexander R, et al. The laryngeal mask airway and the tracheal route for drug administration. *Br J Anaesth.* 1997;78(2):220.
93. Quinn AC, et al. The reinforced laryngeal mask airway for dento-alveolar surgery. *Br J Anaesth.* 1996;77(2):185.
94. Pennant JH, et al. The laryngeal mask airway and laryngeal polyposos [letter]. *Anesth Analg.* 1994;78:1206.
95. Brimacombe J, et al. The Laryngeal mask for percutaneous endoscopic gastrostomy. *Anesth Analg.* 2000;91:635.
96. Brimacombe J. Laryngeal mask airway for access to the upper gastrointestinal tract. *Anesthesiology.* 1996;84(4):1009.
97. Salvi L, Pepi M. Pressure-assisted breathing through a laryngeal mask airway during transesophageal echocardiography. *Anesth Analg.* 1999;89:1585.
98. Hamaguchi S, et al. Use of a fiberscope and closed-circuit television for teaching laryngeal mask insertion. *Anesth Analg.* 2000;90:501.

99. Breen PH. Simple technique to remove laryngeal mask airway "guide" after endotracheal intubation. *Anesth Analg.* 1996;82:1302.

100. Pennant JH, Joshi GP. Intubation through the laryngeal mask airway. *Anesthesiology.* 1995;83(4):891.

101. Preis CA, Preis IS. Oversize endotracheal tubes and intubation via laryngeal mask airway. *Anesthesiology.* 1997;87(1):187.

102. Dimitriou V, Voyagis GS. Use of a lighted flexible catheter for guided intubation through the intubating laryngeal mask by nurses. *Br J Anaesth.* 1999;82(1):22.

103. Agro F, et al. Use of a lighted stylet for intubation via the laryngeal mask airway. *Can J Anaesth.* 1998;45(6):556.

104. Asai T, et al. Unexpected difficulty in the lighted stylet–aided tracheal intubation via the laryngeal mask [letter]. *Br J Anaesth.* 1997;78(1):111.

105. Asai T. Use of a lighted stylet and the laryngeal mask for tracheal intubation. *Anesth Analg.* 1998;86:494–500.

106. Hooda S, et al. Acute transient sialadenopathy associated with laryngeal mask airway. *Anesth Analg.* 1998;87(6):1438.

107. Brimacombe J, Keller C. Sialadenopathy with the laryngeal mask airway. *Anesth Analg.* 1999;89:261.

108. Ogata J, et al. The influence of the laryngeal mask airway on the shape of the submandibular gland. *Anesth Analg.* 2001;93:1069.

109. Sullivan M. Unilateral negative pressure pulmonary edema during anesthesia with a laryngeal mask airway. *Can J Anaesth.* 1999;46(11):1053.

110. Devys JM, et al. Biting the laryngeal mask: an unusual case of negative pressure pulmonary edema. *Can J Anaesth.* 2000;47(2):176.

111. Maltby J, et al. Acute transient unilateral macroglossia following use of a LMA. *Can J Anaesth.* 1996;43(1):94.

112. Branthwaite MA. An unexpected complication of the intubating laryngeal mask. *Anaesthesia.* 1999;54:166.

113. Wong DT, et al. Fractured laryngeal mask airway (LMA). *Can J Anaesth.* 2000;47(7):716.

114. Mesa A, Miguel R. Hidden damage to a reinforced LMA-Fastrach™ endotracheal tube. *Anesth Analg.* 2000;90:1250.

115. Nagi H, Brown PC. Undetected hole in a laryngeal mask. *Anesth Analg.* 1999;88:232.

116. Patel SK, et al. Failure of the laryngeal mask airway: an undiagnosed laryngeal carcinoma. *Anesth Analg.* 1998;86:438.

117. Wakeling HG, et al. Large goiter causing difficult intubation and failure to intubate using the intubating laryngeal mask airway: lessons for next time. *Br J Anaesth.* 1998;81:979.

118. Ishimura H, et al. Impossible insertion of the laryngeal mask airway and oropharyngeal axes. *Anesthesiology.* 1995;83(4):867.

119. Parmet JL, et al. The laryngeal mask airway reliably provides rescue ventilation in cases of unanticipated difficult tracheal intubation along with difficult mask airway. *Anesth Analg.* 1998;87:661.

120. Joo HS, et al. The intubating laryngeal mask airway after induction of general anesthesia versus awake fiberoptic intubation in patients with difficult airways. *Anesth Analg.* 2001;92:1342.

121. Shung J, et al. Awake intubation of the difficult airway with the intubating laryngeal mask airway. *Anaesthesia.* 1998;53:645.

122. Fukutome T, et al. Tracheal intubation through the intubating laryngeal mask airway

(LMA-Fastrach™) in patients with difficult airways. *Anaesth Intensive Care.* 1998; 26:387.

123. Langeron O, et al. Comparison of the intubating laryngeal mask airway with the fiberoptic intubation in anticipated difficult airway management. *Anesthesiology.* 2001;94(6):968.

124. Ferson DZ, et al. Use of the intubating LMA-Fastrach™ in 254 patients with difficult-to-manage airways. *Anesthesiology.* 2001;95:1175.

125. A.S.A. Difficult Airway Algorithm. 2002. Available at: www.asahq.org.

126. Benumof JL. Laryngeal mask airway and the ASA difficult airway algorithm. *Anesthesiology.* 1996;84(3):686.

127. Godley M, et al. Use of LMA for awake intubation for caesarean section. *Can J Anaesth.* 1996;43(3):299.

128. Gataure PS, Hughes JA. The laryngeal mask airway in obstetrical anaesthesia. *Can J Anaesth.* 1995;42(2):130.

129. Osses H, et al. Laryngeal mask for difficult intubation in children. *Paed Anaesth.* 1999;9:399.

130. Walker RWM. The laryngeal mask airway in the difficult paediatric airway: an assessment of positioning and use in fibreoptic intubation. *Paed Anaesth.* 2000;10:53.

131. Keller C, et al. The laryngeal mask airway ProSeal™ as a temporary ventilatory device in grossly and morbidly obese patients before laryngoscope-guided tracheal intubation. *Anesth Analg.* 2002;94:737.

132. Brimacombe J. Does the laryngeal mask have a role outside the operating theatre? *Can J Anaesth.* 1995;42(3):258.

133. Pollack CV. The laryngeal mask airway: a comprehensive review for the emergency physician. *J Emerg Med.* 2000;20(1)53.

134. Dimitriou V, et al. Letter. *Anesthesiology.* 1997;86(4):1011.

135. Giraud O, et al. Limits of laryngeal mask airway in patients after cervical or oral radiotherapy. *Can J Anaesth.* 1997;44(12):1237.

136. Asai T, Shingu K. Tracheal intubation through the intubating laryngal mask in a patient with a fixed flexed neck and deviated larynx. *Anaesthesia.* 1998;53:1199.

137. Asai T, et al. Ease of placement of the laryngeal mask during manual in-line neck stabilization. *Br J Anaesth.* 1998;80(5):617.

138. Asai T, et al. Placement of the intubating laryngeal mask is easier than the laryngeal mask during manual in-line neck stabilization. *Br J Anaesth.* 1999;82(5):712.

139. Nakazawa K, et al. Using the intubating laryngeal mask airway (LMA-Fastrach™) for blind endotracheal intubation in patients undergoing cervical spine operation. *Anesth Analg.* 1999;89:1319.

140. Wakeling HG, Nightingale J. The intubating laryngeal mask airway does not facilitate tracheal intubation in the presence of a neck collar in simulated trauma. *Br J Anaesth.* 2000;84(2):254.

141. Moller F, et al. Intubating laryngeal mask airway (ILMA) seems to be an ideal device for blind intubation in cases of immobile spine. *Br J Anaesth.* 2000;85(3):493.

142. Brimacombe J, et al. Laryngeal mask usage in the unstable neck. *Anesth Analg.* 1999; 89(2):536.

143. Kihara S, et al. Segmental cervical spine movement with the intubating laryngeal mask during manual in-line stabilization in patients with cervical pathology undergoing cervical spine surgery. *Anesth Analg.* 2000;91:195.

Index

Page numbers followed by *f* indicate figures; those followed by *t* indicate tables.